BLACK MENTAL HEALTH

PATIENTS, PROVIDERS, AND SYSTEMS

T0176381

BLACK MENTAL HEALTH

PATIENTS, PROVIDERS, AND SYSTEMS

Edited by

Ezra E.H. Griffith, M.D.

Billy E. Jones, M.D., M.S.

Altha J. Stewart, M.D.

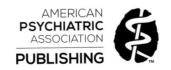

AMERICAN
PSYCHIATRIC
ASSOCIATION

PUBLISHING

Manufactured in the United States of America on acid-free paper
22 21 20 19 18   5 4 3 2 1

American Psychiatric Association Publishing
800 Maine Avenue SW
Suite 900
Washington, DC 20024-2812
www.appi.org

Library of Congress Cataloging-in-Publication Data
Names: Griffith, Ezra E.H., editor. | Jones, Billy E., editor. | Stewart, Altha J.,
    editor. | American Psychiatric Association Publishing, publisher.
Title: Black mental health patients, providers, and systems / edited by Ezra E.H.
    Griffith, Billy E. Jones, Altha J. Stewart.
Description: Washington, D.C. : American Psychiatric Association
    Publishing, [2019] | Includes bibliographical references and index.
Identifiers: LCCN 2018034264 (print) | LCCN 2018034931 (ebook) | ISBN
    9781615372102 (ebook) | ISBN 9781615372065 (pbk. : alk. paper)
Subjects: | MESH: Mental Health—ethnology | African Americans | Healthcare
    Disparities—ethnology | Psychiatry | Health Personnel | Mental Health
    Services | United States—ethnology
Classification: LCC RC451.5.N4 (ebook) | LCC RC451.5.N4 (print) | NLM
    WA 305 AA1 | DDC 616.890089/96073—dc23
LC record available at https://lccn.loc.gov/2018034264

British Library Cataloguing in Publication Data
A CIP record is available from the British Library.

The editors dedicate this book to four black psychiatrists who, while they were in our midst, made their mark with distinguished contributions to the field of psychiatry.

Jeanne Spurlock, M.D.: she was truly the mother of Black Psychiatry, thoughtfully caring and guiding us, while setting standards of professionalism.

Phyllis Harrison-Ross, M.D.: with profound understanding and sensitivity, she taught us about the political and social determinants of mental illness, long before those terms were in common use.

William Arthur Ellis, M.D.: a brother who offered friendship and encouragement, as he supported us with a benign smile and pointed at the realities of being black.

Walter W. Shervington, M.D.: his remarkable insights and intellectual brilliance radiated over us, providing comfort and leadership embellished by humor and laughter.

The editors also express deep appreciation to their spouses, families, and close friends for their ever-present love and support.

CONTENTS

PART II
Patient Care

PART III
Training of
Black Mental Health Care Providers

PART IV
Psychiatric Research and Blacks

PART V
Conclusion

CONTRIBUTORS

Kenneth B. Ashley, M.D., FACLP, DFAPA
Assistant Professor of Psychiatry, Icahn School of Medicine at Mount Sinai; Director of Mental Health Services, Peter Krueger Clinic, Institute for Advanced Medicine, Mount Sinai Beth Israel Hospital, New York, New York

F.M. Baker, M.D., DLFAPA
Professor of Psychiatry, Retired, University of Maryland School of Medicine, Baltimore, Maryland; Consulting Psychiatrist, Deer's Head Hospital Center, Salisbury, Maryland; Consulting Psychiatrist, Harrison Senior Living and Rehabilitation Center, Snow Hill, Maryland

Carl C. Bell, M.D., DLFAPA, FACPsych
Staff Psychiatrist and CL Psychiatrist, Medical/Psychiatric Unit, Jackson Park Hospital, Chicago, Illinois; Chairman of the Department of Psychiatry, Windsor University, Cayon, St. Kitts; Clinical Professor Emeritus of Psychiatry, Department of Psychiatry, University of Illinois at Chicago, Chicago, Illinois

Iverson Bell Jr., M.D.
Assistant Professor and Director of Residency Training, Department of Psychiatry, University of Tennessee Health Science Center, Memphis, Tennessee

Chyrell D. Bellamy, M.S.W., Ph.D.
Associate Professor and Director of Peer Services and Research, Program for Recovery and Community Health, Yale University School of Medicine, New Haven, Connecticut

Curley L. Bonds, M.D., DFAPA
Professor and Chair, Department of Psychiatry and Behavioral Medicine, Charles R. Drew University of Medicine and Science, Los Angeles, California; Health Sciences Clinical Professor of Psychiatry, David Geffen School of Medicine at University of California, Los Angeles; Chief Deputy Director, Clinical Operations, Los Angeles County Department of Mental Health

Ellen S. Boynton, B.A.
Director, Office of Multicultural Healthcare Equity, Department of Mental Health and Addiction Services, Hartford, Connecticut

June Jackson Christmas, M.D.
Medical Professor Emeritus of Behavioral Science, City University of New York Medical School, New York, New York; Past Vice President, American Psychiatric Association, and Past President, American Public Health Association, Washington, D.C.

Frank Clark, M.D., FAPA
Medical Director of Adult Inpatient Services, Greenville Health System/Marshall Pickens Hospital, Greenville, South Carolina; Clinical Assistant Professor, University of South Carolina School of Medicine, Greenville, South Carolina

Tiffany Cooke, M.D., M.P.H., FAPA
Violence Prevention Task Force Director, Physicians for Criminal Justice Reform, Inc., and Owner, Innovations Behavioral Health, LLC, Atlanta, Georgia

Larry Davidson, Ph.D.
Professor of Psychiatry and Director, Program for Recovery and Community Health, Yale University School of Medicine, New Haven, Connecticut

Miriam E. Delphin-Rittmon, Ph.D.
Commissioner, Connecticut Department of Mental Health and Addiction Services, Hartford, Connecticut

Charles Dike, M.D., M.P.H.
Associate Professor of Psychiatry, Yale University School of Medicine, New Haven, Connecticut

Richard G. Dudley Jr., M.D.
Private Practice of Clinical and Forensic Psychiatry, New York, New York

Dexter L. Fields, M.D.
General and Forensic Psychiatrist (Retired), Detroit, Michigan; Former Fellow, Solomon Carter Fuller Institute

Elizabeth Flanagan, Ph.D.
Research Scientist, Program for Recovery and Community Health, Yale University School of Medicine, New Haven, Connecticut

Anderson J. Franklin, Ph.D.
Honorable David S. Nelson Professor of Psychology and Education, Department of Counseling, Developmental, and Educational Psychology, Lynch School of Education, Boston College, Chestnut Hill, Massachusetts; Honorary Professor, Center for the Advancement of Non-racialism and Democracy, Nelson Mandela University, Port Elizabeth, South Africa

Linda N. Freeman, M.D.
Special Lecturer in the Department of Child and Adolescent Psychiatry, College of Physicians and Surgeons at Columbia University, New York; Independent Practice, New York, New York

David Friedlander, M.A.
Graduate Student, University of Hartford Graduate Institute of Professional Psychology, West Hartford, Connecticut

Mindy Thompson Fullilove, M.D., Hon AIA
Professor of Urban Policy and Health, The New School, New York, New York

Derrick M. Gordon, Ph.D.
Associate Professor of Psychiatry, Department of Psychiatry, Yale University School of Medicine, The Consultation Center, New Haven, Connecticut

Ezra E.H. Griffith, M.D.
Professor Emeritus of Psychiatry and of African-American Studies, Yale University, New Haven, Connecticut

Anthony P.S. Guerrero, M.D.
Professor of Psychiatry and Clinical Professor of Pediatrics; Chair, Department of Psychiatry; and Director, Child and Adolescent Psychiatry Division, University of Hawai'i John A. Burns School of Medicine, Honolulu, Hawai'i

Aaron D. Haddock, Ph.D.
Postdoctoral Fellow in Clinical and Community Psychology, Santa Barbara Special Education Local Plan Area, Santa Barbara, California

Sidney H. Hankerson, M.D., M.B.A.
Assistant Professor of Clinical Psychiatry, Columbia University Medical Center, New York, New York

Helena B. Hansen, M.D., Ph.D.
Assistant Professor of Psychiatry and Anthropology, New York University, New York, New York

Nzinga A. Harrison, M.D., DFAPA
Cofounder, Physicians for Criminal Justice Reform, Inc.; Owner, Nzinga A. Harrison M.D., LLC, Atlanta, Georgia

Jacquelyne F. Jackson, Ph.D.
Independent Scholar, Oakland, California

Billy E. Jones, M.D., M.S.
Clinical Professor of Psychiatry, New York University School of Medicine, New York, New York; Past President, Black Psychiatrists of America

William B. Lawson, M.D., Ph.D., DLFAPA
Adjunct Professor of Psychiatry, University of Maryland School of Medicine; Emeritus Professor of Psychiatry, Dell Medical School, University of Texas at Austin, Austin, Texas; Emeritus Professor of Psychiatry and Behavioral Sciences, Howard University College of Medicine, Washington, D.C.

Orlando B. Lightfoot, M.D.
Professor of Psychiatry Emeritus and Former Vice Chair, Community Psychiatry, Boston University School of Medicine; Retired Psychoanalyst, Boston, Massachusetts; Consultant, Greenfield Health Promotion Consortium, International

Lorraine E. Lothwell, M.D., FAPA
Assistant Clinical Professor, Department of Psychiatry, Columbia University; Medical Director, Child and Adolescent Psychiatry Outpatient Clinic, Harlem Hospital Center, New York, New York

Ayesha McAdams-Mahmoud, M.P.H.
Sc.D. Student, Harvard T.H. Chan School of Public Health, Boston, Massachusetts

Patricia A. Newton, M.D., M.P.H., M.A.
CEO and Medical Director, Black Psychiatrists of America; President, Newton and Associates, PA, Baltimore, Maryland

Donna M. Norris, M.D.
Clinical Assistant Professor, Beth Israel/Deaconess Hospital and Children's Hospital Medical Center, Harvard Medical School, Boston, Massachusetts

Melvin Oatis, M.D.
Assistant Professor of Clinical Psychiatry, New York University Langone Child Study Center, New York; Independent Practice, New York, New York

Kenneth Polite, Ph.D.
Executive Director, Champion Counseling Center/Faithful Central Bible Church, Inglewood, California

Annelle B. Primm, M.D., M.P.H.
Senior Medical Adviser, The Steve Fund, Baltimore, Maryland

Jyotsna S. Ranga, M.D.
Assistant Professor, Director of the Child and Adolescent Fellowship, and Psychiatry Clerkship Director, Department of Psychiatry, University of Tennessee Health Science Center, Memphis, Tennessee

Racquel E. Reid, M.D.
Board-Certified Child and Adolescent Psychiatrist, Atlanta, GA

Ruth S. Shim, M.D., M.P.H.
Luke and Grace Kim Professor in Cultural Psychiatry and Associate Professor, Department of Psychiatry and Behavioral Sciences, University of California, Davis, California

Christine Simon, Sc.M.
Graduate Student, Department of Social and Behavioral Sciences, Harvard T.H. Chan School of Public Health, Boston, Massachusetts

Patricia Simon, Ph.D.
Associate Research Scientist, Department of Psychiatry, Yale University School of Medicine, The Consultation Center, New Haven, Connecticut

Altha J. Stewart, M.D.
Associate Professor and Chief, Public and Community Psychiatry, and Director, Center for Health in Justice Involved Youth, University of Tennessee Health Science Center, Memphis, Tennessee

Michael J. Strambler, Ph.D.
Assistant Professor, Department of Psychiatry, Yale University School of Medicine, The Consultation Center, New Haven, Connecticut

Nadia L. Ward, Ph.D.
Associate Professor, Department of Psychiatry, Yale University School of Medicine, The Consultation Center, New Haven, Connecticut

David R. Williams, Ph.D., M.P.H.
Florence Sprague Norman and Laura Smart Norman Professor of Public Health and Professor of African and African American Studies and of Sociology, Harvard University, Boston, Massachusetts

Eunice C. Wong, Ph.D.
Behavioral Scientist, RAND Corporation, Santa Monica, California

The volume editors and authors of this book have no competing interests to report.

INTRODUCTION: FRAMING THE TEXT

THE CONCEPTUALIZATION of this text grew out of conversations among the three of us editors and with other colleagues about recent developments in American psychiatry. We started by considering commentary in a broad cultural context about the possibility of a post-racial phase in American life. Such commentary had been regularly sparked by the election of Barack Obama to the presidency. Intellectuals of all persuasions were suggesting that the old black-white dichotomy was now old news. There was no longer need for concern about political elections in the South. Blacks were about to have the time of their lives. They would occupy high posts in many professions and would feel a part of life in practically every significant arena of the culture. But was this pervasive sense of progress and contentment widespread among blacks? Our conversations gradually took on a more focused and deliberative tone. We asked ourselves what the situation was in the psychiatric branch of medicine. What were black psychiatrists, psychologists, and public health specialists saying about their professional practices, the care of their patients, and their interactions in healthcare organizations? Those deliberations led to our decision to structure a comprehensive look at mental health for black Americans relating to patient care, training, and research in the current context. We also decided to include directions for improvements in the future.

Racism and racial segregation have left their mark on the mental healthcare of black patients in the United States. Racial inequity has had a significant effect on the training of black mental health professionals, on their subsequent integration into American professional organizations, and on their clinical praxis. Racism and segregation have affected formulation of payment mechanisms that underwrite the mental healthcare of blacks, training curricula attuned to the preparation of black health professionals, and research relevant to both black mental healthcare professionals and black patients.

However, the Civil Rights Movement of the 1960s and 1970s in the United States, reinforced by global human rights developments and legal decisions, produced its own effects on the rights of black patients and on the futures of black mental healthcare professionals. Examples of the positive effects are the increased attention to the disparities in outcomes of mental healthcare between blacks and other groups; the significantly improved climate in which healthcare research is carried out with black populations; and the enhanced access of black professionals to a broad spectrum of training and practice facilities throughout the country. These elements have been reinforced by civil rights decisions and by progressive transformation of the secular society. Nevertheless, we agree that in the face of such progress, there are still significant problems remaining.

Taking a narrow look at mental healthcare, we recognize several distinctive developments. First, in 1969, blacks in the American Psychiatric Association (APA) formally called attention to the organization's lack of diversity in its leadership. Those black psychiatrists were also concerned about the APA leadership's minimal interest in black psychiatrists and patients. Second, Dr. Jeanne Spurlock edited a text (Spurlock 1999) that described contributions of black psychiatrists and their collective place in American psychiatry. That book took a historical approach to the work and lives of early black psychiatrists and articulated their reflections and comments on hurdles they had overcome. It also addressed certain matters related to the psychiatric care of black patients. Third, we note that in May 2018, the APA installed its first black president. This was a remarkable event in the history of the organization and for the discipline of psychiatry on a national scale.

Those events of 1969 and 1999, linked to the 2018 change in APA leadership, will lead to this new face of American psychiatry. Spurlock emphasized people and their connection to places where black psychiatrists toiled diligently to contribute to their profession and to the care of black psychiatric patients. Those efforts highlighted the access of black patients to psychiatric care even though the exclusion of black professionals and patients from the mental health marketplace was common. Isabel Wilkerson (2010) described the place of black medical professionals and black patients in her story of blacks' migration from the American South to the North and other regions between 1915 and 1970. In a similar vein, John Hoberman (2012) commented on the traditional conservatism of the American medical organizations that kept black physicians excluded from state medical societies even during the American Civil Rights Movement of the 1960s.

It is therefore time to reflect more comprehensively on what occurred before and is continuing in the present-day context related to black individuals' need of mental healthcare. It is also important to give more thought to the efforts of black psychiatrists and other mental health professionals whose training and clinical, research, and teaching activities are relevant to providing care for blacks and other nondominant groups.

It is evident that preparing a book about mental health professionals from a variety of different disciplines contributing to the care of black psychiatric patients would result in a voluminous text. Thus, we set out to limit the parameters of this book and to extend Spurlock's earlier scholarship while still paying homage to her emphasis on a historical perspective. There is increased emphasis in this new text on the present, suggested pathways to the future, and comparisons with what has gone before. There is explicit recognition that other disciplines, such as psychology and public health, contribute to the clinical care of black patients, to the scholarship enhancing that care, and to the specialty training of black psychiatrists.

With its narrowed conceptual focus, this text permits a clearer view of the terrain concerning black psychiatrists (their training, scholarship, and clinical praxis), buttressed by the contributions of psychologists and public health specialists. The book's other concern is the black patients in need of mental healthcare. In carefully chosen chapters, the text addresses these two central themes. Of necessity, the list of topics is not exhaustive, but the chapters draw attention to this important task of documenting the place of these two constituencies (the professional caregivers and their black patients) in the context of American psychiatric healthcare.

In Part I of the book's five parts, there are five chapters presented as personal narratives. The first three chapters, written by the editors, include the one authored by the individual (A.J.S.) who ascended to the post of president of the American Psychiatric Association in May 2018. The five authors of the reflections are all senior black psychiatrists who have taken different pathways to building their careers in psychiatry. Their stories reflect a personalized view of their experiences over the past 50 years and conceptualize their notions of what the future may hold for the care of the black community. The personal narratives bring a special measure of authenticity to the text, because the authors come from different geographies and cultural contexts. They have participated in the black struggle within American medicine and psychiatry in their unique ways. This use of narrative defines a distinctive dimension of this volume because it adds a qualitative aspect to the more traditional scholarly themes.

Part II (Chapters 6 through 17) focuses on different aspects of patient care. The authors address topics related to their knowledge base and experience. The 12 chapters illustrate the complexity of delivering mental healthcare to the black population. The content of the chapters represents examples that will be useful in teaching about the interaction of blacks and psychiatric care. We recognize that our choices have arbitrarily omitted other important topics.

Chapters 6, 7, and 8 make up the first subgroup. Chapter 6 concerns the public system of care, its payment mechanisms, and the impact of the "recovery" and "citizenship" movements; Chapter 7 examines the role of the criminal justice system in accounting for the predominant presence of blacks in prisons across the country and the organization of psychiatric care in that system; and Chapter 8 focuses on black international medical graduates and their contributions to the care of black patients. This chapter also highlights the adaptation of these black psychiatrists to the task of caring for their patients in the unique American context so defined by the structural features of poverty and racism.

The second subgroup (Chapters 9 through 14) explores the challenges of providing psychiatric care to differentiated groups within the black population: children and adolescents; women; young minority fathers; elders; gays, lesbians, and other related groups; and adults with attention-deficit/hyperactivity disorder. This second subgroup points out several creative ways of addressing groups of black patients who contend with difficulties linked to their psychosocial status and stigmatized characteristics. From reading these chapters, it is hoped that clinicians will come to understand that there is a body of explicit knowledge needed to effectively diagnose and treat black patients and that the knowledge base can be learned, although it is not specifically taught in many training programs. An example is in Chapter 9, where the authors point out that signs of depression in black youth are often misdiagnosed as resistance, thereby delaying treatment and increasing the likelihood for poor outcomes.

The third subgroup (Chapters 15 through 17) focuses on three of the many treatment techniques available: psychotherapy, psychopharmacology, and treatment interventions linked to the black church. These treatments are adapted by skilled caregivers to the cultural parameters of life for blacks in the United States.

Part III, composed of Chapters 18 through 22, contemplates the training of black mental health professionals in subjects of import to the black population. The chapters in this part address the emphasis on cultural psychiatry in new training curricula; workforce problems related to different arenas of clinical praxis; the special needs of black youth; the significance of implicit bias in the work of practitioners; and the present and future roles of historically black medical schools in the training of black psychiatrists and the preparation of black professionals for the new breadth of roles in the mental health professions.

Part IV, containing Chapters 23 through 27, addresses research that is relevant to the care of the black population and provides a window to this unique terrain of specialized professional activity. Chapter 23 explores the problem of attracting and retaining black researchers. The next four chapters describe the empirical scholarship in four arenas: racism and mental health; the pervasive problem of inequality in mental health; trauma among black and other minority adolescents and its effect on their academic and social performance; and the formulation of addiction and drug policy as they relate to black mental health.

The editors conclude the text, in Chapter 28 (Part V), by emphasizing the main themes that emerged in each part of the book. These parts collectively should make it easier to formulate ideas of blacks' place in American psychiatry. It has taken a long time for a black psychiatrist to become president of the APA. However, prestigious training institutions in this country are appreciating the need to expand educational curricula that address the needs of black patients. Blacks are also obtaining graduate degrees in neuroscience, ethics, health law, and business. Thus, there is change in the air, and we wish to emphasize that point as we urge policy makers to think earnestly about the future of black professionals and about the mental healthcare of black Americans.

Even as we prepared the outline of this text, we could envision several themes for consideration in the conclusion. For example, the narratives at the beginning of the text come from experienced academics and administrators who have managed major national agencies with potential impact on healthcare policy. Their stories suggest that despite discrimination, the future for black patients and their caregivers will benefit from thoughtful management of our human and other resources. Yet it also will depend on attending seriously to problems of inequality and workforce difficulties.

Early on in the planning for this text, we discussed the use of the terms "black" and "African American." The editors' use of both terms in their personal and professional writing varied, as did the practice of capitalizing "black." The editorial consensus was that in this text we would use the term *black* (this format also is consistent with established style guidelines) and *African American* interchangeably at the discretion of each contributing author.

The chapters highlight creative models of caregiving focused on defined groups within the black population and consider relatively new concepts such as "recovery" and "citizenship." These developments have transformed the relationship between physician and patient and set new standards for community care that benefit minorities. Our preparatory discussions of the chapters also highlighted broader opportunities for blacks in the profession of psychiatry. Our authors recommended involving blacks in research activities and examining evidence-based solutions to the psychiatric health problems of the black population.

We hope this text will be of substantial interest to all those who are attracted to organized psychiatry and to the understanding of mental healthcare in the United States. Trainees should be informed about this topic, as caring for black and minority populations is now a central concern of those who provide mental healthcare in this country. Practicing clinicians will find clinical utility in the chapters on research advances and treatment modalities, especially those described for various population subgroups within the African American community. Historians, ethicists, educators, and administrators from the healthcare professions all need to understand better how race matters have evolved in these narrow corridors over the past 50 years. This book helps to fill this gap and contributes to knowledge of the relationship between race and mental healthcare.

Ezra E.H. Griffith, M.D.
Billy E. Jones, M.D., M.S.
Altha J. Stewart, M.D.

References

Hoberman J: Black and Blue. Berkeley, University of California Press, 2012

Spurlock J (ed): Black Psychiatrists and American Psychiatry. Washington, DC, American Psychiatric Association, 1999

Wilkerson I: The Warmth of Other Suns: The Epic Story of America's Great Migration. New York, Random House, 2010

PART I
Reflections

CHAPTER 1
THE WELCOME TABLE
IN THE WORKPLACE

Ezra E.H. Griffith, M.D.

I SPENT a long time preparing for when I would join the workforce. I had finished college, spent my 2 years as a draftee in the United States Army, completed medical school and specialized training, and then plunged into my first job at the Yale School of Medicine located in New Haven, Connecticut. Back then, in July of 1977 when I took up my post at Yale, people talked about New Haven in racialized terms. The Civil Rights era had left its mark. The Black Panther Party was known in this small New England city, and everybody talked openly about Yale's being an Ivy League school where blacks had limited access to faculty and student positions.

My assignment was to the Connecticut Mental Health Center, a facility that had benefited from the new emphasis on community psychiatry. The state government had funded construction of the center and contracted with Yale University and its medical school to run it. This meant that I, as a physician, was a university employee. As I settled into this new job, I realized that during the preceding 10 years, I had been absorbed in my craft, learning to be a physician. I was intent on understanding my role in the healing process. However, I had paid minimal attention to the transactions and interactions that transpired in the workplace. One's place of employment only occasionally came up in a few seminar meetings when we were discussing the work of consulting to organizations. The new job forced me into making observations about the people around me. Here I was not referring exclusively to the patients. Staff at all ranks contributed to what went on in the work economy, and that was evident in the weekly community meeting led by the unit director and at the staff meeting.

3

As I considered the geography of this psychiatric unit of fewer than 30 patients, I was intrigued by the way people talked about themselves. I recognized quickly the Yale-state duality in discussions taking place in the small space. Some staff were employed by Yale, and others received a paycheck from the state. Patients and staff were preoccupied with each other. This distinction was crucial, especially to patients who were there against their will. There was also due attention paid to the place of men and women in the organization of the unit. However, the black-white theme was palpably dominant. It was identifiable everywhere, and it drove much of people's concerns about each other.

This latter dichotomy became more apparent to me as I made my observations over time. People told me that I was one of the few black physicians on the entire Yale faculty. I hadn't thought much before about being a curiosity in the workplace, but while some individuals on the unit hid their interest in learning about me, others (both patients and staff) were bold in describing their ideas about how a black doctor lived his life. Leadership in the center and in the School of Medicine had few blacks in its ranks. I was a symbol of black exceptionalism at Yale without having planned it. In this unique work context, this led to about 40 years of intriguing experiences for me.

In this chapter, I concentrate on my experience as a black physician-scholar in a workplace that by any measure was dominated by whites. In this context, I gradually recognized a central concern of black staff, faculty, and students at Yale: whether they might ever develop the feeling of belonging at this highly prized institution, of feeling truly included in its structure. Or as Peter Block (2009) put it, could blacks have the experience of feeling membership in the organization and some sense of emotional ownership of it? Might they even be lucky enough to envisage themselves one day sitting at a symbolic Yale "welcome table"?

My interest in this theme of belonging led me in recent years to an important line of discourse carried on by medical anthropologists and geographers: the intriguing relationship between health and place (Gesler 1992). In forging the connection, we seek opportunities to turn architectural spaces into therapeutic landscapes where people feel better about themselves and function more effectively at confronting the task of daily living (Doughty 2013). This line of scholarship has contributed to our understanding of how useful it is to divide into discrete spaces the places where we spend our time, where we live our lives. For many of us, there are the usual categories of workplace and home-space environments where we spend our leisure time, and sacred spaces where we worship. There are also the unusual spaces occupied by the homeless or those in prison. Still others are temporarily housed in hospitals, boarding schools, and military barracks. Even in conventional spaces like home, the activity of living may extend, with significant impact, into the surrounding community.

The scholarship on health and place has taught us several basic lessons. First, the architecture of the place (both inside and outside) may have an impact on our health. Second, in these places, the interactions among individuals may promote good health, or they may affect our health negatively and sometimes cause us stress. The recognition of this possibility has been pressing scholars to think about the importance of identifying stress linked to places, hence the term *stressed spaces* (Connellan et al. 2013). The third point is that many of us who frequent the space, and especially leaders within the space, should consider the inherent responsibility of improving the space. Ultimately, there is a good chance that manipulating the climate within the space (in biopsychosocial terms) may favor the good health of those within its boundaries. Thus, clinicians and others have been at work diluting the potentially pernicious effects and, when possible, transforming the spaces, such as where we work, into a therapeutic landscape.

The concept of *therapeutic landscapes* has influenced my evaluation of the experiences lived during the long decades in this unique Yale workplace. My reflections in this piece are related to the time I spent in the broad context of the university. They are not limited to the space of the psychiatric facility where I did my clinical work. It is not just the architecture defined by the clinic and hospital but the real and virtual boundaries of this world-class educational arena. The transactional experiences are also linked to my racialized view of life and the black-white dichotomized lens through which I saw Yale.

Like many blacks, I could not stop myself from noticing how few black people were present at the meetings I attended in those early years. Many of us weren't present in that university workplace, and the more serious the discussions on the meeting's agenda, the less diverse the group would be. It was easy to conclude after a few months that blacks had little representation in the seats of power. It was a chilling conclusion, I thought, especially once I learned that New Haven had a black neighborhood, with black churches, and a group of immigrants from the Caribbean island of Nevis. I also met many blacks whose families had come up from the South as participants in the Great Migration. There were even political advocates, some of whom were known to be outspoken, walking around agitating for continuation of the national civil rights agenda. Over the next three or four decades, there would be a black chaplain of the university, a black dean of the college, several black professors in the medical school, and even a black mayor in the city. But that reflected improved access to opportunity, not necessarily solutions to the more complex problem of inclusion.

Early in my career, I decided to study the therapeutic dimensions of a New Haven black church's rituals and knew that no faculty in the medical school had an interest in that subject. However, one day a white professor asked me in a meeting what I was thinking about as a research topic. As I proceeded hesitantly to explain my initial work, he pointed out that it might be helpful for me to consider the church as a healing community. It was a concept that a colleague of his had described in a book some years earlier. The intervention, from this senior white supervisor, saved me months of struggling. First, he showed an interest in my work and encouraged me. He also pointed out the considerable benefit my writing would have for the outside community. He put me on my way to pursuing a scholarly enterprise, one that blossomed.

It took some time for me to recognize the full impact of this mentor's guidance. As we talked during the next months, and as the months became years, some ideas crystallized. He knew better than I did how easy it was for me to become isolated in a predominately white institution. While it would have been desirable for me to seek a mentor and get to work, he knew it would be helpful for some white professor to step forward and offer me guidance. He also told me bluntly that white professors found it easy to offer help spontaneously to white faculty in the junior ranks. He said it without rancor. It was just the way it was. No hostility needed to be read into the matter. So we adopted each other, and I was thankful for it. Another idea was clarified: getting promoted in these competitive universities across the country required at least one or two mentors who could guide and protect, as well as support and correct.

This mentor and I talked of many things that concerned the place where we worked. He helped me understand how to think about the workspace and analyze the numerous interactions going on around me. He demonstrated how we all brought our traditions and cultural prejudices into the workplace and, without recognizing it, tried our best to impose our biases on others. He was interested in helping me learn not only how to manage administrative systems but also how to manage people. He took pains to point out how administrative decisions affected people's lives. I began to see, under his guidance, why whites, constituting the dominant group in places like Yale, took steps to maintain control over resources and space. As I internalized that basic finding, it became easier for me to anticipate the likely outcome of certain discussions long before conclusions were reached. As I eventually grasped it, my mentor's tutorial moved from consideration of individuals to contemplating the concerns of larger communities. With time, greater clarity set in about the interaction of individual and community.

Thinking about the personal level was evident when I found myself encouraging a young black nurse working in a Yale facility to think about pursuing advanced studies in her field. She talked about the lack of confidence in her ability to pass a statistics course, and I asked her boldly who had said she couldn't pass the course. It became clear that she had no reference points to look to, no senior individual in her discipline who effectively insisted that pursuing advanced studies was a possibility for her. Probably worse, no one was stepping forward to ask what her plans were for further professional development. She seemed settled and accepting of the idea that the future was somehow limited, not open or full of promise. I intervened because someone had done it for me. I was delighted when the report eventually came back that the statistics course had been conquered and that the master's degree diploma was in sight. Her personal carriage improved, with a straighter back and head held high and a voice that stated confidently what was possible in the future. This confidence also transformed her view of the surrounding environment, as she saw herself more competent to contend with the slights encountered in the workplace.

One other powerful example of the microlevel served to focus my attention in later years. I was the director of the Connecticut Mental Health Center at the time and professor in Yale's Department of Psychiatry. In those roles, I hosted a holiday party in December and invited everybody who worked in the center. I wanted to solidify a climate of unity that could pervade the workplace. After all, everyone was a valued member of the group, contributing to the mission of providing clinical services to the community and the state. I spread my message that the holiday party would celebrate the cohesion of our unit. I mentioned it in meetings I attended and as I met staff in my walks through the center. One day, a black staff member engaged me in conversation and said that he would not attend the party. No white work colleague had ever invited him out, and he was unaccustomed to socializing with whites. He saw little point in extending the workplace into his home-space. It was an informative, penetrating conversation, without any heat to it. He did his job well, one with supervisory responsibilities that he executed with distinction. Whites did not go out of their way to befriend him, and he had no desire to socialize with them. All he sought was contentment in his home-space and in the other places where he spent his leisure time and worshiped. The transactions at work were limited and simple. He knew his job, and he was pleased he handled it well.

He assured me that he was proud I was the head of a Yale-run facility, and he supported my leadership. He was confident the holiday party would draw a large attendance, and he complimented me on my efforts to be thoughtful and respectful of all the employees, but his going to the party would demand too much of him. Deep down he felt that the whites were only putting on a front. There was no sincere wish on their part to be in a social context with him. At first, I considered this an individualized example. The interaction was between him and me, and it had no policy implications. I could not walk away from the interaction and write a memorandum or instruct the implementation of a broad decision. All I could do was to ponder the depth of my colleague's feelings.

The black-white dichotomized thinking was ingrained, and deeply so. He had defined the boundaries of his workplace. In the context of our conversation, he had clarified the limits of the other places where he spent his personal time. He had found a way to defend himself against the daily slights that he encountered. He had figured out a singular way of living his life in this racialized style, measuring integration in his own fashion. He spiced it up with his form of resistance, tempered and nonthreatening. At the same time, however, I recognized some interaction between individual and broader community in this example. With some legitimacy, he could not see himself as a member of the broader university setting. He could not visualize his children walking through the entrances of the university as enrolled students. While he was making visible contributions to the broader workplace, he felt they were not deeply appreciated by anyone white.

At another time, I was older, and serving as a deputy chair of Yale's Department of Psychiatry. A young black trainee came to discuss an interaction he had recently experienced with a supervisor. He wanted to write a paper on a subject that had to do with blacks. The supervisor discouraged him, pointing out that scholarship focused on blacks had little worth at a place like Yale. The trainee had concluded from the ensuing discussion that blacks' lives had little worth, at least in the eyes of some white supervisors. I quickly put him at ease and helped him examine the assertion that blacks' lives were unimportant. On the face of it, the claim was preposterous. I conceded that some people might believe that there was nothing of merit in black lives. He agreed with me it was the sort of statement that was contradicted by much evidence around us.

We turned to discussing what he wished to study and write about and how I could facilitate his scholarship. He had no desire to file a formal complaint. We chatted further about his being protected from any retaliation possibly contemplated by the supervisor. I wanted to be helpful in healing the scars left by the microinsult, but there was a longer analysis of the environment, an evaluation of whether he was enjoying the workplace. We explored his sense of being empowered to spread his wings and explore the less obvious spaces of this large campus. We discussed his sampling some of what the university offered to people like him who came from far and wide for the experience. I wanted to put some balm on his wounds, while reassuring him that I could easily find him a supervisor to match his scholarly interests. He belonged there at the university like everybody else. I emphasized that I wanted to work with him to preserve his overall health so that he could cope with the strains and stresses he might encounter in the months of his remaining time on campus.

In the olden days, my years at Yale would have been spent struggling against the tyranny of segregation and the impact of earnest and overt racial discrimination. Things have changed. Certainly, access for blacks has improved. The task is now more nuanced, while still requiring energy and tenacity to combat the legacy of yesteryear's traditions. My 40 years in the university's precincts extended long enough to provide me with a view of the changes that took place in that time. The progressive transformation of the black-white interactions, now certainly less caustic, has persuaded me that there is not yet a post-racial phase for U.S. universities like this one. Race is still an important matter, and its impact is palpable and sustained.

Peter Block (2009, p. xiii) likes to talk about the structuring of community and the possibility of creating "the experience of belonging" in places "where people come together to get something done." The academy is obviously such a place.

I believe it is true that many universities have made sincere efforts to fight against the scenario of fragmented communities within their precincts. They have made progress toward establishment of greater cohesiveness and a commitment to the metaphor of the welcome table in characterizing their communities. Drew Gilpin Faust (2014), president at Harvard, has explicitly made clear that her university's commitment to diversity is robust and that the welcome table is securely in place. Yet my feelings of belonging at Yale have an element of insecurity in them.

My state of unsettledness has been partly provoked by Block's (2009, p. xii) definition of belonging, as I mentioned earlier. He recommended as important this fundamental demand of emotional ownership and membership in the space to which one wishes to belong. Yet the brief vignettes I have presented in this chapter, in my view, tarnish the claims that blacks have attained ownership and membership in this academy. The remaining question concerns the commitment of some in leadership to a future for the university that embraces the imagination and dreams of black people.

I feel a bit foolish that current conditions in these distinguished university spaces would prevent me from reporting to Langston Hughes (2004), with reference to the welcome table in his celebrated 1925 poem "I, Too," that all is settled. I could not say to Hughes that the welcome table at Yale is prepared. I also could not state that blacks have been invited with elegant flourishes of ritual to attend and partake of all that is on the table. It is more that a lot of committees have been set up, and those in power are still studying the matter and contemplating how to make sure their places are not overrun by all the newcomers.

References

Block P: Community: The Structure of Belonging. Oakland, CA, Berrett-Koehler Publishers, 2009

Connellan K, Gaardboe M, Riggs D, et al: Stressed spaces: mental health and architecture. HERD 6(4):127–168, 2013 24089185

Doughty K: Walking together: the embodied and mobile production of a therapeutic landscape. Health Place 24:140–146, 2013 24100237

Faust D: To sit at the welcome table (letter). Harv Mag July–Aug:3, 2014

Gesler WM: Therapeutic landscapes: medical issues in light of the new cultural geography. Soc Sci Med 34(7):735–746, 1992 1376497

Hughes L: The Collected Poems of Langston Hughes. New York, Vintage Books, 2004

CHAPTER 2
CALL TO PUBLIC SERVICE

Billy E. Jones, M.D., M.S.

MY FATHER, a factory worker, and my mother, a domestic, struggled and sacrificed to send their three children to college. Both parents had separately migrated to Dayton, Ohio, during the period of black migration from the South (Wilkerson 2010). Though we lived in a black community, my early education occurred in racially mixed schools with 30%–35% black students. However, segregation existed and was modeled in many obvious ways. It was not until several years into high school that I had a black teacher. In high school, I also encountered the existence of separation of races socially. A blatant example occurred in my senior year. Our senior class queen was black, with an academic record of all As. The class king was the captain of the football team, who was white. The problem this created for the first dance at the class party was solved by each having a partner from his or her own race.

It was during the latter part of my high school years that I began to contemplate a future vocation. I had always expected to go to college but had not chosen a career. Until that time, I had tepidly played around with music. I took piano lessons throughout my elementary school years and organ lessons in high school. I liked music, but there was never a passion for it, and even I realized I was not gifted or creative. I had not given any thought to what I could do in the music field. Luckily for me, my aunt was one of the early female graduates of Howard University Medical School, an internist so forward and brash one would have guessed she was a surgeon. She pointed out I would never be able to support a family as a musician. She looked me right in the eyes and commanded,

"You should be a doctor!" I was unclear about the logic, but the idea was appealing, and it stuck. As I would discover later, I was hooked by the thought of humanism, a sense of helping others, and the worthy, honorable intent associated with being a physician.

I became a premed student at Howard University because I wanted to attend a black college outside Ohio, as far away from home as possible. Howard was an excellent choice for me. I loved it and grew from a small-town, protected teenager to a more mature young adult. Along with the growth in other areas, I realized that my sexual orientation was becoming more definitely defined. I had dated girls in high school and was occasionally attracted to some guys, but overall, I was late in developing sexually. Now, as an undergraduate, I began to experience more interest in and feeling for males. While I recognized those feelings, I repressed them, thinking I had more important things to accomplish and this was not the time to get derailed.

I graduated from Howard and attended Meharry Medical College in Nashville, Tennessee. Medical school was much more intense, rigorous, and concentrated. I had to change from taking a laissez-faire approach to studying to adhering to a rigid, scheduled arrangement with almost no outside interruptions. The time was the early 1960s, during the student sit-ins for racial equality in Nashville and throughout the South. Like many Meharry students, I wanted to participate but was strongly advised by faculty not to do so. There was a strong likelihood of being arrested and jailed for extended periods, and that might have threatened my medical career. I have always regretted not joining the movement. I later admired how Congressman John Lewis and my former Howard classmate Diane Nash had physically put their bodies and lives on the line during the protests.

The education, training approach, and philosophy at both Howard and Meharry emphasized serving others and being a service to your community. Meharry's motto was "Worship of God through service to mankind." This augmented my basic reason for wanting to be a doctor and was in harmony with my soul. Around that time, Dr. Lloyd Elam came to Meharry as chair of psychiatry and served as a role model. Six students from our small graduating class chose psychiatry as our specialty. This was very unusual at the time, because most black medical students were men who wanted to be more hands-on, such as surgeons, orthopedists, or gynecologists. Psychiatry, by comparison, was a much younger field of medicine, was not hands-on, and was relatively unknown in the black community. For me, however, psychiatry was it. I liked talking and relating to patients and having to use my mind in diagnosing and treating. In addition, the field of community psychiatry was in its early phase and seemed a perfect match. At the time I was making these choices, my reasoning was not so logically deduced. Now, as I reflect, I can more clearly determine that my interest, training selections, and even future jobs all supported and directed me toward public service in which I would try to make a difference in the lives of people, particularly those from poor, underserved minorities.

I chose New York Medical College/Metropolitan Hospital (NYMC) in New York City for psychiatric residency training. That was where Drs. Alfred Freedman and Harold Kaplan were editing the groundbreaking *Comprehensive Textbook of Psychiatry* (Freedman and Kaplan 1967). However, more important to me were Dr. Freedman's interest in community psychiatry and the fact that a federally funded community mental health center was planned. Psychiatry was beginning to focus less on psychoanalytic theory, long inpatient stays, and the private practice model and more on psychopharmacology, deinstitutionalization, and community-based treatment. These changes were making treatment more available to poor, underserved, and minority populations.

The residents in my program were encouraged to enter psychoanalytic treatment. Most did, including me. I chose to seek treatment not to become an analyst, but for my own benefit and to be a better therapist. Also, I realized this was a much better way to explore and become comfortable with my sexual orientation and feelings. For 2 years of my residency, I had sessions three times per week lying on the couch. The residents in my year also had insight-oriented group therapy weekly. The group taught us how it felt being a member and was therapeutic. It also revealed an interesting occurrence when we taped a group session and played it back for review and discussion. Several of the members commented, "I had forgotten Billy is black." I was the only African American in my residency year. This brief episode was later described in an article I coauthored with other African American residents in other programs on training of blacks in white institutions and given the name "hallucinatory whitening" (Jones et al. 1970).

The most significant event to occur during my training years, however, took place outside the program and psychiatry. I met my partner and spouse for the next 50-plus years. I had spent considerable time on the couch dealing with resistance, but finally I became comfortable with my sexual orientation and accepted it.

Before I could concentrate on building a career, I had a 2-year military obligation to fulfill, incurred while at Howard and renewed yearly. I entered active duty as a psychiatrist the July following my residency training and was in Viet Nam by September 1969.

As I recount my service in Viet Nam I realize there were many interesting lessons for me. A major one was that as a psychiatrist there are many opportunities and expectations for you to intervene and make a difference far beyond the treatment dyad you are taught. Also, society expects you to be able to apply your knowledge of human behavior and actions to an individual, a few people, or a large group.

My main assignment was leading the mental health clinic in the only stockade for U.S. troops, the notorious Long Binh Jail, more popularly referred to as

"LBJ" (a pun related to the 36th president, Lyndon Baines Johnson). Before arriving in country, like most Americans, I did not know there had been a riot in the stockade the previous year led by black soldiers and that much of the stockade had burned down. I immediately understood why I had been assigned to Viet Nam and LBJ. It certainly was not related to the zero forensic experience I had. The prisoners were 75% black soldiers between the ages of 18 and 23 years. Most were there for minor infractions, such as refusing to cut their high afro hairstyle or to stop wearing a black woven bracelet, known as a "slave bracelet." The guards were nearly 100% white enlisted military police between 18 and 23 years of age who had received little or no training in conflict resolution or in how to de-escalate a situation. The racial difference, age, and testosterone created a powder keg. Low-level conflicts were the usual situation. My role rapidly expanded to include serving as a consultant to stockade command. When serious situations arose, I was called on for advice. One such crisis arose when one barrack of prisoners staged a sit-in to protest their treatment. The other barracks were deciding whether to support them. I recall walking around the outside perimeter of the stockade with the commanding officer as he sweated about what actions to take. Obviously, this could quickly get out of hand, leading to a riot, with guards and prisoners hurt and likely the end of his military career. I suggested I try to go in along with a young black lieutenant to talk with the prisoners and determine their grievances, serving as a go-between to command and seeking some resolution. My major aim was to keep the prisoners from being hurt. Part of our meeting with the prisoners was spent interpreting reality to them. They were rambunctious young men who would have been hurt and court-martialed. Contrary to what they thought, no one back home in the world would have heard anything about it. The approach worked.

Another unexpected lesson arose when the medical command in Viet Nam was directed to evaluate the racial tension within its command. I was assigned the task of assessing the situation and left alone to figure out how. I conducted focus groups of black enlisted men, white enlisted men, noncommissioned officers, and mixed integrated groups in four medical locations around the country. In each location I started with a courtesy visit with the hospital commander. I vividly recall one commander voicing his thoughts on the issue as "Let sleeping dogs lie." The assessment and report showed that the racial tension between black and white enlisted men was low but that the tension between black enlisted men and noncommissioned officers was high.

Following military service and back in New York City, I had a conversation with a black psychiatrist friend and colleague, Dr. Walter Shervington (now deceased), that caused me to wonder how completing the remainder of my analysis would be with a black analyst. Of course, that issue came up in my next session with my Jewish analyst, who helped me explore the topic and, more importantly, work though my resistance to changing. I spent the last year of my analysis with a black analyst. One of the major differences I found was obvious, yet profound. It was far easier for me to talk about racial and cultural issues. I did not feel the need to explain or provide a preface for those topics. Now, reflecting on this experience, I am also certain the transference helped strengthen my sense of self-worth and self-esteem.

Working at Lincoln Medical and Mental Health Center (Lincoln Hospital), the city hospital in the South Bronx, was one of the most enjoyable and productive experiences of my career. Lincoln served a diverse population of approximately 500,000 urban minority, poor residents. The South Bronx had large burnt-out areas, heavy substance abuse, high crime rates, and all the ills associated with the worst problems of a poor inner city. I started at Lincoln in 1977 and remained there for more than a decade. For the first 10 years I served as director of psychiatry and planned, fought for, and obtained many services needed for the South Bronx. During that time the department increased its inpatient beds from 12 to 55, expanded the psychiatric emergency room to an emergency service with needed holding beds, initiated a fully accredited psychiatric residency training program, and conducted clinical research. It was at Lincoln that we showed the importance of cultural factors in psychiatry. We hired, trained, and mentored a diverse mental health staff of talented minority members to serve the Latino and black patient populations. In addition, I recruited, mentored, and trained Spanish-speaking residents from U.S.-approved medical schools in Puerto Rico. We demonstrated how, in a public program, minority patients could be treated by staff who looked, sounded, and in many ways *were* culturally like them. We published papers in many academic journals on minorities and clinical issues, such as manic-depressive illness (Jones et al. 1981, 1983); psychotherapy (Jones et al. 1982a); and diagnosis (Jones and Gray 1986; Jones et al. 1982b). During the same time Carl Bell, a black psychiatrist, colleague, and friend, was also writing about similar concerns (Bell and Mehta 1980, 1981). We also studied and wrote about urban psychiatry's major challenge of that era, the homeless mentally ill (Jones et al. 1986).

During 2 of the years I worked at Lincoln I also served as president of Black Psychiatrists of America (BPA). I was elected to be vice president, but the president stepped down early in his tenure and I was moved up to run the organization. It was during my tenure that we started the BPA transcultural meetings, which were held annually in one of the countries in the black Caribbean diaspora. Discussion at these meetings centered on the culture and health problems of the country visited. The first meeting was planned by Andrea Delgado, M.D. (now deceased), a talented colleague and friend.

After about 7 years at Lincoln, I was approached by the chairman of psychiatry at Columbia University about becoming the director of psychiatry at Harlem Hospital. We met, and at the end of the meeting he offered me the position. A day or two later, I called him and accepted. He was pleased, saying we would work out the arrangements. Before any written correspondence was exchanged, I heard from two colleagues and friends who worked at Harlem that the word was out I had been selected to be the director. They informed me that the Harlem psychiatrists had held a meeting to discuss the selection and that some had strongly objected because I was gay. There was no further communication from the chairman. I, of course, was livid. Although this was the first such episode of discrimination I was aware of, unfortunately it was not the last.

Professionally, I remained at Lincoln, where my career continued to thrive, moving more to medical administration in the public sector. I became the medical director of Lincoln Hospital and senior associate dean and professor at NYMC. I also attended New York University's Graduate School of Public Service. My personal life also flourished. My spouse and I expanded our family by adopting a 3-week-old son.

In 1990, when David Dinkins became New York City's first, and to date only, African American mayor, I was asked to serve as commissioner of the Department of Mental Health, Mental Retardation and Alcoholism Services, becoming one of the first openly gay city commissioners. The department was the largest local mental hygiene system in the world, treating 425,000 people through 807 programs with 320 contracts costing $700 million per annum. I enjoyed working in this position because one could make a difference for the populations who needed the services most. I was also able to continue to mentor and train younger minority colleagues.

I had been a member of the New York City mental health community for more than 20 years at that time and felt prepared for most of the tasks that arose. What I had not anticipated, however, were the emergencies that came up from time to time. I started at the beginning of March 1990. The Happy Land Social Club fire occurred in the Bronx on March 25, 1990, killing 87 young club-going Honduran immigrants. The fire occurred in a building with only one exit and a plethora of building and fire code violations (Barron 1990). We needed to arrange for the provision of mental health services for Honduran families. We turned to sociologists to help us better understand the grieving and cultural processes we should anticipate and what might be normal and what might indicate a need for intervention. We worked with some of our Latino mental health provider agencies around the city to provide services as needed for support and direct treatment. Ultimately, we were able to patch together a robust service network.

Another unexpected occurrence took place around the same time we were busy working to develop a mental health service plan and division for children and youth. A tragedy happened at City College of New York. A much-anticipated basketball game featuring celebrity rap stars was being held in the downstairs gym. The street level doors were opened, and there was a stampede, with the crowd rushing downstairs, where the doors were closed. The crowd kept swelling and turmoil occurred, resulting in the death of eight young people from suffocation or trampling, and trauma and injuries to many others (McFadden 1991). I was called to the scene and assigned to talk with the parents and relatives of those who died and were injured. The department provided supportive services and followed and monitored the families.

After several years as commissioner, I was asked by the mayor to become the president and chief executive officer of the New York City Health and Hospitals Corporation (HHC). At that time, HHC was the largest municipal healthcare system in the nation, with a budget of $3.6 billion. As commissioner, I had been on the board of directors of HHC and chaired the Quality Assurance Committee, so I was familiar with the current problems. In addition, having previously worked in several HHC hospitals, I knew the long-standing troubles. It was a sprawling, difficult-to-manage, and underfunded healthcare system that required many hours of the day to get and maintain any semblance of management. The intensity of the work schedule reminded me of medical school, and as in that experience, all my waking hours were consumed by work. I regularly carried home an evening folder of work. On reflection, this was public service and professional healthcare administration at its most taxing, while at the same time being extremely personally rewarding. I, and my team, accomplished some major successes. We established a new financial relationship with the city that increased the budget, negotiated a successful $550 million capital bond offering, negotiated a new master affiliation contract with the medical schools, and successfully managed our acute care hospitals through a series of Joint Commission surveys. I also made several personnel changes, both at the corporate office and among hospital directors.

At one point during my tenure at HHC, I was approached, through a friend, by a senior official at the State University of New York (SUNY), who asked if I had any interest in the position of president at SUNY Downstate Medical College in Brooklyn. A dinner was arranged at a mutual friend's home. The dinner meeting went well, and I left believing there was interest in me for that position as I had been urged to interview. The interview went very well, and I anticipated getting the position. Instead, I never again heard from the medical college's administration. I did not understand what had happened, but I learned much later from a black state legislator that my name had been passed around to the black Brooklyn state legislators, and they had blocked my appointment because I was gay. Once again, I was angry at being discriminated against for a position for which I knew I would have been excellent. I was eager to achieve some important accomplishments in Brooklyn, and all of New York, especially for black New Yorkers.

As I give this accounting of these events in my life and reflect on the accompanying experiences, I more fully recognize important forces that have been at work—forces that have pushed and helped to mold my life and career. My parents and family, through their love and expectations for me, motivated and pushed me to strive toward my potential. Howard and Meharry not only honed my intellectual and medical abilities but also heightened my black consciousness. Psychiatry provided a community-oriented profession as a means of providing service. Discrimination, both racial and sexual orientation, placed obstacles in my career path but strengthened my resolve to succeed. Public service administration provided a channel to give back to my community and an opportunity to mentor younger members of racial and sexual minorities. Most importantly, a long-term, stable, loving relationship provided family and support for career accomplishments.

References

Barron J: Fire in the Bronx; grief deepens as horror of the disaster sinks in. The New York Times, March 27, 1990

Bell CC, Mehta H: The misdiagnosis of black patients with manic depressive illness. J Natl Med Assoc 72(2):141–145, 1980 7365814

Bell CC, Mehta H: Misdiagnosis of black patients with manic depressive illness: second in a series. J Natl Med Assoc 73(2):101–107, 1981 7205972

Freedman AM, Kaplan HI (eds): Comprehensive Textbook of Psychiatry. New York, Williams & Wilkins, 1967

Jones BE, Gray BA: Problems in diagnosing schizophrenia and affective disorders among blacks. Hosp Community Psychiatry 37(1):61–65, 1986 3510956

Jones BE, Lightfoot OB, Palmer D, et al: Problems of black psychiatric residents in white training institutes. Am J Psychiatry 127(6):798–803, 1970 5482873

Jones BE, Gray BA, Parson EB: Manic-depressive illness among poor urban blacks. Am J Psychiatry 138(5):654–657, 1981 7235063

Jones BE, Gray BA, Jospitre J: Survey of psychotherapy with black men. Am J Psychiatry 139(9):1174–1177, 1982a 7114311

Jones BE, Robinson WM, Parson EB, et al: The clinical picture of mania in manic-depressive black patients. J Natl Med Assoc 74(6):553–557, 1982b 7120489

Jones BE, Gray BA, Parson EB: Manic-depressive illness among poor urban Hispanics. Am J Psychiatry 140(9):1208–1210, 1983 6614232

Jones BE, Gray BA, Goldstein DB: Psychosocial profiles of the urban homeless, in Treating the Urban Homeless: Urban Psychiatry's Challenge. Edited by Jones BE. Washington, DC, American Psychiatric Press, 1986

McFadden RD: Stampede at City College: inquiries begin over City College deaths. The New York Times, December 30, 1991

Wilkerson I: The Warmth of Other Suns: The Epic Story of America's Great Migration. New York, Random House, 2010

CHAPTER 3
LONG JOURNEY TO THE TOP OF THE PSYCHIATRIC LADDER

Altha J. Stewart, M.D.

MY JOURNEY to becoming president of the American Psychiatric Association (APA) began in Memphis, Tennessee, where I was born before the Supreme Court decision in *Brown v. Board of Education*. I was 17 years old when a group of black psychiatrists stormed the APA Board of Trustees meeting in 1969 with their demands for changes in the organization, paving the way for all of the now recognized minority underrepresented (MUR) groups to become more fully integrated into the organization. I had no idea then what impact their actions would have on my future in psychiatry or the APA all these years later. Some parts of the story of my training and early experiences have been chronicled elsewhere (Stewart 2012), so I will not repeat them here.

My goal in this chapter is to share my personal experiences and perspectives on external events that converged to create the environment in which I would become the first African American to be elected president of the APA. There are also several other sources of information describing the history of blacks in American psychiatry. They include the biography of Solomon Carter Fuller (Kaplan 2005); a chapter on the formation of Black Psychiatrists of America (Pierce 1973); stories of the experiences of blacks in key positions in American psychiatry (Spurlock 1999); and my own discussion of disparities in psychiatric care (Stewart 2010). My journey to this point has been supported by these and other resources I found along the way.

Although not planned, my path into psychiatry began to come into focus in 1968 with the assassination of Dr. Martin Luther King Jr. in Memphis. The months before his assassination were filled with lots of protests and activities that placed African Americans in prominent roles in what was a growing civil rights movement marching across the South. For a young high school student, it was an exciting time, but I was still too young to really be a part of it. Watching on the local news scenes that might well have been torn right out of the nightly national newscasts was quite an experience. There was even a local chapter of what I am sure we all saw as the Black Panthers (called "the Invaders") right in my neighborhood. Their protests closed the local high school every Friday, sending students out of the school building and home early as a safety precaution. Everything changed in our world, though, on April 4, 1968. I remember clearly being at the dining room table doing homework when the news came over the television. Dr. Martin Luther King Jr. had been shot on the balcony of the Lorraine Motel. Initially the details were sketchy, and then it was finally announced that he was dead. The news started to flash photos from the scene as local news teams made their way there. Breaking news on the three local channels was all about the "assassination," as it was now being called. The manhunt for killers was on, and the local groups of angry protesters, many of whom had turned a peaceful protest violent months earlier, were calling for walkouts and marches to protest the assassination of Dr. King. I did not realize it at the time, but my neighborhood and other mostly black areas of town were quietly being surrounded as the National Guard was called up to maintain calm. The highway and major streets formed perimeters around many of these communities, and armed guardsmen patrolled them, advising everyone to adhere to the curfew or face arrest. A couple of nights after the shooting, groups of young people in my neighborhood began testing the guardsmen, coming off their porches and walking into the street, only to be warned that they had better return to their porches. Needless to say, armed guardsmen made quite an impression on our usually quiet neighborhood.

My parents were strong advocates for getting an education above all else, because it was viewed as the key to "making something of yourself," and that was their sole goal for me. The family agreement was "don't get pregnant or go to jail, but you can do anything else." The regular Friday school closings by the Invaders were interfering with that goal, so by the end of my high school sophomore year, I had determined that I would transfer out of my local public high school to an all girls' Catholic high school an hour across town. After the events of April 1968, it was clear that the opportunity to learn was the only way out, and while the family stories describe a young woman who made the transfer decision without discussing it with my parents, all I can remember is believing that finishing my education and getting out of Memphis was my only goal. I didn't know how to articulate it at the time, but in retrospect I think I saw it as the only way to survive because they were killing good black people who saw injustice and spoke out about it. As a black girl growing up in Memphis I had learned about people like Ida B. Wells, and while I wanted to be one of those outspoken activists, I knew well that the South did not reward that in a black person, and certainly not a black woman.

The transfer was harder than expected for two reasons: although I was Catholic, most of the girls at the school had been together since kindergarten, and I was an obvious outsider, which led to the second reason: there were only a half-dozen black students in the school, and they had also known one another for many years. Fortunately, I was accepted by my "tribe" and, in fact, by the second year was part of the first interracial social group to ever be established at the school. There were a few racial incidents in my 2 years at the school, but by and large it was a fertile training ground for my future interactions with the diverse groups of the world in which I would live and work.

As I had hoped, the educational opportunities were much better than those at my previous high school, and I took full advantage of that. At the time I had no plans for medicine, although I felt a strong attraction to science. I entered senior year believing that I was on the road to becoming a laboratory technician, but I graduated from high school knowing that I wanted more. I had no thought of becoming a doctor, and certainly not a psychiatrist. I did not know any black doctors but had met several laboratory technicians while working as a candy striper at St. Jude Children's Hospital during the summer. By graduation I had received several hundred thousand dollars in scholarship offers and chose a local Catholic college with a good science department because by then I had discovered a love for science (what would be called *STEM* today).

Thus, a part of my "life plan" was forming in sync with the timeline of blacks in American psychiatry without my awareness. In 1969, when the group of black APA members interrupted the APA Board of Trustees meeting in Miami with demands for change in how the organization engaged its "Negro" members (Shenker 1969), I was just finishing my junior year of high school and making decisions about my future—college and beyond. Memphis was not yet the progressive twenty-first-century city it would later become, and the most important decision for a young black woman like me was making a plan to depart as soon as possible. Christian Brothers College (now Christian Brothers University) was an all-male school before the admission of women in 1970. That year, more than 20 young women were formally admitted, and I was among the first to matriculate as a full-time student at the college.

In addition to the excellent education, the years at Christian Brothers College also helped me find my voice as an activist and as a black woman. There were only a few more black students on campus than there were women, so we were a pretty tight-knit group. Our black student association, the Organization of Black Leadership and Brotherhood (BLB), became a place where my views on race, gender, and ethnicity started to take shape. We were a presence throughout the college from the business administration and social sciences to science and engineering departments, proudly wearing our dashikis and afros. It was also during my college years that I became active in the local theater community, taking extra classes in drama and creative writing at a sister university in town. This helped immensely in my gaining comfort in public speaking in challenging situations, which would serve me well in my later professional life.

Through my experience in the Biology Club, I learned about a summer program sponsored by Harvard University for minority students interested in medicine. Encouraged by a group at our local medical school, I applied and was accepted to spend the summer taking biology and chemistry classes with other minority students interested in careers in medicine. That medical school, at the University of Tennessee Health Science Center, would figure prominently later, as I joined the faculty in 2015. There was also another twist with the Harvard experience. A part of the program was a mock medical school admission interview, and my interviewer was noted psychiatrist Dr. Alvin Poussaint. He was the only black psychiatrist whom I had ever heard of, and I was sitting across a desk being mock-interviewed for medical school by him. His no-nonsense approach resulted in my leaving the Harvard University Summer Pre-med Program in Boston determined to become a doctor. Truthfully, it was a challenge he made to me that led to my serious consideration of medicine as a career (all those summers as a candy striper finally paid off!).

After the summer ended I threw myself into preparing for medical school and officially became a premed biology major. After the rejection for early admission to my first choice, Meharry Medical College in Nashville, Tennessee, the only criterion for medical school applications was outside Tennessee. It was the mid-1970s, and my advisor, who was also my biology (pre-med) professor, cautioned me to keep my expectations low, because it might be difficult for students like me to gain entry into some of the schools I wanted. He suggested I focus on the historically black colleges and universities and other non–Ivy League institutions where applications from minority students might be more favorably received. I ignored him and headed north to Temple Medical School, where I had applied and been accepted.

Medical school was challenging on many levels, but mostly it was the cultural change. I had never quite known just how much of a Southerner I was until I went north. The harsh weather was nothing compared with the very different attitude and demeanor of many of the people I met, in and outside the medical school environment. I met my future husband, also a medical student, in medical school, but we divorced early in my residency. My favorite course was neuroanatomy, so maybe I should have guessed psychiatry was in my future. Much like in high school and college, I also found time for extracurricular activities, including class officer, note-taking group, American Medical Student Association, and Student National Medical Association, holding leadership positions in each. There were also experiences with racism and sexism throughout the 4 years, but those are stories for another book, another time. By the end of medical school, however, I had a plan and the courage to carry it out thanks to a group of black psychiatrists in Philadelphia who had shown an interest in me and begun actively recruiting me to the specialty.

Much like the medical school application process, the decision about where I would complete residency was based on very simple criteria. My dilemma was whether I would move from the place that taught me to love psychiatry down the street to a place that had a core group of black psychiatrists ready and willing to contribute to the next phase of my training. I had gone through the first 2 years of medical school convinced that I would become a pediatrician, until completing my psychiatry clinical rotation during the summer of 1976. I was the only student on the rotation; the faculty showered me with attention, and I was like a starving person, taking in all the "food" that psychiatry had to offer. What I did not appreciate until much later was that it was also my first exposure to black psychiatrists and how psychiatry might apply in the lives of people who looked like me. The clinical rotation years solidified for me the fact that I was going to be a psychiatrist, and my only problem was deciding on a location for my residency. Philadelphia had a strong psychiatry presence, with the historical Philadelphia Hospital, several medical schools with thriving departments of psychiatry, and a local public mental health system that actively collaborated with the academic centers. I decided to leave Temple and went to complete my psychiatric residency at the only psychiatry program listed on my match form—Hahnemann Medical College and Hospital (now Drexel University College of Medicine). The Hahnemann recruitment process had introduced me to more than a half-dozen black psychiatrists in the Philadelphia area—adult- and child-trained clinicians, academics, researchers, and administrators. Although initially I was the only black resident in my class (I was later joined by a colleague who completed training with me in 1982), I had a black supervisor each of my 4 years (one year I had a black supervisor at the community mental health center to which I was assigned and another as a psychotherapy supervisor). Along the way I was learning more than just how to be a psychiatrist; I was being trained to be a leader.

The Philadelphia Black Psychiatrists group was one of my early leadership training grounds. I was introduced to key figures in the Philadelphia psychiatric circles and supported in my efforts to compete with my peers at the time for involvement in psychiatric activities at the local and national level. I was encouraged to serve as chief resident and supported in my work with the local psychiatric society. Other aspects of the experience of the early years of my journey to becoming a community psychiatrist included the Falk Fellowship and its focus on leadership in the field of psychiatry; chief resident training; and time spent at the A.K. Rice Institute. One of my supervisors, Dr. Earline Houston, was an advisor and determined administrator, and she welcomed my involvement in her work as the superintendent (first female and first black) at the local state psychiatric hospital. We had worked together early in my residency when she was director of the community mental health center to which I was assigned, so she knew of my interest in the administrative side of psychiatry. She had studied organizational leadership and even written an unpublished paper on challenges for black women in leadership roles that she left for me to finish when she died. I was very proud when the local group for black psychiatrists was renamed the Houston Society in her honor.

I joined the APA in 1980 while I was still a resident. I was awarded a Falk Fellowship and was officially on the path to leadership in the field of psychiatry. My training director and I had a tumultuous relationship because I held him responsible for my not getting the Substance Abuse Mental Health Services Administration Minority Fellowship, which was more coveted at the time. It was where all the minority residents were, and as one of two blacks in my training program, I very much wanted to be with other residents like me, sharing experiences and ideas about how to navigate the often conflicting worlds of gender, race, professional training, and aspiring to leadership in psychiatry. I resolved to make the best of it, however, and ultimately found the Falk Fellowship to be very meaningful to my overall professional development. The fellowship experience set me on the path to more opportunities, including being chief resident, and opened the door to many more things than that little girl from Memphis had ever dreamed possible.

First jobs are always important to future career choices, and mine was certainly that. To pay for medical school I had received a National Health Service Corps scholarship, so although I completed medical school with zero debt, I did have a multiyear service obligation as payback for the financial support. While still in residency I began to negotiate how to remain in the Philadelphia area where I had trained as a community psychiatrist with expertise working with urban, mostly minority populations, and I was ultimately successful. I remained in Philadelphia and took on the job of creating a mental health clinic for a methadone maintenance program, which set me on the path of creating services to meet a demonstrated need in a target population. It was also my first medical director position, and I finally understood how I might use some of the leadership lessons from the fellowship.

There were many significant events along the way from my training in Philadelphia to being elected president of the APA. The experiences with Dr. Houston solidified my interest in administration and led to subsequent high-level administrative positions in the public mental health systems in Philadelphia, New York City, and Detroit over the next two decades. I was encouraged by my residency advisor, Dr. Michael Vergare, to pursue my interest in psychiatric administration, and his support continued to be invaluable throughout my career.

Drs. Samuel Bullock and George Gardiner made me a better "psychiatrist who happened to be black"—aware and comfortable in my black and female skin but not encumbered by the challenges I might encounter due to either. The Falk Fellowship and subsequent opportunities to work with the APA and my local district branch, the Philadelphia Psychiatric Society, led to deeper involvement in the APA, where I served on dozens of components over a 30-plus-year period. There were also opportunities to learn and to become involved in leadership in my areas of interest along the intersection of race and gender in psychiatry through my work with both Black Psychiatrists of America and the Association of Women Psychiatrists. The more involved I became with the APA, however, the more interested I became in its history and the history of blacks in the field.

My first appointment to an APA component was the Committee of Black Psychiatrists. The members at the time included Drs. Earline Houston, Irma Bland, Esther Roberts, and Michelle Clark, all of whom became mentors and over time taught me a lot about the black members of the APA who had made significant contributions to the organization and the field. Beginning with Solomon Carter Fuller, I learned the stories of men and women who had worked in academia, research, and administration in public, private, and government settings going back as far as the 1960s. Learning that black women like Drs. Jeanne Spurlock, Mildred Mitchell-Bateman, and June Jackson Christmas were or had been in key roles in my areas of interest made me more determined to play a leadership role in the field. In fact, it was at a Committee of Black Psychiatrists meeting that I first heard the story of the 1969 confrontation with the APA Board of Trustees (Pierce 1973). I also came to understand the importance of having minority group professional organizations, such as Black Psychiatrists of America and the Association of Women Psychiatrists, and was proud to serve as president of both before the age of 50.

In retrospect, the 20 years between residency graduation and my last government position in Detroit flew by in a blur of increasingly responsible administrative positions in large public behavioral health systems and organizations. Between 1982 and 2002 I served as chief executive officer, executive director, and commissioner of, or in the chief administrative position in, public governmental agencies, publicly funded treatment systems and hospitals, and community-based behavioral health programs. I had the honor of working with excellent role models and mentors, both black and white, throughout this time. My involvement in the APA intensified in the 1990s, and in the 20 years between residency and my work in Detroit, I served on the Managed Care Committee, chaired the Council on Social Issues in Public Psychiatry (during an early reorganization of the APA components), cochaired the steering committee on the APA's response to the first-ever Surgeon General's report on mental health, and was elected deputy representative to the APA Assembly from the Black Caucus during the tenure of Dr. Donna Norris, the APA Assembly's first female and African American Speaker. Outside the APA, I worked with Dr. Walter Menninger in the Group for the Advancement of Psychiatry and, as mentioned earlier, was elected president of both Black Psychiatrists of America and the Association of Women Psychiatrists. I was also honored to be named to the board of directors of the American Psychiatric Foundation, where I later served as president for 4 years.

Throughout all this time, I saw the need to have blacks involved in the APA beyond the traditional minority-focused activities or components. It became clear very early in my work within the APA that there were significant gaps in the general membership's awareness of the APA's racial history. When I was invited to speak at psychiatric meetings and shared the story of APA's racial past, I found that not many people had read the *American Journal of Psychiatry* articles on institutional racism (Sabshin et al. 1970) or the history chronicled by Dr. Chester Pierce and others in the book *Racism and Mental Health* (Willie et al. 1973). My progression upward in the organization was supported by several past APA presidents, including Drs. Paul Fink, Joe English, Mary Jane England, Jack McIntyre, Richard Harding, Harold Eist, Rod Muñoz, Carol Nadelson, Carolyn Robinowitz, and Paul Summergrad, just to name a few.

By 2010, the challenge had become what balance I would strike related to my involvement in the APA as I learned more of the history of psychiatry (and the rest of medicine) related to racist practices in the areas of treatment, training, and research. It was against this backdrop that I had become an APA member almost four decades earlier and worked over the years to work within the organization to address some of those issues raised in 1969. But what was next?

The loss of the nonvoting seat on the APA Board of Trustees for the chair of the Committee of Black Psychiatrists in favor of the Minority/Underrepresented Trustee position (a voting position but open to all MUR groups) was viewed by many black APA members as a serious shift in the APA's relationship with the original minority advocates in the APA. The move from minority affairs to diversity was part of a change in organizational direction, and for many blacks who had been active members for years, it seemed to signal that perhaps the APA was no longer committed to addressing the outstanding and unique issues facing blacks in the organization. It was around this time that the APA launched the Conversations on Diversity series to create a forum for dialogue between the APA leadership and members of the APA's MUR groups and dissipate the growing tension between those groups and the leadership. There was discussion among some in the organization, in which I participated, that it was time for a black to be elected to the organization's highest office. I tested the water with a run for secretary of the APA Board of Trustees and was successful in that bid. As a member of the board for the 2-year term, I continued to work on various APA components that afforded me the opportunity to work closely with others in leadership roles, and for the first time I considered running for president. Beginning with Dr. Charles Prudhomme's election as vice president in 1970, blacks had been elected to national office but never president. My campaign for secretary occurred about 5 years before what would be the 50th anniversary of the 1969 confrontation between the APA black psychiatrists and the APA Board of Trustees, and the symbolism of a presidential run from a historical perspective did not escape me—the election of the first black president might follow the series of "conversations" just as the election of Dr. Prudhomme, the first black officer of the organization, occurred the year after that confrontation (Pierce 1973)—and that's exactly what happened. I was successful in my bid for president, and in May 2018, I was installed as the 145th president of the American Psychiatric Association, the largest psychiatric organization in the world.

In the months since the election, I have thought a lot about the early challenge posed to me by Dr. Alvin Poussaint, the early efforts of Dr. Charles Prudhomme to engage the APA leadership in areas of importance to its black members, the analysis of the historical role of blacks in the APA by Dr. George Mallory, the singular work of Dr. Jeanne Spurlock to institutionalize "minority" affairs in the organization, and the courage of the group of black APA members led by Dr. Chester Pierce who "spoke truth to power" at the APA in 1969. Being "first" comes with great responsibility but also offers great opportunity. So as I consider meeting themes, presidential initiatives, and other responsibilities of the office, I look forward to experiencing the APA described by Dr. Pierce: "The historical tradition of the APA as a learned society must continue without compromise. What is required *in addition* is that the learned society must use itself in the vital and urgent issues of our times" (Pierce 1970, p. 471). This means that issues such as health equity, workforce diversity, and training in the role of culture in diagnostic formulation for psychiatric treatment must be fully integrated into the APA efforts in advocating for high-quality care, appropriate physician reimbursement and regulatory structures, and effective partnerships with the rest of medicine and the people we serve. It is my hope that future black psychiatrists will learn from the history of blacks in the APA (including mine) and continue working to improve the unique relationship that exists between blacks and American psychiatry through the world's largest psychiatric organization. I look forward to being part of that journey.

References

Kaplan M: Solomon Carter Fuller: Where My Caravan Has Rested. Lanham, MD, University Press of America, 2005

Pierce CM: Black psychiatry one year after Miami. J Natl Med Assoc 62(6):471–473, 1970 5493608

Pierce CM: The formation of the Black Psychiatrists of America, in Racism and Mental Health. Edited by Willie CV, Kramer BM, Brown BS. Pittsburgh, PA, University of Pittsburgh, 1973, pp 525–554

Sabshin M, Diesenhaus H, Wilkerson R: Dimensions of institutional racism in psychiatry. Am J Psychiatry 127(6):787–793, 1970 5482872

Shenker I: Racism is called health problem; negro psychiatrists make demands to association. The New York Times, May 9, 1969

Spurlock J: Early and contemporary pioneers, in Black Psychiatrists and American Psychiatry. Edited by Spurlock J. Washington, DC, American Psychiatric Press, 1999, pp 3–25

Stewart A: Determinants of disparities, in Disparities in Psychiatric Care: Clinical and Cross-Cultural Perspectives. Edited by Ruiz P, Primm A. Philadelphia, PA, Lippincott Williams & Wilkins, 2010, pp 10–18

Stewart A: Specializing in the wholly impossible, in Women in Psychiatry: Personal Perspectives. Edited by Norris D, Jayaram G, Primm A. Washington, DC, American Psychiatric Publishing, 2012, pp 161–176

Willie CV, Kramer BM, Brown BS (eds): Racism and Mental Health. Pittsburgh, PA, University of Pittsburgh Press, 1973

CHAPTER 4
BRIDGING THE GAP

Challenges for Mental Health Policy, Research, and Practice

June Jackson Christmas, M.D.

AS I REFLECT on my professional life of more than six decades, I see how my focus evolved from the individual in psychoanalysis, to family and group, to intersecting systems. I believe my choice of psychiatry stemmed partly from significant life experiences: a young woman reared in a middle-class family challenged by northern racism and empowered by African American strengths of survival. Rooted firmly in the black community, I moved, with limitations, in both black and white worlds.

A fourth-generation New Englander on both sides, I grew up in an "integrated but separated" neighborhood in Cambridge, Massachusetts. Of modest means, we were considered middle-class because my father, the breadwinner, was a civil servant and my mother was a homemaker. Northern racism revealed itself along class and race lines. The elite expressed disdain with more civility than my schoolmates, children of the white working class. My parents believed deeply in working hard for education and against racism. Sharing values, they differed in tactics to address racial discrimination. My mother tended to talk each situation through. My father chose his battles. As racial tensions worsened in Cambridge in the 1940s, they both became more involved; their activist roles reflected their personalities. My mother joined a new interracial community relations committee of "town and gown" members. My father was elected head of the chapter of an all-black national organization fighting to redress the grievances of black postal employees, victims of on-the-job discrimination. They shared parenting roles, valued our extended family, and with ingenuity managed to get by in times of economic insecurity (Hill 1973).

Life in the semi-integrated North was confusing in the 1920s and 1930s. Many working-class whites fled as lower-middle-class blacks were let in as tenants on our street. At the nearest Episcopal church, we were among six black families already warmly welcomed to this old Yankee parish. In our public schools serving these mostly white neighborhoods, black children often either got short shrift or were teacher's pets. All teachers were white; some made racist remarks. On "I Am an American Day," all teachers would call on their classes to take part. Row by row, each student would name her or his ancestry (all European) and then proudly proclaim, "But I am an American." Each teacher passed over every black child every time! Slavery was all *our* background was; we must be ashamed of it. Yet I thank my eighth-grade teacher. Different from others, she listened and crossed the color line to inspire. She reinforced my mother's adage about things well done.

Citywide Cambridge High and Latin School (CHLS) brought my Latin teacher, whom I also cherished, into my life. As my father did, he challenged me to be intellectually curious. The 1930s saw labor and racial unrest. As chair of the teen club at the black YWCA, I led our "sit-down" at a local skating rink. When white Southern college teams refused to play a local college unless it benched its sole black player, my two circles of friends (one black, one interracial) expressed indignation. My magazine writing partner, a white friend from our Sunday School, and I thought of writing our column as an interracial team but doubted that we would get our advisor's permission. Regretfully, we did nothing more.

Interracial friendships in a school with black students in the minority had little impact on our all-white teachers and their racist practices. CHLS did not, as a policy, permit black students to attend any social functions, such as proms. Third in my class, I qualified for the National Honor Society but did not expect to be invited because the society did not accept Negroes. At graduation, my favorite teacher presented me with the prize for overall academic achievement. Classmates had asked me to write a poem for the class graduation song; a classmate wrote the music. We all sang together. Our families—one white, one black—gathered in the lobby to share congratulations after the ceremony, a rare sight even in liberal Cambridge.

My family and I had always assumed I would go to nearby Radcliffe College, where my paternal aunt had graduated cum laude in 1919. She was one of only a few black graduates in its 40 years as the women's college of Harvard. I was shocked when the older sister of my high school writing partner, who was a senior at Vassar, sent me word that Vassar was finally going to accept Negroes. (Unlike in my aunt's day at Radcliffe, they would not be forbidden to live on campus.) They wanted students who could succeed academically and socially. She urged me to apply.

Vassar and Radcliffe both accepted me and offered partial scholarships. Eager to travel, though only to New York, I chose Vassar. The president of the Vassar Club of Boston wrote me a courteous note to suggest that it might be better for me, as a freshman, to withdraw my previously submitted request for a roommate. Northern racism, politely expressed! Accepted to a cooperative dormitory at Vassar, I was assigned a single room. My first surprise was that almost every Vassar student had been at the top of her senior class. The second was that the national search to integrate had yielded only two Negro students in a class of more than 500!

The more I did social and laboratory research and met classroom challenges, the more certain I was that I wanted to be a physician. After freshman year, I was accepted into an innovative cooperative dormitory where 24 young women lived. We were of many backgrounds and came from places ranging from the deep South to the Alaska Territory. I integrated this living situation and made lifelong friendships, including with my roommate. Questions about Negroes from many people I met helped me educate my white fellow students. Growing up in Cambridge had prepared me both for interracial relationships and for what were later called microaggressions (Pierce 1974). I had to determine my response: avoidance, education, and occasionally confrontation. Overall, college was a positive experience of intellectual, social, and emotional growth for me. I have remained involved with Vassar all my life, as student and alumna, mentor and trustee, supporter and critic.

By graduation in December 1944 (after our class accelerated to 3.5 years because of World War II), I had decided on psychiatry, to understand and to heal. I wanted to explore human behavior and improve race relations. However, I wanted to go back home. Accepted by Tufts and Boston University, I chose Boston University, with its strong psychiatry and community health programs. I began in the fall of 1945, one of only seven women in our class. Boston University School of Medicine (BUSM) emphasized both the science and the art of medicine. Our innovative senior year exemplified an effort to better serve our South End neighborhood of poor and working-class Negro and Irish people. After junior year clinics, all seniors were required to work full-time as family doctors in a home-health service with teaching faculty who were family physicians. From this introduction to *community health*, I saw how socioeconomic and psychological factors limit or promote health.

Learning firsthand about racism in health, I joined the fight for equity in healthcare. In my junior year I was elected as chair of our chapter of the Association of Internes and Medical Students, a national, progressive, interracial advocacy organization. We pushed to enact national health insurance, open the restrictive American Medical Association to Negro physicians, eliminate racial segregation on wards in hospitals, improve the health status of Negroes and poor people, and increase the number of Negro and women physicians. For most of us across the country, including me, this commitment to informed action in health continued all our lives.

In addition to community health and health activism, BUSM cemented my choice of psychiatry as a specialty. Our psychiatric faculty spanned the ideological distance from Freudian psychoanalysts with patients on the couch to clinicians working in near-drudgery caring for patients warehoused in old state hospitals. My curiosity was piqued as to how such different therapeutic techniques might be effective and what role the psychiatrist played in each.

A 2-year rotating internship at Queens General Hospital in New York City was my choice to gain experience in general medicine before psychiatry. At this small, busy public hospital I learned everything from emergency appendectomies to comforting patients trapped in iron lungs due to the polio epidemic. I was pleased to be accepted for a 3-year residency at Bellevue, the large public hospital synonymous with psychiatry. This was a crucial time; new antipsychotic drugs such as Thorazine were being developed. Along with antidepressants they would replace lobotomies, electroconvulsive therapy, and insulin shock for schizophrenia and depression. As a resident and outpatient staff member, I learned the old and new.

The 1950s were the beginning of the modern Civil Rights Movement. We few black psychiatrists displayed racial solidarity and activism in the face of discrimination in our lives, our practices, and the lives of our mostly black patients. White colleagues initially rarely referred patients to us; they treated few blacks as private patients. Yet some downtown white-owned private clinics hired young psychiatrists across racial lines. We were expected to draw our first private patients from this roster, regardless of race. Working in these settings and in small free clinics in Harlem such as Harriet Tubman and Lafargue reinforced my decision to be a psychiatrist. With added training in group therapy and family therapy, I began working with children in foster care (in the all-black child welfare system) and with couples.

Like many colleagues, I wanted to become a psychoanalyst. I followed the neo-Freudian precepts of Harry Stack Sullivan, who developed the theory of interpersonal psychoanalysis. It held that fundamental to the psychoanalytic process is *the person as a social being within the surrounding culture*. In 1955, after 5 years of study, personal and training psychoanalysis, and supervised practice, I graduated, the second black person and first black woman to receive a certificate in psychoanalysis from the William Alanson White Institute in New York City.

For the next decade, I practiced mainly psychoanalytically oriented psychotherapy, as well as psychoanalysis and group therapy. Although private practice was fulfilling, I came to wish I could reach more people. So I did not hesitate when, in the early 1960s, Elizabeth B. Davis, M.D., a Columbia University–trained psychiatrist, asked me to join her team. An African American New Yorker, she was founding the first full-fledged department of psychiatry at Harlem Hospital, in affiliation with Columbia University, in the heart of the black community. She asked me to set up the group therapy program and teach these techniques to staff. Soon she urged me to do something so that chronically mentally ill patients did not overwhelm our planned community mental health center (CMHC), for which we hoped to obtain federal funding.

With its demographics of poor, working-class, and middle-class populations, Harlem had among the lowest per-capita incomes in the city. It ranked among the highest in rates of discharges from state psychiatric hospitals, with hundreds of patients being released each week into our streets. My proposal to build rehabilitation into our CMHC plans was rejected, with a challenge that we find funds. (Federal CMHCs listed rehabilitation as "optional.") Surveys and visits to the few existing rehabilitation programs in big cities showed that they had almost no black patients and knew no culturally relevant techniques effective with mentally ill black people. One prospective funder at first feared that research in Harlem would be "pouring money down a bottomless well." Yet we succeeded. The National Institute of Mental Health, Rehabilitation Services Administration, New York State Department of Mental Hygiene, and New York Division of Vocational Rehabilitation eventually awarded 7 years of research funding. I was principal investigator on major interrelated grants to study the effectiveness of group methods in psychiatric rehabilitation in an urban ghetto. Paraprofessional workers would be the primary agents (Wade et al. 1969).

Consistent with the Sullivanian principle of the centrality of the individual in society, I read, brainstormed, and imagined a program that would help black middle-aged men and women move from years in psychiatric hospitals to living new lives in and out of the Harlem community. I visualized a graduated approach, both psychiatric and social in orientation, that assumed an intrinsic developmental nature and that recognized the interaction between human beings and society in a social systems approach. Furthermore, because of the historical and current experiences of black people in a society with institutionalized racism, this approach acknowledged that black patients are placed in a devalued imposed social position because of both their illness and their racially oppressed status. Improved coping is a goal. I called this approach *sociopsychiatric rehabilitation*. It is characterized by multidisciplinary interventions directed toward helping individuals achieve optimal social, psychiatric, educational, and vocational roles within their capacities and potentialities (Christmas 1969; Richards and Daniels 1969).

Harlem Rehabilitation Center (HRC) was set up in a newly renovated building about a half mile from the hospital. The primary staff were members of the local community. Identified for their skills in coping constructively and potential for empathy, among other talents, they were hired and trained by us as paraprofessional rehabilitation workers. Many of the women had been welfare recipients; the men were all ex-offenders. All were black. A small interracial professional staff served as supervisors and trainers. On-the-job training followed paid full-time training. A four-rung "rehabilitation worker ladder" went from trainee to supervisor. Workers conducted group activities along a continuum in three full-day rehabilitation programs (psychiatric, transitional, and prevocational). Each program provided social work, community organization, and community action; family casework, counseling, and aid; educational evaluation; literacy training; health services (psychiatric, medical, nutritional); and remediation activities. Music, dance, drama, and art were expressive vehicles.

Findings from structured psychiatric interviews by the research unit were that in contrast to comparison groups (patients attending the hospital clinic for monthly medication), patients in all HRC programs showed (among others) greater improvement in mood, psychiatric status, self-esteem, and community contacts. They had fewer hospitalizations with shorter stays. Research showed that this approach worked. Fortunately, efforts for permanent funding brought our work as an innovative program to the attention of Mayor John Lindsay. Shortly thereafter, in 1972, I accepted his offer to appoint me as deputy commissioner of the Department of Mental Health. For more than 35 years, the rehabilitation workers and professionals provided services as HRC developed this effective model of mental healthcare.

Six months after I was appointed deputy commissioner, Mayor Lindsay swore me in as commissioner of the New York City Department of Mental Health and Mental Retardation Services (DMHMRS). DMHMRS was the largest locally administered system of mental hygiene services in the United States, yet it did not provide direct services. Its mandate was to plan, fund, contract with, and supervise services provided by (at that time) 118 nonprofit agencies and hospitals, 14 municipal hospitals, the Departments of Courts and Corrections, and the Bureau of Child Guidance of the Board of Education. Mental health, mental retardation, and alcoholism services were under its aegis. (Addiction services were under the Health Department.)

My first policy paper, presented in 1973 (Christmas 1999), stated three goals:

1. To develop a single, integrated service system, unifying public (municipal and state) and private (not-for-profit) services, whether preventive, therapeutic, or rehabilitative.
2. To provide care for a defined geographic population. Priority was to be given to populations at risk. The goal was to make high-quality, effective services accessible, available, and responsive to locally identified needs.
3. To include residents of these defined areas and staff members of the institutions and agencies serving these areas in the planning and decision making concerning mental hygiene programs and policies.

Despite fiscal and systemic barriers, in my administration we were able to make progress in extending and improving services for the mentally and developmentally disabled.

In this policy paper after 9 months with the department, I assigned top priority to the goal of *unified services*. I saw state duality as the barrier to a rational mental health system. Being both provider and funder prevented coordination, collaboration, and appropriately shared responsibility. Deinstitutionalization policy kept the bulk of funds in empty buildings while new money was not made available to the locality for CMHCs.

The exposure of terrible conditions of neglect of people with developmental disabilities at Willowbrook State School led to emergency state and city funding. We, city and state, took this opportunity to develop joint mental retardation plans, programs, and staff. Despite this successful collaboration, we could not develop comparable informal agreements with state psychiatric hospitals. Despite working with county commissioners statewide, it still took 4 years for state unified services legislation to pass. Only two counties joined (excluding New York City). Limited new state funds came mainly after political calls to "get the homeless off the streets." Nonetheless, in the spirit of the law, we continued to push the priority of supportive housing.

Needs assessment showed major gaps in allocation of resources, distribution and range of services, and quality. African Americans, Latinos, and Chinese Americans were underrepresented as both providers and mental hygiene consumers. Children of all ethnicities, adolescents, elderly people, and residents of the outer boroughs were underserved as well. We systematically began building on available resources and allocating funds for new models of culturally appropriate community mental health services, often without specific federal CMHC funding.

We ensured that the city equal employment opportunity policy was an actuality. Adding to our ranks, we cast our net widely and increased the number of persons of color in positions of responsibility. Several black middle managers already on board whose skills had been overlooked in the past earned the opportunity to contribute to a renewed department. Young psychiatrists (women and men; black, Latino, and white), promoted from inside and/or hired from outside, went on to head agencies and succeed in other leadership positions.

The relative financial plenty of the first 3 years allowed growth. Task forces developed programs for children, for the elderly, and for youth in foster care and the legal system, as well as programs for rehabilitation and alcoholism. We added mental health services to small clinics led by people of color in underserved communities (Harlem, the South Bronx, Chinatown, and Bedford-Stuyvesant). The Mental Health Worker career ladder was established under the Civil Service. Inpatient and outpatient services were strengthened. Interagency connections were fostered and collaboration improved. We expanded and/or improved services in all underserved boroughs.

During the fiscal crisis of 1975, contracts with mental health and alcoholism agencies required reductions through personnel cuts imposed on all city departments except police and fire. Given the option, we refused to impose uniform cuts across the board. As far as possible, we wanted to be consistent with policy and plans and do the least damage to the most needy. Otherwise, some older, more traditional nonprofit agencies would have willingly eliminated all their Mental Health Worker lines (essential to their program) and used the funds to keep another psychiatrist (needed or not). City Budget once even suggested it would be easier to eliminate a group of smaller agencies (headed by people of color) than labor over individual cuts in each older, larger, established agency (with, incidentally, white administration). We found a nonracial alternative.

Our demand for greater accountability meant that we were able to reallocate funds toward greater need as well as demand efficiencies from agencies of all sizes. We instituted the first contract (rather than a letter of agreement) with the Health and Hospitals Corporation and with the Board of Education. We had funded them for years. Filling gaps, we moved *toward* a system of services. People in need of services could more readily and easily get quality care. Yet a major regret is that we continued past failures to adequately address the poor quality of mental health services in prisons, where young men, many black, continued to suffer from mental illness.

Strong program and administrative staff helped our hard work succeed. Our Mental Hygiene Advisory Board, composed of mayor-appointed outstanding citizens and experts, provided support. As we created a new body of providers and consumers, we moved forward successfully to plan with citizen participation. The Federation for Mental Health, Mental Retardation, and Alcoholism Services was empowered to assist us in project review, plan development, and program evaluation. Organized on a catchment area, regional, borough, and citywide basis as well as across specialties, this structure of providers and citizens not only made recommendations for new services and for the annual plan but also was represented in the city health planning agency and on our advisory board. As we used media and open meetings to inform the city on mental hygiene, federation families and consumers also educated the public.

Developmental disability participation in the federation became a model because of family participation and joint city and state staffing. Other consumer representatives and families joined, including once-reluctant citizens and providers in alcoholism programs. A model for effective planning, this structure was incorporated into the city charter. The federation was one of our activities for which we proudly received local, state, and national recognition.

After 8 years as commissioner, I stepped down, now a breast cancer survivor, buoyed by the support of my husband and three young adult children. Providing mental health services for black patients and leading a city mental hygiene department were hard tasks. I needed to be part of something larger than myself, besides family, such as the 1969 "rebellion" by our small group of black psychiatrists, which had led to structural changes in the American Psychiatric Association (APA) and the National Institute of Mental Health and to greater attention by psychiatry to racism and mental health. In the early 1970s the APA Black Caucus and the newly established Black Psychiatrists of America supported my election as they had those of the two prior black vice presidents, Dr. Charles Prudhomme and Dr. Mildred Mitchell-Bateman. In the late 1970s the American Public Health Association (APHA) was pushed to focus on environmental racism and on narrowing the racial gap between black and majority populations. Support for my APHA presidency came from across the membership. In each position I advocated for mental health as a public health concern and for policies to decrease racial disparities. The 1980s required effort just to stay in place or manage crises. Early in the 1990s I brought a dozen colleagues together to see what the decade would demand of us.

We established a research institute, the Urban Issues Group (UIG), to conduct policy analysis from the perspectives of New Yorkers of African descent. Coming together had been stimulated in part by the 1990 election of the first black mayor, David N. Dinkins, but UIG was nonpartisan. We were leaders in health, family, and child welfare; economics, law, and industry; communications and the arts; education; and research and policy analysis. Our mission was to contribute to developing and implementing public and private policies affecting the quality of life of people of African descent.

Our strategies were to conduct research, perform policy analyses, publish reports, hold policy symposia and conferences, and promote development of African descent policy analysts (Christmas 1994). Walter Stafford, Ph.D., a political scientist at the Wagner School at New York University, and Leith Mullings, Ph.D., an anthropologist at the City University of New York, joined me as cofounders. I was then clinical professor of psychiatry (PT) at Columbia University College of Physicians and Surgeons and I soon became the UIG executive director. Our proposals received foundation interest and funding. We held research workshops led by the Research Advisory Council, symposia and conferences, focus groups, and community conversations. *Urbanscope* was our quarterly newsletter with invited commentary. Young researchers, mainly of African descent, developed and conducted surveys, interviews, and analysis of primary and secondary data under the supervision of our research codirectors. Reports on our studies included topics such as health policy and the health of black New Yorkers, the health of black children and adolescents, foster care, education vouchers, the state of the black family, how black families view trends in health, and welfare reform.

Bedford-Stuyvesant in Brooklyn was the community of our interest for several studies. I interviewed formal and informal community leaders and led focus groups of people with or affected by HIV/AIDS, teenagers aging out of foster care, and families struggling without health insurance and with illness. When grant support decreased in a changing environment, we reluctantly closed after 10 years.

In psychotherapy we listen. In rehabilitation we challenge. I have added to my training the listening that my mother modeled for me, to hear what people say or do not say. Similarly, as my father did, as administrator I have had to choose between righteous confrontation and challenge and what is right for the situation at this time.

As a black student in near-white educational settings, I had to decide how to respond to microaggressions even before they had a name. Living in a certain time and place, I experienced individual and institutionalized racism from that vantage. Yet the North also exposed me to the good: diversity and interracial relationships as equals. Black and white people helped me on the way. White church friends gave me information about Vassar ending racial exclusiveness. Two men, a black physician expert in addiction and a white psychologist theoretician, each brainstormed with me as I conceived HRC. A white psychiatric colleague volunteered to manage my successful campaign for the APA vice presidency. Dr. Elizabeth Davis, a black woman, gave me freedom to create.

I deplore racism, North or South. Yet the need to cope with the challenges of northern racism and the gift of being empowered by African American strengths of survival (as exemplified by the lives of my parents) have *both* influenced my work. I have tried to implement the values of equity, autonomy, and community in a way that enhances my practice of psychiatry and works to decrease the gap that separates and devalues.

References

Christmas JJ: Sociopsychiatric rehabilitation in a black urban ghetto, I: conflicts, issues, and directions. Am J Orthopsychiatry 39(4):651–661, 1969 5803599

Christmas JJ: About UIG. New York, UIG Report, 1994

Christmas JJ: Community psychiatry and work in the public sector, in Black Psychiatrists and American Psychiatry. Edited by Spurlock J. Washington, DC, American Psychiatric Association, 1999, pp 57–59

Hill RB: The Strengths of Black Families. New York, Guilford, 1973

Pierce CM: Psychiatric problems of the black minority, in American Handbook of Psychiatry. Edited by Arieti S. Washington, DC, American Psychiatric Association, 1974, pp 512–523

Richards H, Daniels MS: Sociopsychiatric rehabilitation in a black urban ghetto, II: innovative treatment roles and approaches. Am J Orthopsychiatry 39(4):662–676, 1969 5803600

Wade R, Jordan G, Myers G: Sociopsychiatric rehabilitation in a black urban ghetto, III: the view of the paraprofessional. Am J Orthopsychiatry 39(4):677–683, 1969 5803601

CHAPTER 5
BLACK PSYCHIATRISTS OF 1969 SURVEY THE SCENE, THEN AND NOW

Orlando B. Lightfoot, M.D.
Dexter L. Fields, M.D.

IN MAY 1969, at the American Psychiatric Association (APA) annual meeting in Miami, 16 senior black psychiatrist members made a series of demands for a change in the status quo to the APA hierarchy. They demanded that the APA use its considerable influence to change the function of the National Institute of Mental Health (NIMH). Additionally, they demanded that the APA take a national stand with them against hospitals and educational facilities that practiced racial discrimination. At this same meeting, five young, black, male psychiatrists in training, or who had recently completed training, shared their experiences ("Racism is Called Major Problem of Mental Health in the Nation" 1969).

The demands made and the responses of the APA began a dialogue that resulted in significant changes in the inclusion of blacks within organized psychiatry and reduced racial discrimination in mental health facilities. This chapter comprises a series of reflections and recollections from a select participating group of psychiatrists about that action 50 years ago, the changes that it precipitated, and the realities confronting blacks in psychiatry, now and in the future.

Black psychiatrists making demands on the hierarchy of the APA did not develop within a vacuum. They stood on the shoulders of largely unidentified blacks, mute and vocal, indentured or enslaved, who over four centuries in the United States had resisted enslavement, Jim Crow practices, physical assault, and discriminatory laws (Grier and Cobbs 1968; Peters 1996). Racism/white supremacy can be documented throughout all aspects of civil discourse in the lives of black and white Americans. Black psychiatrists were aware that the psychiatric theory, clinical practice, and social psychology of that time deemed black people inferior, devalued, angry, intellectually deficient, hypersexual, incapable of introspection, and products of dysfunctional families and poor childrearing practices. All of these negative and untrue perceptions contributed to blacks having reduced access to psychiatric services and less effective psychiatric interventions (Lightfoot 1974; Thomas and Sillen 1972; Willie 1973). These misperceptions needed to be changed through intentional redress and reformulation with black participation and direction (Harrison and Butts 1970; Pinderhughes 1969).

Race has always been an undeclared organizing factor in American life, although most often unacknowledged (Katznelson 2005). No area of civil discourse is untouched, including health, education, housing, social welfare, politics, religion, law, criminal justice, the environment, sports, entertainment, and media (Lightfoot 1971; Stevenson 2014; Wallis 2016; Welsing 1991).

The senior black psychiatrists, men and women, making demands on the APA were united in purpose, although different in age, personality, background, style, and undergraduate, medical school, and postgraduate training. They found strength in working together to improve the services delivered to black patients and wanted to increase the number of blacks throughout the entire educational, service delivery, and research continuum. Because of racial exclusion by the American Medical Association, the National Medical Association (NMA) was founded in 1895 to ensure black physicians received comprehensive training (Spurlock 1999).

The "Young Lions," five young, black, male psychiatrists participating in the program, were all friends, educated together either in undergraduate school, medical school, and/or training programs. Psychoanalytic theory and psychoanalysts dominated each of the three separate training programs. The Young Lions discovered that if a patient was a person of color, by definition he or she did not meet the gold standard for being selected for individual psychotherapy but received primarily medication management (White 2011). Their recommendations to predominately white training programs included more education regarding cultural and racial identity issues for all staff, including supervisors and particularly first-line intake workers; broadened admission policies for individual psychotherapy, with emphasis on inclusion of community residents; increased recruitment of black supervisors; the requirement that all staff work in a community facility managed and directed by a black professional; and recruitment of more black trainees to minimize racial isolation ("Racism is Called Major Problem of Mental Health in the Nation" 1969; Jones et al. 1970).

Much has changed in the world since 1969 when black psychiatrists made their formal demands in Miami Beach. 2018 is a reasonable time to initiate a retrospective survey of those black psychiatrists, allowing them to consider and offer longitudinal reflections on the past 49 years. The following survey evolved from that basic idea. The task was to offer an open-ended format for response using a few guidelines to ensure uniformity of approach to all participants.

Survey Design

Senior psychiatrists who presented the demands at the APA annual meeting in Miami were Hugh F. Butts, M.D.; J. Alfred Cannon, M.D.; June Jackson Christmas, M.D.; James P. Comer, M.D.; Elizabeth B. Davis, M.D.; Lloyd C. Elam, M.D.; Hiawatha Harris, M.D.; Phyllis Harrison-Ross, M.D.; Mildred Mitchell-Bateman, M.D.; Chester M. Pierce, M.D.; Charles A. Pinder-hughes, M.D.; Alvin F. Poussaint, M.D.; Charles Prudhomme, M.D.; Jeanne Spurlock, M.D.; Frances C. Welsing, M.D.; and Charles B. Wilkinson, M.D.

The Young Lions were Billy E. Jones, M.D.; Orlando B. Lightfoot, M.D.; Don Palmer, M.D.; Raymond G. Wilkerson, M.D.; and Donald H. Williams, M.D.

For this project, four senior psychiatrists and four Young Lions were interviewed. The interview format is included with each interview. All contacts were tailored for the convenience of the interviewee. The following talking points were used as general guidelines for the interviews:

- General comments about 1969 and 2017.
- Who were you professionally, privately during that time? Family life?
- How were you included in the group of senior psychiatrists or Young Lions? Invited? Included early in formation process or later?
- What were your "burning issues"? Clinical work, research, education or other?
- How did you understand the relationship between black psychiatrists and the APA?
- What was your involvement in local or national APA issues? Role?
- What was your personal response to the presentation of demands to the APA? Expectations or wishes for the APA's response?
- Was your personal or professional trajectory altered after 1969?
- What do you feel has been accomplished since 1969? What started? What stalled or faltered?
- What needs to be done in the future?
- Any other items that flowed organically from the interview.

Both the authors and interviewees were excited about the opportunity to review that period in their lives and the aftermath despite interview scheduling issues. The authors made editorial decisions as to how the interviews would be reported. Although there was much rich material produced, all could not be reported because of time constraints and contextual factors. What may appear stilted or sterile in the reporting is no reflection on the relaxed, collegial exchanges that took place while renewing old contacts with Dr. Lightfoot or establishing new ones with Dr. Dexter L. Fields. The authors thank each participant for their involvement and for making this chapter possible.

Results: Interviews 1–6
Interview #1

- *Subject:* Alvin F. Poussaint, M.D., Professor of Psychiatry and Associate Dean of Student Affairs, Harvard University School of Medicine, Boston, Massachusetts
- *Interviewers:* Drs. Fields and Lightfoot
- *Location:* Dr. Poussaint's office, Boston, Massachusetts
- *Interview:* 1.5 hours

Dr. Poussaint graduated from Cornell Medical School in 1960 but did not "feel welcomed." He was the only black student in his class. He was encouraged to apply for residency in psychiatry at UCLA by Dr. J. Alfred Cannon, who had trained there. Poussaint recounted numerous racist acts toward him, including being called the "N-word" and being physically assaulted by a patient. Supervisors gave little support and said, "If you can't take it, you shouldn't be in psychiatry." During his years of training, he was the only black resident. Few black patients were treated there because the white staff stereotypically assumed they were angry, acting out, and not wanting or accepting of psychiatric intervention. His support came from two black psychiatrists in the community—Dr. Cannon and Dr. Hiawatha Harris, who had begun an outpatient clinic for blacks who were not welcomed at UCLA or other predominantly white facilities. Poussaint had also expressed an interest in research at UCLA and was encouraged. Dr. Chester Pierce, at the University of Oklahoma, supported his interests and connected him with enuresis research—Pierce studying naval recruits and Poussaint children. The interviewee also spoke about his interest in social justice and his support from the Student Nonviolent Coordinating Committee (SNCC), the local NAACP, Dr. Martin Luther King Jr., Rev. Jesse Jackson, and from various psychology and social work groups active during that era. Leaders of the Black Power movement and the Congressional Black Caucus were all involved in discussing and demanding cultural relevance. Dr. Poussaint worked as the Southern Field Director of the Medical Committee for Human Rights in Jackson, Mississippi (1965-1967). While there, he met Dr. Robert Coles, who was writing about the impact of racism and segregation on child development.

Currently, Dr. Poussaint continues to advocate for studies that focus on children and child development. He also supports improved diagnosis and more culturally relevant interventions for black children.

Interview #2

- *Subject:* James P. Comer, M.D., Professor of Psychiatry and Associate Dean, Yale University Medical School; Director, Comer School Development Program, New Haven, Connecticut
- *Interviewers:* Dr. Lightfoot face-to-face; Dr. Fields via telephone patch-in
- *Location:* Dr. Comer's office, New Haven, Connecticut
- *Interview:* 1.75 hours

Dr. Comer began by recalling that in 1969, the United States had "civil unrest in the air." He thought black psychiatrists had to make a statement and be involved in those changes. He adamantly thought white psychiatrists, who were using a variant of benign neglect, would not articulate our position for ourselves or our black patients. Comer gave a passionate recollection of growing up in a small Indiana town with God-fearing parents who, though largely unschooled, pushed for a better life for their children through education and strong religious underpinnings. Early parental training was a solid framework for his future development. It has carried him into public health, psychiatry, academia, research, and educational contributions in child development. Comer recalled childhood friends who did not fare well in school until positive personal traits were identified (e.g., utilized by the individual and the system) and toxic environmental elements ameliorated (Comer 2014). He wishes for a future black-inspired organized study group/structure/multidisciplinary entity that includes as many perspectives as possible that could address some of the basic issues of early childhood development in order to provide appropriate interventions. Dr. Comer fondly recalled contacts with the other black psychiatrists from 1969.

Interview #3

- *Subjects:* "Young Lions" Raymond G. Wilkerson, M.D., Retired Psychoanalyst and Clinical Assistant Professor of Psychiatry, University of Illinois Medical School, Chicago, Illinois; Donald H. Williams, M.D., Professor and Chairman of the Department Emeritus, Michigan State University, East Lansing, Michigan; Orlando B. Lightfoot, M.D., Professor of Psychiatry Emeritus and Former Vice Chair, Community Psychiatry, Boston University School of Medicine, and Retired Psychoanalyst, Boston, Massachusetts

- *Interviewers:* Dr. Fields, with Dr. Lightfoot as interviewer and interviewee
- *Location:* The apartment of Dr. Williams
- *Group interview:* 2.75 hours. A group format was suggested by Dr. Williams, who thought it might more readily stimulate recall.

The interview began with reflections on the residency years. It was clear that these three men liked one another and were compatible as well as competitive, in the healthiest way. They had been in residency training together at the University of Illinois, Chicago, with Dr. Williams 2 years ahead of the others. The subject of race was a daily part of their training experience. These psychiatrists discussed, particularly, how even today racism/white supremacy shapes and influences their lives as people and professionals. During residency they traveled together to APA, NMA, and other conventions. They knew many senior black psychiatrists as mentors and found them accessible as people. The trio also talked about the complexity of race and the formation of individual concepts influential on the way they would practice in the future. Recalling the 1969 meeting, one member of the trio was impressed by the conference room–to–conference room negotiations between the black psychiatrists and APA leadership. Observing the mentors in that real-life role filled him with pride. Another member of the group became acutely aware of the origins of some of his ideas about how a practicing psychiatrist functions—in particular, his approach to administrative decision making that was a combination of experiences gleaned in the residency and the discussions the Lions had had among themselves. That incredible insight became clear only during this interview in 2017. Another in the trio recalled the discussion of their paper by their training director, Dr. Melvin Sabshin, who modeled for his white colleagues how one respects another person's efforts, point of view, beliefs, and passion by intentionally withholding harsh criticism. Sabshin was a mentor and role model who blended personal and professional traits the Lions all emulated and admired. He espoused multidisciplinary inclusion, attentiveness, and awareness of issues of racial differences and the need for engagement around them. In addition, he demonstrated how one encourages thinking about racial and ethnic isolation and the need for a critical density of people in order to effect change in a system (Jones et al. 1970).

Interview #4

- *Subject:* Billy E. Jones, M.D, Clinical Professor of Psychiatry, New York University School of Medicine, New York; Former Commissioner, New York City Department of Mental Health, Mental Retardation, and Alcoholism Services; Former President, New York City Health and Hospitals Corporation

- *Interviewers:* Dr. Lightfoot; Dr. Fields via telephone patch-in
- *Location:* Dr. Jones's home in Harlem, New York
- *Interview:* 2 hours

Concerning his training, Dr. Jones was acutely aware of being racially isolated even though there was a black woman, admitted previously, whom he never met and who later left the program. He got along well with many of the "liberal, Jewish whites" whom he considered friends. Interestingly, many residents viewing a video of a group therapy session had "hallucinated [him] white," as they did not remember him as black. He was mentored by the then chairman of the department, Alfred Freedman, M.D. His main support in the hospital came from black staff—nurses, secretaries, maintenance workers, cafeteria workers, and security officers. The interviewee was comfortable with other Young Lions because he attended medical school with two and interned with one of those. While at Meharry Medical College, Dr. Jones was taught by Dr. Lloyd Elam, whom he saw as a mentor and role model. Dr. Robert Sharpley, former director of the Solomon Carter Fuller Institute, was also in that class. Early on, Jones recognized the need for a critical density of black physicians because of his racial isolation (Jones et al. 1970). Regarding the 1969 presentation by the Young Lions, the interviewee was in favor of participating because doing so could be useful for future black residents. He was aware also of advantages for blacks as active participants in the APA committee structure and in the NIMH grant-funding mechanism. Another change brought about by the black psychiatrists' action was the appointment of Dr. James Ralph as chief of the Center for Minority Group Mental Health Programs at NIMH. Dr. Jones expressed concern that structural changes, initiated by the black psychiatrists' action in both institutions, were not sustained. Dr. Altha J. Stewart became APA President in 2018, exemplifying the positive result of many years of inclusion within the organization. In the face of intractable racism/white supremacy, Jones is interested in contributing to the development of a comprehensive black study group/institute/program that focuses on adult and child development by a multidisciplinary team that understands power, management, financing, program development, and related issues.

Interview #5

- *Subject:* June Jackson Christmas, M.D., Clinical Professor Emeritus of Behavioral Science, City University of New York Medical College; Former Commissioner of Mental Health, Mental Retardation and Alcoholism Services, City of New York; Former Clinical Professor of Psychiatry (PT), Columbia University College of Physicians and Surgeons, New York; For-

mer Executive Director, Urban Issues Group, New York; Retired Psycho-
analyst; Former Director of Rehabilitation Psychiatry, Harlem Hospital
Center, New York
- *Interviewers:* Dr. Lightfoot face-to-face; Dr. Fields via telephone patch-in
- *Location:* Dr. Christmas's home, New York City
- *Interview:* 2 hours

Dr. Christmas graduated from college in 1944 and completed medical school
in 1949. At the time she completed psychiatry training and psychoanalytic studies, there were very few blacks in psychiatry. In the United States there was "a
comradeship among black people fueled by the Civil Rights and the Black Power
Movements." In the 1960s, black psychiatrists within the APA gravitated to
one another and formed an informal support group that by 1969 became action
oriented. She identified as leaders Dr. Jeanne Spurlock, a wise and forceful presence; Dr. J. Alfred Cannon; and Dr. Chester Pierce. In making demands for
change within the APA and NIMH, Dr. Christmas fully understood the need
for enlightened white support like the support she had received from Dr. John
Spiegel, Dr. John Talbott, and others. One outgrowth of these demands was
the appointment of Dr. Robert Phillips as Director of Minority Programs at
the APA. She pointed out that in successive APA national elections in the early
1970s, blacks were elected vice president: Dr. Charles Prudhomme, Dr. Mildred
Mitchell-Bateman, and herself. The joy of those elections was tempered by the
pain of living through the defeat of three excellent blacks who were not, in subsequent years, elected president: Dr. Charles Wilkinson, Dr. Chester Pierce, and,
later, Dr. Donna Norris, twice!

Dr. Christmas also recognizes the strength in numbers afforded her by joining two other black women psychiatrists in the mid-1960s at Harlem Hospital—Dr. Elizabeth B. Davis as chair and Dr. Margaret M. Lawrence as head of
the adolescent and children's unit. She had other black mentors and colleagues,
including Dr. Frances J. Bonner, a psychoanalyst, and Dr. Charles Bonner, an
internist in the Boston area. She recalls growing as a rehabilitation psychiatrist
when she directly observed the strength and wisdom exhibited by parents and
other community residents, who soon became valued members of her extended
treatment team. Despite positive and regressive changes over the years at the APA
and NIMH, the interviewee still yearns for the development of a study unit that
focuses on the qualities needed for young, talented, black college students to
succeed. She indicates that identifying, articulating, assessing, and teaching those
qualities are a valid focus of study for the future. Dr. Christmas is appreciative
of the scholarships given in her name at Vassar College and Boston University
School of Medicine, from which she graduated; however, she feels that both financial and emotional support are vital.

Interview #6

- *Subject:* Hiawatha Harris, M.D., Current Director, Pathways to Wellness, Oakland, California; Former Director of the South Central Mental Health Center, Los Angeles, California
- *Interviewers:* Dr. Fields and Dr. Lightfoot, telephone conference
- *Interview:* 45 minutes

Dr. Harris describes himself as one of the younger psychiatrists who were mentored by Drs. Chester Pierce, J. Alfred Cannon, Jeanne Spurlock, and Charles Prudhomme. Dr. Prudhomme knew Dr. Solomon Carter Fuller, the first black psychiatrist in the United States and contemporary of Sigmund Freud. Fuller also did early research into Alzheimer's disease. After graduating from Meharry Medical College and completing an internship at San Francisco General Hospital, Harris was encouraged to apply for psychiatric training at Metropolitan State Hospital, in Norwalk, California, by Dr. Price Cobbs, who knew the program was receptive to black trainees. The director, Dr. Arnold Beisser, became a mentor who invited him to coauthor a paper (Beisser and Harris 1966). There were two other black trainees in the program during Dr. Harris's tenure at Metropolitan State. He had been alerted that the University of California, Berkeley, and Langley Porter in San Francisco were not accepting black trainees. South Central Mental Health Center in the Watts Community of Los Angeles, where Dr. Harris worked in concert with Dr. J. Alfred Cannon, became a major center for services and training on the West Coast. He feels that the greatest result of the 1969 confrontation was opening the door for blacks in training and expanded advancement within the APA and NIMH. These opportunities, forged by blacks, opened up the gates for other minority and underrepresented groups. The interviewee feels that reparations for blacks should be made in the form of educational access and financial support so that dreams can become a reality without financial millstones.

Dr. Harris was active in APA programs and committees for many years but later shifted his activism to the California black psychiatric community that included Drs. Rose Jenkins, George Mallory, and Herbert Robinson. Dr. Harris laments the absence of a think tank in concert with other blacks, across multiple disciplines.

Findings: Main Themes

1. The 1969 event was recalled differently by all responders, with some having great details of the time and others having few memories. The talking points

did stimulate memories; however, all the interviewees were current with 2017 psychiatric and political issues.

2. Racism/white supremacy is as pernicious today as it was in 1969.

3. Managing, dealing with, and educating ourselves and others about racism/ white supremacy is a *never-ending process*. The temptation to deny this reality is enormous.

4. Accepting the powerful magnitude of racism/white supremacy helps one to marshal resources to more readily manage its impact and to share the methods used with other professionals over time.

5. To help manage the ongoing racism/white supremacy during training or practice, one might consciously organize personal and professional environments to reflect the following:

   • Having a critical density of consulting black professionals available
   • Using mentors, regardless of race or ethnicity, and assessing their ability to enhance one's skill, which will occur over time
   • Respecting the value of a multidisciplinary team for consultation
   • Remaining respectful and consciously inclusive with regard to others
   • Establishing, encouraging, and maintaining relationships with various entities—that is, in health, educational, welfare, economic, legal, and related areas (Pierce 1970)

6. The responders acknowledged that the APA and NIMH have made uneven progress managing racism/white supremacy over the past 50 years. The APA has downsized and restructured to a point that few blacks are in relative positions of power. The Center for Minority Group Programs within NIMH no longer exists in its original form. In 2018, 49 years after 1969, a black psychiatrist, Altha J. Stewart, M.D., began leading the APA.

7. There is a need to develop and fund a think tank/alliance/consortium/ forum for continued in-depth collection and study of the many dimensions of racism/white supremacy in the areas of health, medicine, psychiatry, psychology, science, economics, finance, welfare, social services, education, politics, law, criminal justice, religion, sports, media, the environment, and other areas across the life span of black individuals. Such a think tank/ alliance/consortium/forum should strive to be inclusive of all ideas and concepts about black people.

Discussion Points

Racism/white supremacy, confronted by black psychiatrists in 1969, is still alive in 2018 against our patients and us. Because its presentation constantly changes, a major task is to accurately identify it. Its tentacles extend into various components of civil discourse: health, economics, housing, education, law, criminal justice, politics, religion, the environment, sports, entertainment, the military, media, and other areas (Tweedy 2015). Managing this massive, insidious, overwhelming, immutable force requires a mind-set that emphasizes infinite patience and focuses an attack on one small aspect at a time.

Tools exist for professionals managing ongoing racism/white supremacy either in training or in practice and must be utilized consistently by 1) helping to create a climate that encourages the inclusion of other black professionals as colleagues and consultants; 2) using mentors, regardless of race or ethnicity, realizing that the ability to recognize a kindred soul requires time and experience; 3) working with a multidisciplinary team of colleagues and consultants; 4) valuing others in spite of different ideas, orientation, or point of view; 5) establishing, encouraging, and maintaining relationships in health, education, welfare, economic, legal, and allied affiliates.

Recommendation/Action Item

A national entity in the form of a think tank/alliance/consortium/forum should be developed and funded by black psychiatrists and other professionals across multiple disciplines. This entity would have educational and research capabilities with implications for clinical practice. It would also study the multiple dimensions of racism/white supremacy and the coping mechanisms required to manage it in all areas of civil discourse.

This recommendation is a dynamic, vital issue that requires continued attention and review. An assessment of progress regarding the implementation of this recommendation should be initiated within the next 5 years.

References

Beisser AR, Harris H: Psychological aspects of the civil rights movement and the Negro professional man. Am J Psychiatry 123(6):733–737, 1966 5927597

Comer JP: Leave No Child Behind: Preparing Today's Youth for Tomorrow's World. New Haven, CT, Yale University Press, 2014

Grier WH, Cobbs PM: Black Rage. New York, Basic Books, 1968

Harrison PA, Butts HF: White psychiatrist's racism in referral practices to black psychiatrists. J Natl Med Assoc 62(4):278–282, 1970 5423387

Jones BE, Lightfoot OB, Palmer D, et al: Problems of black psychiatric residents in white training institutes. Am J Psychiatry 127(6):798–803, 1970 5482873

Katznelson I: When Affirmative Action Was White. New York, WW Norton, 2005

Lightfoot OB: To be used or useful. The question for black professionals, Cairo, Illinois, USA, 1969. J Natl Med Assoc 63(5):365–371, 1971 5121154

Lightfoot OB: Book review of Racism and Psychiatry by A. Thomas and S. Sillen. Int J Psychiatry Med 5(1):82–89, 1974

Peters JW: Introduction to the 1995 edition, in Black Laws of Virginia: A Summary of the Legislative Acts of Virginia Concerning Negroes From Earliest Times to the Present (1936). Edited by Guild JP. The Plains, VA, Afro-American Historical Association of Fauquier County, 1996, pp 5–20

Pierce CM: Offensive mechanisms, in The Black 70s. Edited by Barbour FB. Boston, MA, Porter Sargent, 1970, pp 265–282

Pinderhughes CA: Understanding black power: processes and proposals. Am J Psychiatry 125(11):1552–1557, 1969 5776864

Racism is called major problem of mental health in the nation. Medical Tribune and Medical News, May 16, 1969, pp 1, 18, 19

Spurlock J (ed): Black Psychiatrists and American Psychiatry. Washington, DC, American Psychiatric Press, 1999

Stevenson B: Just Mercies: A Story of Justice and Redemption. New York, Spiegel & Grau, 2014

Thomas A, Sillen S: Racism and Psychiatry. New York, Brunner/Mazel, 1972

Tweedy D: Black Man in a White Coat: A Doctor's Reflection on Race and Medicine. New York, Picador, 2015

Wallis J: America's Original Sin: Racism, White Privilege, and the Bridge to a New America. Grand Rapids, MI, Brazos Press, 2016

White AA III: Seeing Patients: Unconscious Bias in Health Care. Cambridge, MA, Harvard University Press, 2011

Willie CV (ed): Racism and Mental Health. Pittsburgh, PA, University of Pittsburgh Press, 1973

Welsing FC: The Isis Papers: The Keys to the Colors. Chicago, IL, Third World Press, 1991

PART II
Patient Care

CHAPTER 6
BLACK AMERICANS AND PUBLIC SECTOR SYSTEM-DESIGN STRATEGIES PROMOTING HEALTH EQUITY

Miriam E. Delphin-Rittmon, Ph.D.

Elizabeth Flanagan, Ph.D.

Chyrell D. Bellamy, M.S.W., Ph.D.

Ellen S. Boynton, B.A.

Larry Davidson, Ph.D.

DISCUSSING THE OMISSION of culture from mental health care, the President's New Freedom Commission on Mental Health, in its 2003 final report (President's New Freedom Commission on Mental Health 2003), noted that mental health care systems have failed to incorporate the histories, traditions, beliefs, values, and language systems of culturally diverse groups, resulting in minorities' having to shoulder a greater disability burden than their white peers. As a result, black Americans and other populations of color in the United States fare less well than nonminority groups on a number of health indicators (Institute of Medicine 2002; U.S. Department of Health and Human Services 1999). For instance, studies show that black Americans are less likely to seek formal behavioral healthcare and more likely to rely in times of distress on informal sources of support such as family, friends, or faith communities. Among those who do access treatment, research further has shown that black Americans may be more likely to be misdiagnosed or overdiagnosed and to experience additional healthcare disparities along the care continuum, from decreased retention in outpatient care to increased discharges against medical advice from inpatient care. Explanations for these patterns have included such factors as help-seeking preferences, provider stereotyping, and system-design factors that perpetuate disparities. Because of these findings (as well as similar findings among other minority communities), the subsequent Substance Abuse Mental Health Services Administration (SAMHSA) Federal Action Agenda followed the lead of other federal reports and panels (e.g., U.S. Department of Health and Human Services 2001) in recommending identification and elimination of healthcare disparities as a major goal for the foreseeable future (Substance Abuse Mental Health Services Administration 2005).

In Connecticut, the Department of Mental Health and Addiction Services (DMHAS) manages a statewide system of care in which developing and continuing to evolve a system that is culturally and contextually responsive and that works to advance recovery, citizenship, and health equity have long been priorities. In this chapter we describe key service and system-design strategies and approaches that have been implemented to promote health equity for black Americans and all individuals seeking DMHAS services.

Developing a Culturally Responsive System

DMHAS envisions a system of high-quality behavioral healthcare in which services and supports are culturally responsive; attentive to trauma; built on personal, family, and community strengths; and focused on promoting each person's recovery, wellness, and full citizenship. The services and supports are integrated, responsive, and coordinated. As a result, DMHAS ensures that persons will have maximal opportunities for establishing, or reestablishing, safe, dignified, and meaningful lives in their chosen communities. For a system such as DMHAS to realize this vision, we recommend seven key principles for developing and sustaining a culturally responsive system of care: 1) foster patient, community, and stakeholder participation and partnerships; 2) provide executive-level support and accountability; 3) conduct organizational cultural competence assessments; 4) develop incremental and realistic cultural competence action plans; 5) ensure linguistic competence; 6) diversify, develop, and retain a culturally competent workforce; and 7) develop an agency or system strategy for managing staff and patient grievances (Delphin-Rittmon et al. 2013b).

Hearing From and Partnering With Black Americans

Hearing from the people we serve is one of the essential ingredients to developing a culturally responsive approach in mental healthcare. The following illustrative quotes were taken from a study involving 22 focus groups (7 of which were composed entirely of black Americans) conducted around the state of Connecticut about cultural responsiveness in clinical care (Delphin-Rittmon et al. 2013a).

The individuals spoke about being misunderstood by clinicians because of their race/ethnicity. Many said they leave discussions about their culture and community at the door when they walk into community mental health centers. As one participant noted,

> I never really discuss that with my clinician. I discuss more of how can we get things done as far as my situation, as far as my housing, my social security, bills that needs to be paid, how my depression is coming along. These are the things that we talk about. As far as being African American and race, we never really discuss that. (p. 148)

Another participant said,

> I think the services are okay, right, but do they get to the core of the matter about how things truly affect the community we live in? Not even a drop. Not even a drop in the bucket. (p. 148)

Participants in the study suggested the following priorities for system reform (Delphin-Rittmon et al. 2013a):

- Connect with community.
- Develop peer-based services and supports.
- Develop additional services and supports focused specifically on cultural groups.
- Enhance direct care.
- Offer more provider education and training.
- Offer service user education and training.
- Enhance agency/environment physical space.

A multilevel approach to infrastructure development has been necessary in enabling us to begin to implement these suggestions.

Infrastructure Supporting Multiculturalism

DMHAS's first key service and system-design strategy has been fiscal and policy alignment with the values of multiculturalism, cultural competence, and the reduction of health disparities. For almost 20 years, resources have been dedicated to an Office of Multicultural Healthcare Equity (OMHE). The OMHE director reports directly to the DMHAS commissioner and addresses issues of multiculturalism, cultural competence, and health equity and disparities reduction among DMHAS services, providers, and staff. Through the work of the OMHE, DMHAS has developed and continues to evolve a statewide infrastructure focused on implementation of the Culturally and Linguistically Appropriate Services (CLAS) standards and provision of culturally competent and contextually responsive care in an effort to promote health equity.

A key component of this infrastructure is the Multicultural Advisory Council (MCAC). MCAC members either are employed at DMHAS state-operated or -funded private nonprofit facilities or are family members or people with lived experience of mental health or substance use conditions. Efforts are made to achieve diverse representation from providers, managers, and peer staff. Diversity in membership is also sought from underrepresented minority groups, including black Americans, Asian Americans, Hispanic Americans, LGBTQI persons, and persons with physical disabilities. The MCAC meets monthly and is charged by the commissioner to develop and implement a strategic plan focused on continuing to enhance recovery and health equity throughout the DMHAS system of care. An additional charge for the MCAC is to advise the commissioner on matters related to strengthening the cultural responsiveness of care staff, system strategies for promoting health equity, and approaches to improving the cultural climate and dynamics among staff. Currently, the MCAC has subcommittees focused on data collection and analysis; training and education; and instituting best cultural competence practices across all DMHAS-funded agencies.

Another component of the DMHAS infrastructure supporting multiculturalism is that each state-operated agency is charged with having a diversity committee. Each diversity committee works with its agency leadership to address agency needs related to multiculturalism and implementation of the CLAS standards. Specifically, each diversity committee is charged with agency self-assessment and staff development related to multiculturalism, including hosting guest speakers, lunch and learns, Chicago dinners (i.e., community discussions about diversity-related issues usually focused on a specific theme or national event), and agency-wide trainings. Finally, each diversity committee chair is asked to inform the MCAC about his or her agency's needs and any barriers that have been identified related to multiculturalism and implementation of the CLAS standards. Usually the chair of each diversity committee serves on the MCAC.

A current initiative of the OMHE is the Multicultural Enhancement Project (MEP). The first stage of the MEP is an assessment of each state-operated DMHAS facility using the Organizational Multicultural Competence Assessment (OMCA), which has been developed by the OMHE through its academic partnership with the Yale Program for Recovery and Community Health

(PRCH). The OMCA is under review for publication and consists of 40 questions asking about an agency's compliance with the CLAS standards. Areas assessed by the OMCA include 1) governance, policies, and procedures; 2) staff training and service delivery; 3) addressing stigma and discrimination; 4) accessibility of services; 5) community relationships; 6) quality, monitoring, and evaluation; and 7) human resource development. All staff in an agency (including providers, peer support specialists, administrative assistants, custodial staff, food service, public safety) are asked by their chief executive officer to fill out the survey online. An overall score and scores for each of the seven subscales are created for each agency.

After the survey is completed, the overall scores, subscales, and averages for each item are shared with the agency in a feedback form comparing the agency scores to state averages. The feedback forms are shared with the agency leadership, members of the diversity committee, and clinical leadership (e.g., medical director, director of clinical services) in a meeting in which the agency can discuss with OMHE staff their survey responses, staff concerns related to diversity, and training and human resource needs related to survey responses. OMHE staff, agency leadership, and the agency diversity committee are then charged with implementing a plan to address the training, human resource, or other organizational needs identified in the survey. The survey is repeated every 2 years to assess progress related to implementing the CLAS standards.

Currently, one area of focus of the MEP and the OMHE is ensuring language access for all DMHAS clients who have language support needs related to speaking another primary language or being deaf or hard of hearing. This process involves each agency assessing its language access strengths and needs through the OMCA as well as its resources including staffing to support language access. Bilingual staff are tracked, assessed for language competence in the second language, and offered stipends to be available for translation as part of their other work at the agency. DMHAS administrative data collected on each client at least every 6 months are used to track the number of DMHAS clients needing language support.

Infrastructure Supporting Disparity Reduction

A Health Disparities Initiative has been conducted by the OMHE of DMHAS and Yale PRCH since 2002. Through this initiative, we have used data to better understand patterns and trends in the DMHAS system related to diversity and disparities as well as to track progress in reducing identified disparities. First, we conducted an initial assessment of racial-ethnic differences in DMHAS inpatient mental health and substance abuse agencies in 2002–2005 (Delphin-

Rittmon et al. 2012, 2015) and repeated this analysis in 2010–2011 (Cruza-Guet et al., in press; Flanagan et al. 2017). These analyses are now ongoing and include multiple data sources, including the DMHAS administrative data collected on all clients every 6 months as well as data from numerous grant-funded initiatives (O'Connell et al. 2017; Tondora et al. 2010). Currently we are analyzing the data collected through our Behavioral Health Homes initiative (described later) to identify underserved groups. Analyzing data has been a central mechanism for all DMHAS initiatives, including the continual collection and analysis of data to investigate changes in disparities over time in response to various DMHAS system-wide initiatives.

With regard to African Americans, logistic regression analysis of differences among African Americans, Hispanic Americans, and white Americans who were admitted to DMHAS mental health inpatient units in 2002–2005 found multiple differences (Delphin-Rittmon et al. 2012). Regarding referral to mental health inpatient services, African Americans were more likely than Hispanic Americans to have to self-refer for admission, less likely than Hispanic Americans to be referred by criminal justice settings, and less likely than white Americans to be referred by other inpatient units. Once admitted to the mental health inpatient units, African Americans were more likely to have shorter lengths of stay and more likely to leave against medical advice. African Americans were more likely than both whites and Hispanics to have primary Axis I diagnoses of schizophrenia and substance use disorder at admission and less likely to have a primary Axis I admission diagnosis of a mood disorder or other disorder (e.g., anxiety, cognitive, eating). African Americans were also more likely than whites to have a primary Axis II admission diagnosis of mental retardation or borderline intellectual functioning (DSM-IV [American Psychiatric Association 1994] diagnoses were used at the time). African Americans also were more likely than Hispanic Americans to have a diagnosis of personality disorder not otherwise specified at admission.

In the focus group study about people's experience of receiving care (Delphin-Rittmon et al. 2013a), an African American male's description of his experiences may help to account for these findings:

> One time I had a do-rag, and they all jumped back and they were ready to arrest me. And they said "What is that on? Are you in some type of gang? Are you acting like those gangs out there, those black guys in gangs?" I said "No, you've got it wrong. You need to take some courses on African American culture and behavior. When black men groom, they always brush their hair" and they had this blank look on their face, like "What is he talking about? He's got an attitude." They are uneducated about African American males the way they dress, their gait, their walk, the way they talk with their hands. They are very intimidated any type of address activity. I'm an alpha black male. Any type of aggression or assertiveness is viewed as hostility. (p. 149)

Thus, for some individuals, feeling misunderstood or stereotyped may contribute to leaving treatment against medical advice and subsequently a shorter length of stay.

When these same variables in mental health inpatient units were reanalyzed in 2010–2011, we found that African Americans were still more likely than other groups to self-refer and were less likely to be referred by other inpatient settings (Flanagan et al. 2017). Yet there were no significant differences for African Americans in length of stay, leaving against medical advice, or primary Axis I diagnosis of schizophrenia. The only diagnostic difference that remained was that they were still less likely to have a primary Axis I diagnosis of mood disorders or other disorders (e.g., anxiety, cognitive) and more likely to have a primary diagnosis of substance use disorder or mental retardation at admission. The quantitative findings over time suggest a reduction in stereotypic diagnoses and differential outcomes for African Americans compared with other groups, perhaps as a result of staff training and a continual prioritization of enhancing systemic cultural competence.

Evaluation, Quality Management, and Improvement of Internal Reports

Through our internal DMHAS Evaluation, Quality Management and Improvement Division (EQMI), we also publish a series of reports each year that assess the DMHAS system on a variety of indicators. One report analyzes the entire DMHAS state-operated system, offering crucial information to agencies and providers about which groups are underserved and in what ways. A consumer survey conducted each year assesses client satisfaction as well as quality of life across the system and can be analyzed based on race, ethnicity, and other factors. In addition, this survey includes questions that directly ask about clients' experiences of culturally competent care and the extent to which their recovery plans integrate natural supports and other community resources important to them. The DMHAS EQMI also creates an "outlier report," which is an outcome-driven internal tool that allows us to look at differences across racial-ethnic groups by program, levels of care, and agency. These reports are useful to DMHAS in tracking data over time so that important policy and system-design changes can be informed and evaluated using population-level data.

Addressing Disparities Through Integrated Care

An important initiative that addresses disparities in the DMHAS system includes multiple projects related to integrating primary care and behavioral health to address the finding that people with serious mental illnesses are dying 25 years earlier than the general population, as well as the dramatic racial-ethnic disparities for black Americans that have already been documented. DMHAS has received multiple primary care behavioral health integration grants from SAMHSA to integrate behavioral health and primary care at multiple agencies. Chyrell Bellamy, a coauthor of this chapter, also received a grant from the Patient-Centered Outcomes Research Institute to conduct further data analysis of a primary care behavioral health integration initiative at a DMHAS state-operated service. This project seeks to determine which evidence-based treatments offered by the primary care center improved which outcomes, for whom, and under what circumstances. The funding also supported developing a peer-led wellness enhancement for DMHAS clients whose health outcomes were not improving as a result of the primary care behavioral health integration initiative.

A key DMHAS mechanism for integrating primary and behavioral healthcare is through Connecticut's participation in the national Behavioral Health Homes (BHH) initiative. DMHAS has been part of the federal BHH initiative since 2015. The BHH initiative is an innovative, integrated, healthcare service–delivery model that is recovery-oriented and person- and family-centered and promises better patient experience and outcomes than those achieved in traditional services. The BHH service delivery model is an important option for providing a cost-effective, longitudinal "home" to facilitate access to an interdisciplinary array of behavioral healthcare, medical care, and community-based social services and supports for both adults and children with chronic conditions. The BHH initiative works to be culturally and context sensitive and to address multiple social determinants of health faced by DMHAS clients, especially as related to accessing healthcare. Analyzing health outcomes by disparity indicators is an important priority of this initiative, with DMHAS devoting considerable effort and funding to developing the data infrastructure to measure and track physical health and behavioral health outcomes over time for people enrolled in the BHH. Given the goals of the BHH initiative, it is a promising approach to improving the social determinants of health for clients in the DMHAS system.

Integrative or Alternative Modalities to Address Disparities

DMHAS has multiple integrative or alternative modalities to improve personal and mental health. DMHAS offers mind-body modalities, including mindfulness, meditation, yoga, labyrinth meditation, hypnosis/biofeedback and guided imagery, mindfulness-based psychotherapy (dialectical behavior therapy, eye movement desensitization and reprocessing, acceptance and commitment therapy), dance/movement, art/music, pet therapy/animal-assisted treatment, mas-

sage, supported spirituality, and energy therapies, through DMHAS state facilities as well as through Toivo, a peer-run community-based whole-health
center run by Advocacy Unlimited Inc. These integrated and alternative modalities are available for individuals to utilize in their recovery plan to improve
their own personal wellness and community connections. Research has shown
that a substantial number of black Americans use complementary and alternative medicines. In one study, most commonly, prayer was used for treatment of
specific conditions as opposed to prevention (Brown et al. 2007).

Moving Toward Citizenship-Oriented Care

Citizenship-oriented care is an approach that considers collaboration with
communities essential to addressing systemic structural barriers and social determinants of health (Ponce and Rowe 2018; Rowe 2015; Rowe and Davidson
2016). This approach offers a conceptual framework for thinking about mental
health in the context of broader environmental and structural conditions and
barriers. It highlights practical guidelines for care and for specifically organizing with communities to develop strategies to overcome inequities. Citizenship
builds on recovery principles, which have been successfully disseminated through
behavioral healthcare settings in the United States and have to some extent become part of routine practice. While incorporating recovery principles has
made significant differences to care delivery, principles of recovery have focused
mainly on the individual. The citizenship concept builds on recovery by offering a way of thinking about "a life in the community" for people with psychiatric
difficulties. The citizenship approach argues that people need a strong connection to the "5 Rs": *rights, responsibilities, roles,* and *resources* that society makes
available to its members, and *relationships* involving close ties and supportive
social networks. People need a sense of belonging that is validated by others'
recognition and acknowledgment that they are valued and needed. We are incorporating the citizenship approach in the development of an intervention to
work with black churches in the four major cities in Connecticut to respond to
the opioid crisis. We are also offering a learning collaborative on citizenship-
oriented care for DMHAS agencies.

Recommendations

In conclusion, we offer the following recommendations for increasing the cultural competence of mental health services offered to, and decreasing the behavioral health disparities experienced by, persons of African American origin:

- Make strategic investments in infrastructure and personnel development to increase the multicultural composition of the workforce. In our system, 1) a state-level office; 2) a multicultural advisory council comprising managers, providers, and service users; and 3) diversity committees at each state-operated agency have been foundational components of our infrastructure in addressing disparities.
- Use data from multiple sources analyzed in multiple ways by multiple departments to identify existing disparities and to track changes in disparities over time in response to strategic system-level initiatives such as staff development, integrated care initiatives, and person-centered care planning.
- Offer an array of culturally based integrative and alternative modalities from which service users may choose in order to improve their personal wellness and strengthen their community connections.
- Infuse the recovery orientation of services and outcome measures with cultural competence values and principles. The goals, action steps, and recovery supports identified in clients' individualized recovery plans should include consideration and incorporation of the cultural supports and perspectives that are important to them and their social networks.
- Enhance citizenship within clients' chosen communities. Individualized recovery plans should include a systematic consideration of, and targeted efforts to address, such social determinants of health as housing, income, meaningful occupation, and senses of purpose and belonging. Recovery plans should identify those rights, roles, relationships, resources, and responsibilities that clients value or aspire to as foci of their own efforts, as well as those of their multidisciplinary care teams.

References

American Psychiatric Association: Diagnostic and Statistical Manual of Mental Disorders, 4th Edition. Washington, DC, American Psychiatric Association, 1994

Brown CM, Barner JC, Richards KM, et al: Patterns of complementary and alternative medicine use in African Americans. J Altern Complement Med 13(7):751–758, 2007 17931068

Cruza-Guet M-C, Flanagan E, Tharnish S, et al: An evaluation of racial and ethnic differences in state substance abuse service use: 2004–2005 versus 2010–2011. Psychiatr Serv (in press)

Delphin-Rittmon M, Andres-Hyman R, Flanagan EH, et al: Racial-ethnic differences in referral source, diagnosis, and length of stay in inpatient substance abuse treatment. Psychiatr Serv 63(6):612–615, 2012 22422017

Delphin-Rittmon M, Bellamy CD, Ridgway P, et al: 'I never really discuss that with my clinician': US consumer perspectives on the place of culture in behavioural healthcare. Divers Equal Health Care 10(3):143–154, 2013a

Delphin-Rittmon ME, Andres-Hyman R, Flanagan EH, et al: Seven essential strategies for promoting and sustaining systemic cultural competence. Psychiatr Q 84(1):53–64, 2013b 22581030

Delphin-Rittmon ME, Flanagan EH, Andres-Hyman R, et al: Racial-ethnic differences in access, diagnosis, and outcomes in public-sector inpatient mental health treatment. Psychol Serv 12(2):158–166, 2015 25961650

Flanagan EH, Greig A, Tharnish S, et al: An evaluation of racial and ethnic health differences in state mental health inpatient services: 2002–2005 versus 2010–2011. J Behav Health Serv Res 44(2):242–262, 2017 28000013

Institute of Medicine: Unequal Treatment: Confronting Racial and Ethnic Disparities in Health Care. Washington, DC, National Academies Press, 2002

O'Connell MJ, Flanagan EH, Delphin-Rittmon ME, et al: Enhancing outcomes for persons with co-occurring disorders through skills training and peer recovery support. J Ment Health 10:1–6, 2017 28282996

Ponce AN, Rowe M: Citizenship and community mental health care. Am J Community Psychol 61(1–2):22–31, 2018 29323416

President's New Freedom Commission on Mental Health: Achieving the Promise: Transforming Mental Health Care in America. Bethesda, MD, Substance Abuse Mental Health Services Administration, 2003

Rowe M: Citizenship and Mental Health. New York, Oxford University Press, 2015

Rowe M, Davidson L: Recovering citizenship. Isr J Psychiatry Relat Sci 53(1):14–20, 2016 28856875

Substance Abuse Mental Health Services Administration: Transforming Mental Health Care in America. The Federal Action Agenda: First Steps. Bethesda, MD, Substance Abuse Mental Health Services Administration, 2005

Tondora J, O'Connell M, Miller R, et al: A clinical trial of peer-based culturally responsive person-centered care for psychosis for African Americans and Latinos. Clin Trials 7(4):368–379, 2010 20571133

U.S. Department of Health and Human Services: Mental Health: A Report of the Surgeon General. Rockville, MD, U.S. Department of Health and Human Services, 1999

U.S. Department of Health and Human Services: National Standards for Culturally and Linguistically Appropriate Services in Health Care: Final Report. Rockville, MD, Office of Minority Health, 2001

CHAPTER 7
AFRICAN AMERICANS AND THE CRIMINAL JUSTICE SYSTEM

Richard G. Dudley Jr., M.D.

IT IS AN UNDISPUTED fact that African Americans are overrepresented in the criminal justice system. Blacks are incarcerated at more than five times the rate of whites, and in some state prison systems the disparity is more than 10 to 1 (The Sentencing Project 2016). Although blacks and whites use drugs at similar rates, the imprisonment rate of blacks for drug charges is almost six times that of whites (National Association for the Advancement of Colored People 2017). While the lifetime likelihood of imprisonment for white men is 1 in 17, the lifetime likelihood for black men is 1 in 3; and while the lifetime likelihood of imprisonment for white women is 1 in 111, the lifetime likelihood for black women is 1 in 18 (Bonczar 2003).

Many noted historians, sociologists, psychologists, and legal scholars have studied and written about the various factors that have contributed to this overrepresentation. Viewed collectively, David Oshinsky's *Worse Than Slavery,* Douglas Blackmon's *Slavery by Another Name,* and Michelle Alexander's *The New Jim Crow* describe how the overrepresentation of African Americans in the criminal justice system is rooted in our country's history of slavery and ultimately represents a modern, redesigned alternative for controlling and subjugating black people (Alexander 2012; Blackmon 2009; Oshinsky 1996).

This convergence of evidence suggests a system of policies, sentencing guidelines, and other structural elements of our criminal justice system that intentionally or unintentionally target black people for harsher punishment. It lends support to the argument that the continued existence of systemic racism is a major factor that contributes to the overrepresentation of African Americans in the criminal justice system. For example, studies of the "school-to-prison pipeline" have revealed how various policy changes in our educational system have resulted in a disproportionate number of black students leaving school and entering the criminal justice system (Redfield and Nance 2016) due to the fact that black students are treated more harshly and are subjected to "disciplinary" practices that have been found to be racist. Disparities in sentencing for crack and powder cocaine possession, part of the "War on Drugs," have significantly contributed to blacks serving substantially more time in prisons for drug offenses than whites (National Association for the Advancement of Colored People 2017), and this targeting of black Americans for criminal prosecution is particularly striking when compared to the more recent conceptualization of the "opioid crisis" in white America as a public health crisis.

Research on implicit bias, defined as hidden unconscious bias, has shown that it, too, contributes to the disproportionate incarceration of African Americans even when decision makers are well intentioned, attempting to be fair and objective. Each year, the Kirwan Institute's *State of the Science: Implicit Bias Review* summarizes and integrates the most significant findings of studies of implicit bias, with a section devoted to criminal justice (Kirwan Institute for the Study of Race and Ethnicity 2014, 2015, 2016, 2017). Over the years, these studies have shown that implicit bias results in significant racial disparities with regard to the frequency and nature of police stops and police use of force, prosecutorial charging, the work of defense attorneys, assorted courtroom dynamics, judicial decision making, jury instructions, the decisions of jurors, and sentencing. These racial disparities, occurring at every stage of the criminal justice process, build upon each other, thereby collectively having an impact on the disproportionate incarceration of African Americans that is far greater than any one of these factors might suggest.

Many studies of the role of implicit bias in the disproportionate incarceration of African Americans have included an exploration of interventions designed to minimize its effects, and the results of such studies have been quite promising (Kirwan Institute for the Study of Race and Ethnicity 2014, 2015, 2016, 2017). These intervention studies have shown that education, including education about implicit bias, can dramatically decrease its role in decision making. The identification of policies, sentencing guidelines, and other structural elements of our criminal justice system that are inherently biased, labeling them as such, and then intervening has been shown to decrease the roles of explicit and implicit bias in decision making.

Of course, there are those who argue that the disproportionate incarceration of African Americans is primarily due to the fact that black people commit more crimes than white people, despite the fact that studies of the impact of explicit bias/racism and implicit bias have shown that similarly placed black and white people are treated differently. Although this argument is overly simplistic, it is important to acknowledge that about 62% of African Americans are born and raised in and continue to live in communities characterized by structural disadvantages such as poverty, poor educational systems, and unemployment that are known to be associated with a range of problems, including high rates of crime (The Sentencing Project 2016). However, it is important to note that the persistence of these disadvantages is also a manifestation of American society's failure to address a long-standing pattern of discrimination based on race and class.

Distorted Perceptions of and Responses to African Americans

Explicit and implicit bias also impact perceptions of and responses to African Americans, including regarding their mental health. One of the most relevant areas that have been extensively studied is the perceived relationship between criminality and blackness. The early studies focused on shooter/weapons bias, where study participants, who eventually included police officers, were instructed to shoot at individuals wielding a threatening object and to refrain from shooting when the object was innocuous. These studies consistently showed that it took participants longer to correctly refrain from shooting black unarmed targets (Kirwan Institute for the Study of Race and Ethnicity 2014). More recent studies have revealed that many individuals also associate black males with characteristics such as subhumanness (Kirwan Institute for the Study of Race and Ethnicity 2017). Clearly, this tendency to perceive black men as criminal/antisocial subhuman or as animals makes it all the more difficult to even consider an alternative explanation for any alleged criminal behavior, including mental illness, and thereby contributes to the overrepresentation of African Americans in the criminal justice system.

Observations of many of American society's differing responses to black and white people lend further support to the argument that distorted perceptions of black people contribute to the overrepresentation of African Americans in the criminal justice system. For example, when there is a killing or other violent act at or near a school in a white community, mental health professionals are immediately and quite appropriately called in to evaluate and address the needs of the children who attend the school. In contrast, black children who are living in a violent neighborhood and thereby frequently witness comparable violence are generally not given access to such assistance from mental health professionals, despite the fact that untreated trauma-related symptoms increase their risk of later coming into contact with the criminal justice system. For example, black youth in the juvenile justice system are much more likely to be adjudicated and placed in a juvenile facility or transferred to and convicted and sentenced by an adult criminal court, whereas white youth are much more likely to be placed on probation or placed in a diversion program where they can receive services, including mental health services (Redfield and Nance 2016).

Role of Racial Bias in Forensic Mental Health Evaluations

Given that explicit and implicit bias are implicated in all the noted factors that have been found to contribute to the overrepresentation of African Americans in the criminal justice system, it is reasonable to explore the question of whether forensic mental health evaluations, reports, and testimony might also be influenced by biases and negative perceptions and thereby contribute to the overrepresentation of African Americans in the criminal justice system. Although there are no studies that have attempted to answer this specific question, healthcare-focused implicit bias studies have shown that the implicit bias of nonblack physicians against blacks can have a negative impact on doctor-patient interactions in a variety of ways, resulting in differential treatment, and can impair patient well-being (Kirwan Institute for the Study of Race and Ethnicity 2015). Among the more interesting and relevant findings was that nonblack physicians with high levels of bias against blacks were much more likely to view black patients as superhuman, more able to tolerate pain and suffering, and therefore in less need of pain medication than comparable white patients. Studies of mental health professionals showed that counselors with antiblack implicit bias perceived black patients as less bonded to them (Kirwan Institute for the Study of Race and Ethnicity 2015), which potentially could have an impact on their sense of reciprocal engagement with black patients and a range of clinical opinions and decisions.

In the absence of specific studies that have attempted to determine the extent to which the work of forensic mental health professionals is influenced by explicit or implicit bias, and whether such work contributes to the overrepresentation of African Americans in the criminal justice system, there is anecdotal evidence that can be examined. For this purpose, I narrow my focus to the role of forensic mental health professionals in capital litigation. I do this for a variety of reasons.

First, since 1976, when the death penalty was reinstated, racial disparity with regard to the outcomes of capital litigation has continued to be quite dramatic (Death Penalty Information Center 2017). The most recent statistics indicate that even though blacks make up only about 13% of the population whereas whites make up about 63%, the percentage of black death row inmates is the same as the percentage of white death row inmates. The statistics further indicate that the race of the victim is determinative of who gets executed. Specifically, a defendant is much more likely to be executed if the victim was white. Furthermore, although 20 white defendants who murdered black victims have been executed, 287 black defendants who murdered white victims have been executed.

Second, the results of studies that have examined the role of bias in capital litigation have been particularly alarming and are relevant to the question presented here. For example, Eberhardt et al. (2006) have shown that the perceived stereotypicality of black defendants predicts capital-sentencing outcomes, in that the more stereotypically black a defendant appears to be, the more likely the defendant is to be sentenced to death. For example, the same research group found that the historical representation of blacks as apelike continues to exist in the unconscious and is an element of implicit bias that contributes to the dehumanization of black defendants, and thereby makes them more likely to be sentenced to death (Goff et al. 2008).

Third, capital litigation involves several steps, and forensic mental health professionals are usually involved in each of those steps as experts for the prosecution or the defense. There are pretrial considerations, such as whether the defendant is competent to proceed with the trial. Then there is the first phase of the trial, focused on whether the defendant is guilty of a crime that is eligible for the death penalty, where various affirmative mental health defenses might be proffered, including an insanity defense. If the defendant is found guilty, there is then a second trial phase, focused on whether the defendant should be given the death penalty or life in prison. In this phase, the prosecution presents aggravating factors that argue for the death penalty, and the defense presents mitigating factors, including mental health issues that have impaired the defendant's ability to function, despite the fact that they do not rise to the level of an affirmative defense, that would offer the decision maker reasons why death is too harsh a penalty. In addition, many legal teams seek advice from consulting mental health professionals who do not testify (e.g., to help them identify jurors who have more enlightened views of mental health testimony that will be presented, or who might help them conceptualize the mental health issues in order to select the most culturally competent experts to evaluate their clients and testify). These roles for mental health professionals might be particularly important given that studies have shown that citizens who meet the requirement to be on a death-qualified jury exhibit stronger implicit racial biases than those who are excluded (Kirwan Institute for the Study of Race and Ethnicity 2015).

Fourth, there has been mental health–focused litigation that has resulted in U.S. Supreme Court decisions limiting those who can be given the death penalty. More specifically, in *Atkins v. Virginia* (2002), the court decided that individuals with "mental retardation" were no longer eligible for the death penalty. In

Roper v. Simmons (2005), the court decided that those who committed capital crimes when they were juveniles were no longer eligible for the death penalty.

Fifth, given the severity and irreversibility of the death penalty, there are opportunities to challenge the finding of guilt and the sentence of death that is unique to capital litigation. These postconviction remedies have given mental health professionals, such as myself, an opportunity to review the professional quality of original trial-level work of numerous other forensic mental health professionals and to consider, among other things, the impact of explicit and implicit bias on their work. The anecdotal reports that inform my discussion here are drawn from my own work in such postconviction capital litigation and that of other African American and non–African American forensic mental health professionals.

Before we proceed any further, it is important to note that in capital cases, what type of mental health professionals are retained, when mental health professionals are retained, and what collateral information is provided to retained professionals are determined by the defendant's legal team. Obviously, all of these factors can influence the nature and quality of the expert mental health evidence that is ultimately presented. Evolving constitutional law, the 2003 revision of the "American Bar Association Guidelines for the Appointment and Performance of Defense Counsel in Death Penalty Cases," and the 2008 "American Bar Association Supplementary Guidelines for the Mitigation Function of Defense Teams in Death Penalty Cases" have made this clear and described a standard of practice for defense teams (American Bar Association 2003, 2008). In capital litigation, defense teams must develop a full social history based on collected records, documents, and information gathered from the defendant, family members, and others with intimate knowledge of the defendant. The legal team must also include a member with enough knowledge about mental health issues to help focus the development of that social history and then help assess what type of expert(s) should be retained. In addition, the social history and supporting records, documents, and other collateral sources of information then become part of the informational base for the forensic mental health evaluation(s) (Dudley and Leonard 2008).

Furthermore, it is also important to note that the trial attorney must be intimately involved with and fully familiar with the forensic mental health evaluation(s) that has been performed, its outcome, and the basis for the opinions rendered in order to adequately direct the examination of the expert at trial and effectively integrate the findings of the expert into the overall trial strategy. The importance of this is obvious when one considers the overwhelming evidence that the most effective trial presentation of mental health evidence is one where there is the integration of a narrative presentation of the defendant's social history, presented by lay witnesses, with expert mental health testimony that explains the significance of that history, especially regarding the defendant's ability to function (O'Brien and Wayland 2015). Given what has been learned about addressing implicit bias, in many instances, the attorney might also have to ask the mental health expert to directly address issues of implicit bias and/or educate decision makers about their other preconceived notions that run counter to the mental health testimony being presented, to undo conscious or unconscious beliefs that might otherwise be incorporated into the decision-making process.

The following are several examples, based on anecdotal reports, of the types of error seen in forensic mental health evaluations that appear to be influenced by explicit and/or implicit bias. For each example, evidence that supports the role of bias is described. In addition, for each example, the impact of the error on outcome is noted.

Intellectual Disability and Other Cognitive Deficits

In "Culturally Biased Expert Testimony in Criminal and Family Proceedings," a paper presented at the Symposium on the Structures of Inequality and Race in New York City: Looking Backward and Forward, which is part of New York University's Walter Stafford Project, Woods and Greenspan (2016) described and discussed "cultural-overshadowing" and "cultural under-shadowing" and their consequences for people of color within the legal system. They noted that cultural overshadowing occurs when culture or race is used to minimize or ignore important person-based qualities, such as brain damage, mental illness, or physical illness, and cultural undershadowing occurs when such person-based qualities are relied on excessively, without sufficient or any attention to the explanatory role of cultural and environmental factors.

The diagnosis of intellectual disability and other cognitive deficits is among the examples of cultural overshadowing by forensic mental health experts detailed in Woods and Greenspan's paper. They described cases in which poverty, poor education, and gang affiliation were offered as the explanations for poor social functioning of black defendants, despite a history of brain injury and/or indications of intellectual disability, including longstanding impaired adaptive functioning. They also noted how a black defendant's capacity to perform extremely simple tasks is often used as evidence of normal cognitive capacity, despite obvious, significantly impaired executive functions. In addition, they noted how in many cases a black defendant's history of brain damage is never identified or is identified and ignored. Woods and Greenspan made it clear that during forensic mental health evaluations, the impaired intellectual or cognitive capacity of blacks is often either normalized or minimized and attributed to cultural factors, both of which are a form of race-based discrimination.

Even before *Atkins,* a finding of intellectual disability and/or other clinically significant cognitive deficits could be offered as mitigation against receiving the death penalty. Since *Atkins,* a finding of intellectual disability takes the death penalty off the table. Therefore, failure to recognize intellectual disability or other clinically significant cognitive deficits in black defendants can mean the difference between life and death.

Childhood Trauma and Its Effects

It has been clearly established that repeated exposure to violent, traumatic experiences during childhood, especially in the absence of the type of parental nurture and support that might mitigate its effects on the child, can result in psychological trauma-related symptoms, impaired brain development, and other developmental difficulties (Dudley 2015). Both black and white defendants in capital cases often have a childhood history of such exposure that may include child physical and sexual abuse and exposure to domestic violence. Many black defendants also have a history of repeated exposure to street violence due to having spent their childhood years in neighborhoods plagued by violence.

A postconviction review of numerous trial-level mental health evaluation reports and testimony, coupled with postconviction mental health examinations of defendants, indicates that in many cases the trauma history of black defendants was never uncovered at the trial level, either because the defendant was not asked about trauma or because the evaluator failed to develop the type of working relationship with the defendant that would allow the defendant to talk about early traumatic experiences. In many other cases, an uncovered history of trauma was characterized as the normal experience of children who grow up in violent neighborhoods, who instead of being traumatized by their experiences simply learn to accept and even embrace violence. In cases such as these, school records, social service records, and/or juvenile records that attribute hyper- and overreactive childhood behavior to attention-deficit/hyperactivity disorder or conduct disorder are often simply accepted without questioning the accuracy of the diagnoses or considering whether traumatic experiences and trauma-based responses to those experiences account for the observed behaviors. Such errors are clearly indicative of a lack of ethnocultural competence in the performance of mental health evaluations and/or explicit or implicit bias.

As noted earlier, in capital cases, expert mental health testimony has been shown to be more effective when integrated with a narrative presentation of the defendant's social history, presented by lay witnesses. When there is a significant history of childhood trauma, the mental health expert's role would be to educate the jury about childhood trauma and its effects, address any preconceived beliefs jury members might have about the experiences of black children, and describe to what extent the defendant's behavior is a product of the unaddressed childhood trauma that he or she endured. Although childhood trauma and its effects are not an affirmative defense against guilt, when properly presented and defended, this part of the social history can have a significant mitigating effect against the death penalty.

The Overdetermined Finding of Antisocial Personality Disorder

Much has been written about how the failure to perform an ethnoculturally competent mental health evaluation and explicit and implicit bias can result in the misdiagnosis of black people. An early example is the misdiagnosis of black people who have mood disorders, especially bipolar disorders (Jones et al. 1982). The misdiagnosis of bipolar disorders can be particularly damaging in the context of capital litigation, especially when the black defendant's manic episodes are characterized by irritability, grandiosity, and behaviors such as sexual indiscretions or foolish, risky hustles, which for the defendant might be comparable to the foolish business deals described in DSM diagnostic criteria. Such a black defendant may be misdiagnosed as having an antisocial personality disorder—an evaluator might have readily rushed to that conclusion given the defendant's race and the criminal context of the evaluation—and for a death-qualified jury, such a diagnosis can help define the defendant as part of the group of inherently bad and frightening black people who deserve the death penalty.

An opinion that a black defendant is malingering intellectual disability or some other type of mental illness not only is an argument against a claim of illness but also is often used as evidence that the defendant is antisocial. There is evidence that false positives for malingering are especially likely to occur when minority subjects are being evaluated (Bordini et al. 2002). Culturally influenced clinical presentations that are unfamiliar to an evaluator are often viewed as malingering, and, of course, even if a defendant is exaggerating a symptom(s), that does not mean that the defendant is not ill and impaired; in fact, the nature and quality of the exaggeration might be an indication of the defendant's impairment.

There are many indications in cases such as those noted here that the lack of ethnocultural competence and explicit and/or implicit bias contribute to frequent misdiagnoses and overdetermined findings of antisocial personality disorder in black defendants. The rush to make that diagnosis without a full history that confirms that the defendant's presentation meets the diagnostic criteria and/or the failure to consider more likely alternatives for the defendant's behavior given his or her history and other symptoms/behaviors further confirm the fact that race is an issue here. However, in addition, circumstances that surround the evaluation, such as the ability of defense teams to obtain funding for and identify competent mental health experts for indigent black defendants, may also contribute to such misdiagnosis.

Conclusions and Recommendations

There are no formal studies that have specifically explored the extent to which the work of forensic mental health professionals is influenced by explicit or implicit bias, and whether such bias contributes to the overrepresentation of African Americans in the criminal justice system. However, given that studies have determined that no one is free of implicit bias, and because anecdotal evidence regarding the impact of bias on forensic mental health evaluations is troubling, such formal studies are clearly indicated. There are reliable research methods that can be used to explore this issue. These methods range from those that look at differing outcomes of forensic mental health evaluations of comparable persons from different ethnocultural groups, to protocols that take an extremely nuanced look at how mental health professionals question and otherwise interact with people from different ethnocultural groups and the implications of such differences.

Tested interventions aimed at minimizing the impact of implicit bias would suggest, among other things, that increasing the diversity of the pool of forensic mental health experts would be helpful. It is important to note, however, that even if there is an increased presence of people of color in the forensic mental health expert pool, all the responsibility for addressing the issue of implicit bias cannot be assigned to them. Although they may have valuable knowledge and skills to share, the challenge to minimize the negative impact of bias on forensic mental health evaluations must be championed by all, or at least most, forensic mental health experts if any progress is to be made. Therefore, professional training programs, continuing education programs, and other formal and informal interactions between mental health professionals must become vehicles for raising and addressing these concerns.

Finally, there is the fact that even the most ethnoculturally competent forensic mental health evaluation must be heard and understood by the ultimate decision maker, who is not a mental health professional and who may or may not be aware of personal biases. Therefore, the presentation of expert mental health testimony may have to include an explicit discussion of the ways that racial biases can distort one's understanding of the defendant and the defendant's mental health issues. Of course, this will require mental health experts and attorneys who are comfortable talking about race and racial biases and who have identified ways to help judges and/or jurors identify their biases and minimize their harmful effects. Therefore, legal teams and their mental health experts must always be mindful of and openly discuss issues of race and racial bias, so that by the time of trial they are prepared to appropriately and effectively address such issues.

References

Alexander M: The New Jim Crow. New York, The New Press, 2012

American Bar Association: American Bar Association guidelines for the appointment and performance of defense counsel in death penalty cases. Hofstra Law Rev 31:913–1090, 2003

American Bar Association: American Bar Association supplementary guidelines for the mitigation function of defense teams in death penalty cases. Hofstra Law Rev 36:677–692, 2008

Atkins v Virginia, 536 United States 304, 319 (2002)

Blackmon DA: Slavery by Another Name. New York, Anchor Books, 2009

Bonczar T: Prevalence of Imprisonment in the United States Population, 1974–2001. Washington, DC, Bureau of Justice Statistics, 2003

Bordini EJ, Chaknis MM, Ekman-Turner RM, et al: Advances and issues in the diagnostic differential of malingering versus brain injury. NeuroRehabilitation 17(2):93–104, 2002 12082236

Death Penalty Information Center: Facts About the Death Penalty. Washington, DC, Death Penalty Information Center, 2017

Dudley RG: Childhood Trauma and Its Effects: Implications for Police. New Perspectives in Policing Bulletin NCJ 248686. Washington, DC, U.S. Department of Justice, National Institute of Justice, 2015

Dudley RG, Leonard PB: Getting it right: life history investigation as the foundation for a reliable mental health assessment. Hofstra Law Rev 36(3):963, 2008

Eberhardt JL, Davies PG, Purdie-Vaughns VJ, et al: Looking deathworthy: perceived stereotypicality of black defendants predicts capital-sentencing outcomes. Psychol Sci 17(5):383–386, 2006 16683924

Goff PA, Eberhardt JL, Williams MJ, et al: Not yet human: implicit knowledge, historical dehumanization, and contemporary consequences. J Pers Soc Psychol 94(2):292–306, 2008 18211178

Jones BE, Robinson WM, Parson EB, et al: The clinical picture of mania in manic-depressive black patients. J Natl Med Assoc 74(6):553–557, 1982 7120489

Kirwan Institute for the Study of Race and Ethnicity: State of the Science: Implicit Bias Review. Columbus, OH, Kirwan Institute for the Study of Race and Ethnicity, 2014

Kirwan Institute for the Study of Race and Ethnicity: State of the Science: Implicit Bias Review. Columbus, OH, Kirwan Institute for the Study of Race and Ethnicity, 2015

Kirwan Institute for the Study of Race and Ethnicity: State of the Science: Implicit Bias Review. Columbus, OH, Kirwan Institute for the Study of Race and Ethnicity, 2016

Kirwan Institute for the Study of Race and Ethnicity: State of the Science: Implicit Bias Review. Columbus, OH, Kirwan Institute for the Study of Race and Ethnicity, 2017

National Association for the Advancement of Colored People: Racial Disparities in Incarceration. Baltimore, MD, National Association for the Advancement of Colored People, 2017

O'Brien SD, Wayland K: Implicit bias and capital decision-making: using narrative to counter prejudicial psychiatric labels. Hofstra Law Rev 43(3):751–782, 2015

Oshinsky DM: Worse Than Slavery. New York, Simon & Schuster, 1996

Redfield SE, Nance JP: School-To-Prison Pipeline, Preliminary Report. Chicago, IL, American Bar Association Joint Task Force on Reversing the School-to-Prison Pipeline, 2016

Roper v Simmons, 543 United States 551, 570, 573 (2005)

The Sentencing Project: The Color of Justice: Racial and Ethnic Disparity in State Prisons. Washington, DC, The Sentencing Project, 2016

Woods GW, Greenspan S: Culturally biased expert testimony in criminal and family proceedings: an overlooked yet pervasive form of race-based discrimination. Presented at the symposium Structures of Inequality and Race in New York City: Looking Backward and Forward, under the auspices of the Walter Stafford Project, New York University, Wagner School, New York, New York, 2016

CHAPTER 8
BLACK INTERNATIONAL MEDICAL GRADUATES AND THE CARE OF BLACK PATIENTS

Charles Dike, M.D., M.P.H.

INTERNATIONAL MEDICAL GRADUATES (IMGs) are physicians who graduated from medical schools outside the United States and Canada. Approximately 20% are U.S. citizens, and most of them are trained in medical schools in the Caribbean. The rest come predominantly from developing countries of Asia and Africa. A much smaller proportion are from Western countries. In the United States, 15% of the U.S. active physician workforce are IMGs from lower-income countries (Torrey and Torrey 2012). In this chapter I focus mostly on foreign-born black IMGs.

Most IMGs who immigrate to the United States for residency training are on J-1 Exchange Visitor visas and, to a lesser extent, H-1B visas or a green card. Individuals on a J-1 visa must return to their home country for a period of 2 years after completion of residency or obtain a waiver from the federal government. The waiver stipulates that the IMG agree to work in an underserved area for 3 years, after which he or she is free to stay and work in any part of the country.

There is ample evidence that IMGs disproportionately specialize in primary care (family medicine, internal medicine, and pediatrics) and, to a lesser extent, psychiatry (American Association of Medical Colleges 2013). This finding probably reflects the relative accessibility of these specialties to IMGs compared with other specialties more sought after by U.S.-trained medical doctors. Some of the best-prepared IMGs from developing countries arrive with the initial goal of going into a surgical or medical specialty. However, many of them apparently end up in primary care or psychiatry because of the difficulty they have matching into those other specialties. One reason may be the lack of financial resources available to IMGs to pursue research or other advanced graduate degrees and the engagement in volunteer/community service activities necessary to be a competitive applicant.

Psychiatry is not an attractive subspecialty for African medical students, because the stigma of mental illness in Africa seems to extend to psychiatrists. Psychiatrists are not accorded the same respect as other doctors. The diminished status of psychiatrists in society and their low financial remuneration compared with other specialties make psychiatry unattractive to medical students. Upon arrival in the United States, however, many more African physicians specialize in psychiatry, owing to a combination of factors, including more respect for psychiatry as a profession in the United States and improved earning potential.

Coming to America

The journey, literal and figurative, of black IMGs (especially those from Africa) to the United States is long, tortuous, and arduous. It starts at the completion of medical school. Although some IMGs migrate directly to the United States from their home country, many others finally arrive in the United States after having transited through one or more other countries outside of their country of origin. Stories of the adventures involved in this kind of migration are sometimes fascinatingly rich and sometimes frightening. In a nutshell, some IMGs have endured and overcome considerable hardship before setting foot in the United States. Yet final arrival may not be the end of their suffering; for some, it is in fact the beginning of a new chapter of untold challenges.

Some of the IMGs who immigrate to the United States have been out of medical school for approximately 6 years before the start of residency in the United States (Tankwanchi et al. 2013). Some of those years have been spent practicing medicine or completing a residency program or other postgraduate programs within their country of origin or in a different country outside the United States. It is not infrequent for some to have completed residency in a specialty of medicine and practiced for a few years before coming to the United States. On arrival here, IMGs strive to complete a postgraduate course of study in healthcare or business in the United States to bolster their chances of being accepted into residency. Those who have completed a residency program outside the United States are often expected to start over and repeat their residency in this country. Thus, these doctors, as they begin this new phase of training, are generally more experienced as a group than their U.S.-trained counterparts.

Although they are likely to be married and have children, the circumstances of their immigration could be such that they arrive in the United States without their nuclear family, hoping to bring them over once they settle in the new country.

The process of stabilization, which begins with obtaining a residency position, could take several years, during which the IMG cannot travel outside the United States to see his family for fear of not being able to return.

Many IMGs arrive without personal or family resources while completing the examinations needed to apply for residency; they end up working odd jobs to support themselves. These doctors work as security guards, cleaners, waiters/waitresses, cashiers/clerks, taxi drivers, and so on. It is difficult to capture the psychological humiliation experienced by a qualified physician who commands respect in his own country but now works as a cleaner, bouncer, or cabdriver in the United States. Some may be too ashamed to disclose their true work situation to their family and friends back home or to maintain contact with them, thereby increasing their isolation from their support systems.

Adapting to U.S. Culture and Race Relations

It does not take long for IMG immigrants to discover that the United States is not all they fantasized about back home. An African physician colleague who migrated first to Europe and later to the United States was surprised by how ordinary some boroughs of New York City (NYC) looked in contrast to his picture of what America was supposed to be—big, grand, and opulent. He was rudely disappointed. His friend, another African immigrant who was completing residency at an NYC hospital, could only afford to live in a small apartment in a relatively dodgy part of town. Signs of poverty around the neighborhood, with its ramshackle buildings and cars, crumbling homes, and homeless people in tattered clothes, reminded him of shantytowns in his home country, a far cry from what was portrayed in Hollywood movies about America. He had erroneously built his expectations on these fantasies.

The main challenge for this IMG, however, was adapting to a change of status and dealing with discrimination. In the IMG's home country, almost everyone was black. The IMG's primary and high school teachers were black, his respected and revered professors in college and medical school were mostly black, newscasters were black, media outlets were owned and operated by black people, and the government, at regional, state, and national levels, was run by black people. His status as a respected first-class citizen was assured and never in doubt. His physician status amplified the respect usually accorded to professionals as a class. His skin color did not dictate the potential for success; only hard work and a bit of luck (and connections) did. There were many successful black male and female role models to imitate.

The shift in status once a black IMG arrives in the United States is swift. A black IMG colleague once expressed discomfort with the observation that all the teachers in her daughter's elementary school were white, as were those in her son's high school. The same picture continued in colleges and universities, where black professors were rare. Except for sports and music, all other spheres of human endeavor showed the same propensity. Even in sports, where the majority of athletes were black, the coaches and owners of the clubs/organizations were white. The irony was not lost on the IMG.

A black IMG psychiatrist hired by a Veterans Administration hospital in a large city was surprised when a group of black, nonprofessional staff members of the hospital came to see him. They were happy that in their decades of working at the hospital, they had finally seen someone who looked like them in a position of authority. They thanked him for granting them some dignity. The psychiatrist was nonplussed. He could not believe that this would be the case in a large government hospital located in a major urban area of the United States. This unsettling experience spoke volumes about the status of blacks in the United States.

The media's portrayal of blacks in the United States is so consistently negative that a recent immigrant black IMG was surprised to learn, in one of her early classes in residency, that among adolescents, blacks abused alcohol and illegal drugs at rates less than those of Native Americans, multiple-race adolescents, whites, and Hispanics (Wu et al. 2011). Also surprising was that adult blacks and whites engage in drug offenses—possession and sales—at roughly comparable rates, but blacks are arrested nationwide on drug charges at rates relative to population that are 2.8–5.5 times higher than white arrest rates (Human Rights Watch 2009).

Another striking observation that confronts a recent black IMG immigrant is the level of poverty and marginalization apparent in black communities as well as the mass incarceration of black men. The consequences of these social ills are immense. The author recalls the case of a bright teenage boy whom he saw in therapy as a resident whose view of life was entirely fatalistic; at 15, he was sure he would not live to be 20, and therefore he wanted to father a child as soon as possible despite having no financial, emotional, or psychological means to support the child. A particularly difficult event that arose in therapy was his inability to find a responsible man in his neighborhood to cosign a form attesting to his character and pledging adult male support for a scholarship to attend a leadership program. He stated that he had many aunts and other women in his neighborhood who could sign the form, but no men. This was as incredible sounding as it was unfathomable, for there to be no black man of repute in an entire neighborhood to sign a form. It was a complete role reversal and a situation totally unfamiliar to the black IMG, who came from a country where black men were in charge. It became apparent that some of the black U.S. population had been stripped of citizenship privileges commonly enjoyed by blacks in the IMG's own country.

Other Challenges

One of the greatest challenges of foreign-born black IMGs is understanding the nuances of American culture and language. Lines from classic movies are used in regular discourse to describe a situation, feeling, mood, or event as if the meaning should be apparent to all. Interaction styles with all cadres of staff can be brusque and direct in a manner that could be perceived as disrespectful to the IMG. A thick accent may create uncomfortable situations between the IMG and his peers, and between the IMG and patients, which could in turn cause the IMG to lose confidence. Likewise, characteristics such as a loud voice and physical gesticulations so natural to black IMGs could be interpreted as aggressive and attract complaints. In the clinical arena, issues of patients' empowerment to challenge the authority of physicians/psychiatrists could be jarring to IMGs, and patient-centered interviewing and certain ethics dilemmas may be difficult for IMGs to master quickly.

To compound the problem, there may be difficulty finding mentors who understand the IMG's specific challenges and can provide supervision and career guidance. Only 3% of medical school faculty are black/African American, compared with 63% white, 14.6% Asian, and 3% multiple race/non-Hispanic, some of whom could be presumed to be black (American Association of Medical Colleges 2016).

Issues of discrimination and bias come in various forms: from patients who tell the IMGs frankly they would rather see "an American doctor," to patients (and sometimes staff) who hurl racial epithets at the IMGs, to colleagues who exude an air of superiority over IMGs and address the IMGs condescendingly, to junior colleagues who take offense when their IMG bosses hold them accountable but not when non-IMG physicians do the same. This discrimination and bias also plays out when IMGs are passed over for promotions or denied fellowship positions for which they are clearly qualified. An IMG colleague once described the situation as being made to feel like a second-class citizen.

Limitations of being on a visa create their own sets of challenges. The stress of making sure training is completed before expiration of the visa, and concerns about when and where to waive a J-1 visa are paramount. In addition, the pressure to start earning money quickly and to maximize earning potential could lead to lack of interest in additional training in research, and even in fellowships, and ultimately decrease the chances of taking up leadership positions in academia. The status of being on a visa restricts the IMG's ability to take on moonlighting positions part-time to earn extra income to support family in the United States and at home. This could lead to frustration and depression. Perhaps the most challenging issue with being on a visa concerns traveling abroad. Some IMGs are unable to travel home for family emergencies for fear of being stuck in the home country. One IMG described the anguish of not being able to attend his father's funeral, and his feelings of isolation and guilt for not being present for family members in their time of need.

Benefits of Black International Medical Graduates

African American patients' distrust of physicians has been noted and often blamed on the negative fallout from the Tuskegee experiments, in which blacks were the subjects of research experiments that took place without their consent. This was recently highlighted in the movie *The Immortal Life of Henrietta Lacks*, based on the book of the same title. This distrust of physicians is said to inhibit care-seeking and promote nonadherence with recommended treatment (Jacobs et al. 2006). African Americans also identify expectations of racism (being treated with disrespect and looked down upon) and financial discrimination by physicians (owing to lack of or substandard insurance) as reasons for distrusting physicians (Jacobs et al. 2006). It has been observed that compared with patients whose regular doctors are of a different race, patients who are of the same racial or ethnic group as their physicians were more likely to use needed health services and less likely to postpone or delay seeking care, and reported a higher volume of use of health services (LaVeist et al. 2003). These same use patterns were said to be also true for mental health services. A meta-analysis (Cabral and Smith 2011) highlighted conclusions from previous research: African American clients tend to mistrust mental health services provided by white American therapists, and there is a strong preference by clients for a therapist of one's own race/ethnicity and a small tendency to perceive therapists of one's own race/ethnicity as better than others.

These findings support the belief that ready access to black physicians and psychiatrists is likely to lead to improvement in the health status of African Americans. However, access to black physicians remains a significant problem, as only 4% of the physician workforce in the United States is black or African American (American Association of Medical Colleges 2014), despite African Americans accounting for approximately 13% of the U.S. population (U.S. Census Bureau 2010). This number has remained relatively stagnant for years and is not likely to change significantly in the future, given the small proportion (5.7%) of medical school graduates who were black or African American in 2015 (American Association of Medical Colleges 2016). The numbers are even more abysmal for psychiatrists; according to the American Psychiatric Association (APA), 2% of American psychiatrists identify as black (Bailey 2016). For psychologists, less than 2% of American Psychological Association members are black/African American (American Psychological Association 2014).

The American Psychiatric Association does not have accurate data on the number of APA-IMG members who identify their race as black. In response to this author's recent query, the APA cautioned that although 293 members self-identified in their membership profiles as being both black and IMGs (in December 2017), the data were likely incomplete, because there is a substantial subset of members who have not completed their profiles and for whom the APA does not have complete demographic information on file.

Data from a 2011 American Medical Association Physician Masterfile (Tankwanchi et al. 2013) on IMGs from Africa practicing in the United States could give an approximate understanding of the number of black psychiatrist IMGs in this country. There were 8,693 IMGs from sub-Saharan Africa (SSA-IMGs), and 6,557 from North Africa, for a total of 15,250 IMGs from the African continent in the Masterfile in 2011. Psychiatry accounted for approximately 345 (5%) of the 7,298 SSA-IMGs with identified specialty. This latter number includes white South African physicians but excludes black IMGs from North Africa and the Caribbean countries. Although the number of black IMG psychiatrists is difficult to quantify, it is safe to conclude that they are, at least, in the hundreds, and they provide critical access to care for black/African American patients.

Perhaps the most significant contribution of IMGs is in the provision of care in low-income neighborhoods and to those with limited access to care, the socioeconomically disadvantaged populations (Hart et al. 2007). A New York State study found that the percentage of J-1 visa waiver IMGs planning to practice in shortage areas was triple that of U.S. medical graduates (Salsberg and Nolan 2000). Another study, from Washington State, showed that IMGs on a J-1 waiver to serve low-income and underserved populations remained with their J-1 waiver employers a median of 23 months longer than their required commitment periods of 3 years, and that they remained in practices serving primarily underserved populations for, on average, 34 consecutive months after fulfilling their commitments (Kahn et al. 2010), providing much-needed physician presence in these areas. Critical access hospitals in the United States also rely heavily on IMGs, including in "persistent poverty" rural counties. IMGs make up more than half of the medical staff at 16% of these hospitals (Hagopian et al. 2004).

Although IMGs constitute one-quarter of the U.S. physician workforce, approximately 41% of practicing active IMGs are in primary care disciplines as defined by the Association of American Medical Colleges, including internal medicine, family medicine/general practice, pediatrics, internal medicine/pediatrics, and geriatrics. Psychiatry follows, with 6% of IMGs (American Association of Medical Colleges 2013). A greater proportion of office-based IMG primary care physicians, compared with U.S. medical graduates, practiced in areas with physician shortages where Medicare and Medicaid patients are overrepresented (Hing and Lin 2009). Notably, some states list psychiatry as a primary care specialty.

It is important to note that the benefits of black IMGs transcend patient care and access to care. Black IMGs are as important for patients as they are for junior colleagues of color. They can serve as mentors and role models for medical students, residents, and junior colleagues as well as for nonmedical staff and elementary/high school students of color.

Ethics Considerations

The migration of physicians (and other professionals) from resource-poor and developing countries to industrialized, resource-rich countries (often referred to as "brain drain") has raised important questions of equity and fairness in the distribution of doctors. Physicians represent a scarce, prized resource that impoverished nations of the world can ill afford to lose. Often, these doctors are trained at considerable expense to their countries and, in contrast to doctors in the United States, graduate without much debt. The injustice of subsequently enticing these doctors away from their country at no cost to the benefiting country may ultimately have dire consequences. For example, whereas the United States has 12.4 psychiatrists per 100,000 population, no African country has more than 1 psychiatrist per 100,000. The situation has in fact gotten worse from 2011 to 2014, with countries like Cameroon, Chad, Congo, and a few others reporting no psychiatrist per 100,000 population in 2014 (World Health Organization 2015). Hence, according to Hooper (2008), "brain drain" creates a large gap in the workforce of some countries that leaves their healthcare in tatters (Hooper 2008).

Conclusion

Black IMGs play a crucial role in the healthcare delivery system in the United States, often providing a critical link to care for the poor and underprivileged, most of whom live in underserved and rural areas. Although some of these black IMGs lack the historical legacy of slavery, they share deep ancestral bonds with African Americans by being black. Like African Americans, they experience discrimination, bias, and other negative effects of racism.

It has long been understood that increasing the number of black physicians would improve the health status of African Americans by increasing access to preventive care, health education, and other elements of primary healthcare. Unfortunately, the number of U.S.-trained black doctors has not risen to meet the needs of not just black patients, but also a swath of poor and underprivileged people, many, but not all, of whom are members of ethnic minorities. The consequences of low numbers of U.S.-trained black doctors extend to lack of mentors and role models for children in black and other ethnic minority communities, a dearth of faculty at academic institutions, and a lack of support and mentorship for young college and medical school students and for residents. It is important to emphasize the impact of black IMGs in the U.S. society, especially in the black community. Their presence increases diversity in training and professional environments and enriches the practice of medicine and promotion of health to all, especially those with limited access to care.

References

American Association of Medical Colleges: 2013 State Physician Workforce Data Book. Center for Workforce Studies. Washington, DC, American Association of Medical Colleges, 2013. Available at: https://www.aamc.org/download/362168/ data/2013statephysicianworkforcedatabook.pdf. Accessed January 6, 2018.

American Association of Medical Colleges: Diversity in Physician Workforce: Facts and Figures 2014. Washington, DC, American Association of Medical Colleges, 2014. Available at: https://www.aamc.org/data/workforce/reports/439214/ workforcediversity.html. Accessed on January 6, 2018.

American Association of Medical Colleges: AAMC Facts and Figures 2016: Diversity in Medical Education (website). Washington, DC, American Association of Medical Colleges, 2016. Available at: http://www.aamcdiversityfactsandfigures2016.org/. Accessed January 6, 2018.

American Psychological Association: Demographic characteristics of APA members by membership characteristics. Washington, DC, American Psychological Association Directory, 2014. Available at: http://www.apa.org/workforce/publications/ 14-member/table-1.pdf. Accessed January 6, 2018.

Bailey RK: Working With African American/Black Patients (video). Arlington, VA, American Psychiatric Association, 2016. Available at: https:// www.psychiatry.org/psychiatrists/cultural-competency/treating-diverse-patient-populations/working-with-african-american-patients. Accessed January 6, 2018.

Cabral RR, Smith TB: Racial/ethnic matching of clients and therapists in mental health services: a meta-analytic review of preferences, perceptions, and outcomes. J Couns Psychol 58(4):537–554, 2011 21875181

Hagopian A, Thompson MJ, Kaltenbach E, et al: The role of international medical graduates in America's small rural critical access hospitals. J Rural Health 20(1):52–58, 2004 14974436

Hart LG, Skillman SM, Fordyce M, et al: International medical graduate physicians in the United States: changes since 1981. Health Aff (Millwood) 26(4):1159–1169, 2007 17630460

Hing E, Lin S: Role of International Medical Graduates Providing Office-Based Medical Care: United States, 2005–2006 (NCHS Data Brief No 13). Hyattsville, MD, National Center for Health Statistics, 2009. Available at: http://www.cdc.gov/ nchs/data/databriefs/db13.pdf. Accessed January 6, 2018.

Hooper CR: Adding insult to injury: the healthcare brain drain. J Med Ethics 34(9):684–687, 2008 18757641

Human Rights Watch: Decades of Disparity: Drug Arrests and Race in the United States. New York, Human Rights Watch, 2009. Available at: https:// www.hrw.org/sites/default/files/reports/us0309web_1.pdf. Accessed January 6, 2018.

Jacobs EA, Rolle I, Ferrans CE, et al: Understanding African Americans' views of the trustworthiness of physicians. J Gen Intern Med 21(6):642–647, 2006 16808750

Kahn TR, Hagopian A, Johnson K: Retention of J-1 visa waiver program physicians in Washington State's health professional shortage areas. Acad Med 85(4):614–621, 2010 20354376

LaVeist TA, Nuru-Jeter A, Jones KE: The association of doctor-patient race concordance with health services utilization. J Public Health Policy 24(3–4):312–323, 2003 15015865

Salsberg E, Nolan J: The posttraining plans of international medical graduates and US medical graduates in New York State. JAMA 283(13):1749–1750, 2000 10755507

Tankwanchi AB, Ozden C, Vermund SH: Physician emigration from sub-Saharan Africa to the United States: analysis of the 2011 AMA physician masterfile. PLoS Med 10(9):e1001513, 2013 24068894

Torrey EF, Torrey BB: The US distribution of physicians from lower income countries. PLoS One 7(3):e33076, 2012 22457735

U.S. Census Bureau: QuickFacts. Washington, DC, U.S. Department of Commerce, 2010. Available at: https://www.census.gov/quickfacts/fact/table/US/PST045216. Accessed January 6, 2018.

World Health Organization: Global Health Observatory Data Repository (website). Geneva, Switzerland, World Health Organization, 2015. Available at: http://apps.who.int/gho/data/node.main.MHHR?lang=en. Accessed January 6, 2018.

Wu LT, Woody GE, Yang C, et al: Racial/ethnic variations in substance-related disorders among adolescents in the United States. Arch Gen Psychiatry 68(11):1176–1185, 2011 22065533

CHAPTER 9
PROVIDING HIGH-QUALITY PSYCHIATRIC CARE FOR BLACK CHILDREN AND YOUTH

Linda N. Freeman, M.D.
Melvin Oatis, M.D.

COMPARED WITH WHITES, black children and youth are less likely to initiate care or be referred for psychotherapy and more likely to terminate treatment prematurely, attend fewer sessions, and therefore receive lesser quality of psychiatric care (Alegría et al. 2008). This does not imply that black and other minority youth are in less need of these services. Results from the National Comorbidity Survey Replication—Adolescent Supplement (NCS-A; Merikangas et al. 2010) indicated that 46.8% of racially diverse youth experienced mental health disorders before age 18, and 7% of those youth had serious emotional disturbance that significantly impaired their functioning in the past year. The most prevalent disorder was anxiety disorder (32%), followed by mood disorder (14%). The prevalence of substance abuse was 11%, with drug use accounting for 8.9% of that category. Compared with whites, black youth have an increased rate of anxiety disorder and lower rates of substance use disorder.

Even when black children and youth enter treatment, they encounter obstacles that make their improvement difficult. Disparities in the use of both psychotherapeutic and psychopharmacological treatments suggest that black children are also less likely to receive adequate treatment than white children. These differences are observed across diagnoses. Black youth are significantly less likely than Latino or white youth to receive psychotherapy or counseling, even when family income and parent education are controlled for (Kodjo and Auinger 2004). Both having private insurance or having no insurance are associated with lower access to psychotherapy. This suggests that other factors are associated with the difference in therapy utilization.

Since the predictor of substance abuse treatment in adults is receipt of any mental health treatment, one can assume that the same disparity holds for substance abuse treatment for black youth. The process of evaluating, treating, and engaging black youth and families can be complex and requires clinicians to have special expertise and approaches. In the subsequent sections in this chapter, we address key ways for culturally competent clinicians to provide high-quality care to black children, youth, and their families.

Recommendations for Clinicians

Conducting Assessments and Formulating Treatment Plans Consistent With the Family's Values and Beliefs

Clinicians should identify and utilize individual and traditional strengths of the black child and family in assessment and formulate treatment consonant with the family's values and beliefs. A high-quality assessment of a black child and family appraises many strengths; it does not just identify and label pathology. In addition to evidence-based assessment; a thorough history of presenting problems; a complete developmental history of pregnancy, birth and early development; family psychiatric history; and other standard parts of a child psychiatric assessment, the process of helping to expose and examine the child's and family's strengths is of itself therapeutic because it makes self-help possible. Strength-based assessment allows the child, family, and clinician to join in the therapeutic work and deepens the clinician's understanding of the child. An attitude of positive expectation by the clinician—in which we ask about every child we evaluate and treat, "Is he the one who will contribute to his own and society's reconstruction?" (Lawrence 1976)—stimulates the child's, family's, and clinician's search for latent strengths. This process of identification and freeing of strengths can provide energy to the child, parents, and family and permit them to join in the clinical work of evaluation and treatment. It is a humanizing approach—compared with one examining only pathology, which calls for setting up defenses against painful, overwhelming emotions—one that recognizes the humanity of clinician, patient, and family and thereby creates a positive alliance among them.

Assessment of the child's strengths include the following (Lawrence 1976):

- Can he use his body gracefully for his age?
- Does he have age-appropriate manipulative skills and fine and gross motor coordination?
- Are his visual and auditory perception intact?
- Into what familial and social setting was he born and in what setting does he currently live?
- What ideal images are available for him to identify with?
- What does his name mean, and whom is he like?
- What is right about him in the eyes of his family and of his teachers?
- What is his temperament, and how does he use it to get a response from others?
- Can he express his needs in language?
- Can he express himself creatively?
- Does he show social ease with others?
- Can he self-direct in sustained work?
- Does he know "what is right about him" as a person and as a member of his family and community?
- Can he help himself, protect himself, and share in the common aid of his community?
- What is the role of the child in the context of the family for good or ill?
- With what feelings does he respond to family conflicts?
- How are the child's dynamics related to the parents' own developmental dynamics?
- To what extent are ancestral and group strengths represented in the family and the family's image of the child?
- Is there an adaptive meaning in the pathological symptoms?

Factors in the social environment, social stressors, and culturally relevant social supports should also be identified in an assessment. These include awareness of the effects of exposure to violence (Freeman et al. 1993) that can lead to depressive and anxious symptomatology. Identification of the comfort that may be received by the child and family through spiritual advisors may add resilience toward stressors and aid in the treatment process. There is a plethora of information that could be provided by other influential family members, such as grandparents or nonbiological kin, that will improve assessment and treatment.

Assessing families presents special challenges to clinicians who are not familiar with the diversity of black families. Black families often have different family structures, childrearing practices, gender and family roles, and relationships to community. Failing to appreciate these differences may yield an incomplete assessment of the family, especially regarding family strengths. Misinterpreting a cultural norm or consequence of poverty as evidence of abuse or neglect could lead to removing a child from home and all the accompanying social and emotional losses for the child and family. As Phyllis Harrison-Ross and Wyden (1973, p. xxi) emphasize, "What do blacks want for their children and youth? Nothing more than every parent in every latitude and longitude wants for his child. And nothing less." Clinicians must understand the strengths and protective factors in a family while simultaneously identifying risk factors. Black families regardless of social class have developed strengths in response to a need to survive in a racist society. Parents place a high priority on developing self-esteem in their children and in preparing their children to survive in a racist society. Family strengths need exploration to counteract the general bias toward defining the black family as deficient or pathological.

Clinicians should assume families are motivated to behave as they do by a desire to achieve competence. Basic assumptions should be that parents try to raise their children competently, that they will be successful at some aspect of child care, and that they can use their strengths to improve their situations. This approach can lead to discovering all possible strengths within the family system and redefining the presenting problems as manifestations of a drive for mastery of the environment gone awry rather than as personal or family dysfunction.

Most black parents, across socioeconomic status and different family structures, are involved in activities to promote the well-being of their children. They routinely place a high value on engaging in multiple activities with children, and these activities are used as opportunities to teach values or behaviors and to communicate with their children. Parents receive support for parenting from external caregivers, including grandparents, friends, godparents, and great-grand relatives. There is considerable male involvement in the lives of black children. Most black children have male relatives or friends who at least periodically participate in activities with them. Fathers, whether living at home or not, are the most common male influence on their lives. Other male relatives are next most common. Even children without male relatives interact regularly with other male role models, such as church members, coaches, bus drivers, a mother's boyfriend, Big Brothers, and school personnel. These men not only engage in activities with children but also help with educational or occupational skills and, most importantly, communicate and establish trust with children. The following values are commonly held by black parents (Hurd et al. 1995):

- *Connection with family.* Relatives serve as role models and provide support and affection. Most black children, when asked about their role models, mention a relative.
- *Emphasis on effort and achievement.* Black parents commonly believe that success is related to self-actualization or "growing up to be somebody." Most be-

lieve that occupational success is more difficult for blacks but still encourage children to work hard, understanding they will have to overcome barriers. "You will need to be twice as good [as whites] to achieve the same thing."

- *Importance of education.* Most black families adamantly want their children to receive a high-quality education. The generationally passed-on expression "Get a good education. They can never take that away from you" sums up black families' recognition of education as a key to freedom.
- *Spirituality.* Many parents and caregivers receive comfort and guidance from religious activities and therefore want to nourish the spiritual dimension of their children's lives. In addition, there is social support from church and mosque members, who are often considered extended family.
- *Respect for others.* Respect for elders, helping others, and honesty—"being straight with people"—are highly valued qualities.
- *Self-reliance.* Survival skills such as problem solving, safety at home and outside, self-defense, conflict resolution, housekeeping, planning for the future, and sex education reflect aspects of self-reliance that most parents impart. Additionally, black parents try to prepare their children to survive racism. Developing assertiveness and making a superior effort are coping strategies taught to deal with discrimination. "You need to work twice as hard [as others] to achieve the same thing."
- *Facing reality and acceptance of pain in life.* Instead of overprotecting, black parents teach enduring of life's pain: "God won't give you more than you can handle" as well as the message that success comes not from avoiding pain but by conquering it.
- *Self-respect and racial pride.* Black parents want their children to respect themselves and to have high self-esteem. Parents often share their own personal and family triumphs over racism and teach their children black history and culture to instill their children with pride in being black.

Recognizing family strengths will not undo the effects of racism, violence, inadequate education, poverty, or ill health, but it does promote cultural competence in psychiatric practice and can improve engagement. Knowing what is valued in black families, clinicians are better able to empower parents and caregivers. By focusing on the drive for parental competence, practitioners will more likely remember to reward efforts as well as achievements in childrearing.

Assessments need to include external caregivers, especially fathers, who may not live in the household but are important elements of the family system. These external caregivers can play a vital role in family counseling, providing respite for at-risk parents, and supply psychologically comfortable placements for children who must be removed from home. Practitioners must advocate with educational, legal, and medical systems so that proper recognition is accorded to these external caregivers. It is essential to understand the values, competencies, and behaviors related to raising children that parents ascribe to themselves. Ask parents, if they do not volunteer such information, about their strengths and whether they share these commonly held values. Clinicians can promote self-esteem in parents by sharing their assessment of perceived parental competencies. Parents do experience problems with their childrearing and may not be perfect parents. Yet parents who experience parenting problems do possess strengths, even if these strengths are not being used effectively. Interventions with parents can be tailored to draw on their desire for successful childrearing and that desire can serve as a powerful motivator for treatment and for change. The strength-based approach can reveal the specific hopes parents hold for themselves and their children and lead to personalized goals for change by identifying the barriers that keep parents from mastering the parenting process. Families can better engage and remain in services designed to enhance family strengths rather than to focus only on severe psychosocial problems.

Identifying Barriers Preventing Black Children and Families From Accessing Care

Clinicians should identify and address barriers preventing black children and families from accessing care. Stigma of mental illness remains high in black communities. This is possibly due to the fear of the double stigma of being in a marginalized group and being perceived as someone who has a mental illness. Clinicians must address this fear of stigma as well as educate youth and families about the benefits of mental health treatments. Families can mistrust mental health clinicians and agencies given their history of discrimination or disregard for black culture (Suite et al. 2007). Clinicians who acknowledge their awareness of this history of racism in psychiatry can better engage black parents. Commonly children are referred to mental healthcare by the school. Parental or teachers' lack of recognition of psychiatric symptoms or misperceiving black youth's symptomatic behavior as hostile or aggressive requiring discipline, not treatment, can delay referral until the behavior is unmanageable. This may in part explain why mentally ill black youth often receive their mental health treatment via the juvenile justice system.

Acknowledging and Addressing Implicit and Overt Racial Biases

Clinicians should acknowledge that racial biases can interfere with clinical judgment and work toward addressing implicit and overt biases. The quality of assessment, diagnosis, and treatment can be impaired by clinician biases. Clinical interviews are the most widely used tools for diagnosis and psychiatric assessment. Blacks are far more likely to be misdiagnosed when this method is used than are whites. Stereotyping, biases, and uncertainty of clinicians can lead to poor and unequal treatment. When a presentation is unclear, clinicians who do not identify with minority youth and families may inadvertently overly rely on stereotypes instead of focusing on the child's unique experience or social context and misinterpret information observed or reported during the interview (Whaley and Hall 2009). This often occurs unconsciously even among clinicians who do not believe themselves to be prejudiced. There is considerable evidence in the United States for this type of implicit bias (Dovidio et al. 2002). Clinician biases and discrimination contribute to reducing the quality of the patient-provider relationship and lowering the child's and family's perceived or actual quality of care. The clinician needs the ability to observe himself or herself as a stimulus to how the child or family reacts. As Charles Pinderhughes (1974) said, "Clinicians enjoy positive projections upon people with whom we do identify and negative projections with people with whom we do not identify."

Clinicians must stretch their professional capacity for identification. The Harvard Implicit Association Test (Greenwald et al. 1998) is a useful tool for clinicians to begin examining their own unconscious racial bias and can effectively give clinicians a starting point to explore the subject of racial identity and the myriad ways discrimination has a negative impact on the lives of black youth in dimensions the youth may be unaware of or unable to verbalize and discuss. Clinicians can assist black youth in understanding their feelings of anger, powerlessness, and fear and their recognition of unjust treatment as a consequence of their race by explaining society's historical reluctance to address the relevance of race as a negative stressor that has been shown to cause physical and psychological distress (Jernigan and Daniel 2011). Clinicians' articulation of these issues provides validation for these vulnerable youth and can make an enduring impact in their lives. Black children develop their identity as a result not only of the racial education provided by parents and teachers but also of the positive and negative imagery reflected by society at large. Advancing in school, they undoubtedly become aware of black students' poorer performance on standardized examinations, including IQ tests, compared to others. Lacking knowledge of systems contributing to this outcome, they may make faulty conclusions about their academic abilities. Steele (2010) defined the term *stereotype threat* as underperforming in a situation in which a negative stereotype about an identity is relevant. Stereotype threat has been shown to reduce black youth's performance on academic tests because they reduce their concentration on the task at hand by overactively ruminating about not proving a negative stereotype about their race. The clinician's awareness and attention to this potent factor affecting academic achievement may mitigate the effect of threat in the lives of individual black students.

Applying Knowledge of Cultural Differences in Expressions of Symptoms

Clinicians should apply knowledge of cultural differences in black youth's expressions of distress and in symptom presentation. Idiomatic expressions of emotional and psychological distress vary by culture and do not always correspond to diagnostic criteria. In addition, common patterns of symptomatology presented by black children can differ from others. For example, depression that is classically marked by sadness and helplessness may be expressed by black youth with somatic complaints and irritability taking precedence. Clinicians and culturally incongruent systems may inadvertently mischaracterize irritability and other behavioral manifestations of depression symptoms as aggressive, resulting in more punitive and less treatment-focused interventions. Indeed, research indicates black youth as early as 10–12 years old are significantly more likely to receive harsher judgments, harsher punishments, and disciplinary action as well as to be perceived more negatively than their white peers when exhibiting similar behaviors (Goff et al. 2014).

Evidence-based assessment tools are useful to provide information about a child's or adolescent's functioning compared to normative data. Yet clinicians need to be aware that the reliability and validity of such measures with black youth vary from poor to superior. Clinicians should know the psychometrics of the assessment tool used to diagnose black youth in order to determine that the diagnostic and assessment measures are used in a clinically and culturally appropriate way. To effectively assess black children and youth with evidence-based assessment, clinicians still need to be aware of their own biases and the cultural variation in symptomatology, and to consider black clients' possible mistrust during the assessment process. Clinician interpretation of depressive symptoms of black and white youths can differ. For example, the Children's Depression Rating Scale—Revised (CDRS-R; Poznanski et al. 1985), validated in a racially diverse sample of children, was a principal evidence-based assessment used in the Treatment of Adolescents with Depression Study (TADS). The CDRS-R is a semistructured clinician-administered interview given separately to one parent and to the child, with overall ratings then synthesized by the clinician. Fourteen items are assessed by a semistructured interview, but three items are assessed by behavioral observation. During the TADS, all the evaluators except one Latina evaluator were white. Although there were no racial or ethnic differences in clinician ratings of depression symptoms reported by patient and parent, there was significant difference between Latino and black youth versus whites on ratings of the three observational items. Interviewers rated the behavioral symptoms (observed listless speech, flat affect, hypoactivity) more severely in black youth. As a result, black youth were rated as more severely depressed than the white youth by the predominantly white evaluators on the basis of the more severely rated observational items. This differential rating pattern may have resulted from evaluator bias or the behavior of the youth. Or black children may have entered treatment more depressed than either they or their parents endorsed. Clinicians must consider that cultural factors may affect both their evaluation and the behavior of black youth in clinical settings. Perhaps the black and Latino youth exhibited greater guardedness in their interviews, or perhaps there are cultural reasons such as respect for authority that reduced their activity level and eye contact. Nonetheless, the black youth were rated as exhibiting more severe negative behavioral symptoms than their white peers despite presenting with the same depressive symptoms (Stein et al. 2010). A connection might be made between such subjective observations and the newer literature that suggests that whites tend to view black children and youth as being older than their actual age and with more suspicion, hostility, and negative ascriptions than they do whites of the same age. Black youth may disproportionately experience more negative sequelae associated with depression when depressive behavior is misdiagnosed as severe behavior problems when they are exhibiting the same symptoms of depression as their white peers. Black youth are two times more likely to receive punitive interventions such as punishment or juvenile justice remediation versus remediation with mental health treatment than are white youth (Breland-Noble et al. 2010).

Using Culturally Appropriate Treatment Settings

Clinicians should treat black children in familiar community settings when possible. Because so many children and youth are not receiving the mental health services they require, there is interest in school-based mental health programs. Within urban samples of children in diverse school settings, almost 40% were at risk of psychiatric disorders, but only 11% received treatment in a traditional mental health setting (Zahner et al. 1992). Interestingly, among these at-risk children, 37% received mental health services in the school setting. These programs improve access not only by offering care in convenient locations but also by reducing stigma, reducing financial barriers to care, and offering prevention and screening services to all students, not just those who seek care. There is some evidence that school-based health centers reach students who are more socially disadvantaged and psychiatrically impaired than the general school population as well as students less likely to have prior mental health services. School-based clinics reach students who otherwise would go without mental healthcare (Chatterji et al. 2000).

Using Evidence-Based Interventions Shown to Be Efficacious for Black Children and Families

Clinicians should use evidence-based interventions shown to be efficacious for black children and families. The research on such interventions for black youth is sparse. No well-established treatments have validated outcomes in black children and youth. Of the clinical trials used to create mental health guidelines, few have demonstrated efficacy of the treatment for black youth. Huey and Polo (2008) identified probably efficacious treatments (i.e., those with one high-quality trial comparing treatment with placebo or two trials comparing treatment with no treatment) for black children and youth with anxiety problems, trauma-related syndromes, attention-deficit/hyperactivity disorder, conduct disorder, and substance abuse. Huey and Polo's (2008) comprehensive review of evidence-based psychological treatment with black children and youth described probably efficacious evidence-based interventions, discussed in what follows.

The Multimodal Treatment of Attention Deficit Hyperactivity Disorder (MTA) study found that black children required combination stimulant medication and behavioral treatment to achieve equal outcomes to white children who required only stimulant medication. Group cognitive-behavioral treatment has been modified for black youth in the school setting and found probably efficacious. Multisystem therapy, a family-centered individualized intervention delivered at home or in school, and Coping Powers with a parent training component are probably efficacious for reducing criminal offending by black youth. Multisystem therapy is also efficacious for substance-abusing and for suicidal black youth. For maltreated and abused black children, the trauma-related evidence-based interventions Fostering Individualized Assistance Program and Resilient Peer Treatment met criteria for probable efficacy in the treatment of black children.

There are no published studies of probably efficacious evidence-based interventions for black children and youth for other clinical syndromes. Although there may be a place for the selective use of standard treatments with cultural adaptations, there is no compelling evidence of such culturally adapted treatments' effectiveness in black children and youth.

Conclusion

All psychiatrists can provide high-quality care to black children and families. Successful treatment requires addressing barriers to mental healthcare, including stigma, and recognizing mental health symptoms that may have culturally different expression and presentation among black children, as well as managing the mistrust of mental health clinicians that is often caused by lack of awareness or bias in many clinicians and settings. Focused, culturally relevant, and personalized assessment of child and family and treatment can improve quality of care. Although we are years away from producing large-scale clinical trials of mental health interventions with proven utility for black youth, knowledge and application of a range of evidence-based assessment and therapy techniques validated as likely to be effective for black youth and families improve care. Research is needed to determine which evidence-based assessments and interventions are most effective for black children and families and to develop measures to validate culturally appropriate outcomes. Expanding the scope of black recruitment into clinical trials, achieving appropriate sample sizes, and evaluating race as a moderating factor in all studies can advance psychiatric research for black youth and improve the quality of mental healthcare for the population.

References

Alegría M, Chatterji P, Wells K, et al: Disparity in depression treatment among racial and ethnic minority populations in the United States. Psychiatr Serv 59(11):1264–1272, 2008 18971402

Breland-Noble AM, Burriss A, Poole HK, et al: Engaging depressed African American adolescents in treatment: lessons from the AAKOMA PROJECT. J Clin Psychol 66(8):868–879, 2010 20564682

Chatterji P, Caffray CM, Freeman L, et al: Assessing the costs of school-based mental health programs. The Economics of Neuroscience 2(12):40–46, 2000

Dovidio JF, Kawakami K, Gaertner SL: Implicit and explicit prejudice and interracial interaction. J Pers Soc Psychol 82(1):62–68, 2002 11811635

Freeman LN, Mokros H, Poznanski EO: Violent events reported by normal urban school-aged children: characteristics and depression correlates. J Am Acad Child Adolesc Psychiatry 32(2):419–423, 1993 8444773

Goff PA, Jackson MC, Di Leone BA, et al: The essence of innocence: consequences of dehumanizing Black children. J Pers Soc Psychol 106(4):526–545, 2014 24564373

Greenwald AG, McGhee DE, Schwartz JL: Measuring individual differences in implicit cognition: the Implicit Association Test. J Pers Soc Psychol 74(6):1464–1480, 1998 9654756

Harrison-Ross P, Wyden B: The Black Child: A Parent's Guide. New York, Peter H Wyden, 1973

Huey SJJr, Polo AJ: Evidence-based psychosocial treatments for ethnic minority youth. J Clin Child Adolesc Psychol 37(1):262–301, 2008 18444061

Hurd EP, Moore C, Rogers R: Quiet success: parenting strengths among African Americans. Fam Soc 76(7):434–443, 1995

Jernigan MM, Daniel JH: Racial trauma in the lives of black children and adolescents: challenges and clinical implications. J Child Adolesc Trauma 4(2):123–141, 2011

Kodjo CM, Auinger P: Predictors for emotionally distressed adolescents to receive mental health care. J Adolesc Health 35(5):368–373, 2004 15488430

Lawrence MM: The appraisal of ego strength in evaluation, treatment, and consultation: "Is this the one?" J Am Acad Child Psychiatry 15(1):1–14, 1976 1254841

Merikangas KR, He JP, Burstein M, et al: Lifetime prevalence of mental disorders in U.S. adolescents: results from the National Comorbidity Survey Replication—Adolescent Supplement (NCS-A). J Am Acad Child Adolesc Psychiatry 49(10):980–989, 2010 20855043

Pinderhughes CA: Identification of strengths in young black families. Panel presented at the Transcultural Psychiatry Congress, American Academy of Psychoanalysis, World Federation for Mental Health, Caribbean Psychiatric Association, Kingston, Jamaica, 1974

Poznanski E, Freeman LN, Mokros HB: Children's Depression Rating Scale–Revised. Psychopharmacol Bull 21(4):979–989, 1985

Steele C: Whistling Vivaldi: How Stereotypes Affect Us and What We Can Do. New York, WW Norton, 2010

Stein GL, Curry JF, Hersh J, et al: Ethnic differences among adolescents beginning treatment for depression. Cultur Divers Ethnic Minor Psychol 16(2):152–158, 2010 20438153

Suite DH, La Bril R, Primm A, et al: Beyond misdiagnosis, misunderstanding and mistrust: relevance of the historical perspective in the medical and mental health treatment of people of color. J Natl Med Assoc 99(8):879–885, 2007 17722664

Whaley AL, Hall BN: Cultural themes in the psychotic symptoms of African American psychiatric patients. Prof Psychol Res Pr 40(1):75–80, 2009

Zahner GEP, Pawelkiewicz W, DeFrancesco JJ, et al: Children's mental health service needs and utilization patterns in an urban community: an epidemiological assessment. J Am Acad Child Adolesc Psychiatry 31(5):951–960, 1992

CHAPTER 10
BLACK WOMEN AND MENTAL HEALTH

Psychosocial Realities and Clinical Considerations

Annelle B. Primm, M.D., M.P.H.
Donna M. Norris, M.D.
Ruth S. Shim, M.D., M.P.H.

BLACK WOMEN living in the United States encompass a unique combination of distinct yet shared and universal experiences. These experiences are shaped by the historical landscape of the United States and result in significant implications for the mental health of black women. Within the United States, African American women have existed, thrived, and survived within the dual context of racism and misogyny. This intersectionality has contributed to mental health disparities between African American women and women of other racial/ethnic backgrounds.

To begin to understand the breadth of experience of African American women and the impact of this experience on mental health outcomes, one must understand the historical context that generations of black women have experienced in the United States. This historical context has consisted of structural discrimination, racism, and misogyny but is also rich with resilience and protective factors. The historical context of black women in the United States has served as the foundation for public policies and social norms contributing to an uneven distribution of opportunities to black women (compared to other population groups). This has in turn led to risk factors for poor mental health and ultimately to the morbidity and mortality associated with mental illnesses.

Enduring stereotypes of black women in the United States have become powerful forces in shaping the way black women perceive themselves and how they are perceived, both in society in general and from a psychiatric perspective. In this chapter we present cases that serve to highlight the dangers of these stereotypes and recommend strategies for clinicians to avoid bias that leads to poor mental health outcomes for black women seeking mental health treatment.

Historical Context of African American Women in the United States

The circumstances under which black women arrived in the United States were fraught with trauma and pain, and this has had a distinct impact on the mental health of black women in the United States. History reflects patterns of subjugation, theft of personhood, violence, and devaluing and dehumanizing of black females. In the seventeenth century, African men and women were forcibly taken from their families and homes, transported in inhumane and deeply traumatic conditions, and enslaved in the United States by European Americans. Black women were often separated from their spouses and children and were also frequently victims of sexual assault and exploitation, as illustrated in the heart-wrenching film *12 Years a Slave*.

Following the abolition of slavery in 1865, structural racism continued through Reconstruction and beyond in the form of segregation of black people or Jim Crow laws and "separate but equal" policies. Throughout the period of Jim Crow, violence, including rape, against black women (perpetrated by men of all races/ethnicities) was generally ignored (Broussard 2013).

Beginning in the early twentieth century, approximately 6 million African American people from the rural South moved to other parts of the United States. During this Great Migration, African American women's participation in the labor force created challenges with intimate partners, as their employment in the face of job insecurity for black men threatened the patriarchal order of family and spousal relationships. Furthermore, recent research has shown that between 25% and 50% of African American women who migrated did so without spouses (White 2005).

The Civil Rights Movement of the 1950s and 1960s brought progress toward desegregation and reduced discrimination in the United States. Although African American women like Rosa Parks, Ella Baker, Fannie Lou Hamer, Septima Clark, Diane Nash, and countless others were responsible for major advances in the Civil Rights Movement, the prevailing sexism of the times relegated black women to the less prominent roles. Although African American female entertainers performed at the March on Washington in 1963, black women civil rights leaders did not give speeches, reflecting the sexism that existed even within the Civil Rights Movement. Many black women leaders made great strides, however—for example, the late Honorable Shirley Chisholm was the first black woman elected to Congress, in 1968, and the first black woman to run for president.

Beginning in the 1970s, the "War on Drugs" led to mass incarceration, particularly for nonwhite individuals, despite the fact that rates of substance use did not differ significantly among racial/ethnic groups (Moore and Elkavich 2008). In recent years, black women have been imprisoned at double the rate of white women (Carson and Anderson 2016). Young black women ages 18 and 19 are four times more likely to be imprisoned than white young women of the same age (Dumonthier et al. 2017). Black women are also disproportionately victims of violence. They often underreport interpersonal violence because of inequality in the justice system and expecting that a black person will likely not receive justice (Richie 2012).

Intersectionality and Epidemiology

Intersectionality is defined as the accumulation of race, ethnicity, class, gender, sexual orientation, and other marginalizing characteristics contributing to discrimination or disadvantage. In the last decade, studies have begun to conceptualize intersectionality as it relates to health and mental health outcomes (Bowleg 2012; Seng et al. 2012).

The concept of intersectionality can help in understanding disparities and inequities in mental health outcomes for black women. For example, in the United States, women have higher rates of poverty than men, but African American women have more than double the rate of poverty of white women (Tucker and Lowell 2016). A study reported in the December 10, 2017 issue of the *Boston Globe* highlights the staggering contrast in wealth of black families compared with white families (Spotlight Team 2017). It found that the median net worth of black nonimmigrant families in greater Boston was $8.00 compared with a net worth of $247,500 for white families. In addition, black female single-mother families with children were more likely to live in poverty than were white female single-mother families with children (40% vs. 31%; Tucker and Lowell 2016).

African American Women and the Social Determinants of Mental Health

To better understand the impact of historical and societal factors on black women, it is important to consider the social determinants of mental health—the societal, environmental, and economic conditions that impact mental health outcomes.

As a result of the complex historical pattern of racist and sexist policies and social norms in the United States, African American women often experience discrimination and social exclusion, adverse early life experiences, poor education, poverty and income inequality, unemployment and job insecurity, food insecurity, adverse features of the built environment, housing instability, and poor access to healthcare. These social determinants of mental health impact black girls and women throughout their life-span and contribute to increased vulnerability of black women to mental illnesses and to maladaptive behavioral patterns (Compton and Shim 2015).

Discrimination and Social Exclusion

Discrimination is a powerful social determinant of mental health. Perceived discrimination is closely tied to poor mental health outcomes. Studies have found a robust association between rates of perceived discrimination and major depressive disorder, generalized anxiety disorder, alcohol use disorder, and posttraumatic stress disorder (Krieger 1999, 2014).

As a result of intersectionality, black women have the potential of being discriminated against because of both race and gender. Compared with men and whites, black women are more often discriminated against and excluded from equal participation, are at greater risk of exposure to harm, and are disadvantaged socially and economically. It is unclear if this risk of disadvantage has simple compound or multiplier effects in its impact on mental health and well-being.

Adverse Early Life Experiences

The Adverse Childhood Experiences (ACE) study found a very strong relationship between harmful experiences early in life and a range of poor physical and mental health outcomes and risky behavior patterns (Felitti et al. 1998). In recognition that the original ACE study did not adequately capture adverse experiences of diverse children in the United States, the Philadelphia ACE study expanded the range of negative experiences considered (Table 10–1; The Research and Evaluation Group 2013).

Black women in the United States are vulnerable to this expanded range of adverse early life experiences. For example, black children are twice as likely as white children to be placed in foster care before age 5 and are at greater risk for frequent changes in residence and educational settings, which can impede their ability to learn.

Housing Insecurity and Homelessness

Poor housing quality, such as infestation, mold, and deterioration, is associated with poor mental health outcomes, including depression, anxiety, and psycho-

TABLE 10–1. Types of adverse childhood experiences in the original and the Philadelphia Adverse Childhood Experiences (ACE) study

Original ACE study	Philadelphia ACE study
Abuse	Witnessing violence
Physical abuse	Living in unsafe neighborhoods
Emotional abuse	Experiencing racism
Sexual abuse	Living in foster care
Neglect	Experiencing bullying
Physical neglect	
Emotional neglect	
Household dysfunction	
Family member with illness	
Incarcerated household member	
Mother treated violently	
Household substance abuse	
Parental divorce	

logical distress, particularly among black women (Suglia et al. 2015). The Fragile Families and Child Wellbeing Study found higher rates of depression and anxiety in mothers experiencing housing instability or housing quality issues than in those who did not (Suglia et al. 2011).

There are striking racial disparities in homelessness among families in the United States. In 2010, African American families were seven times more likely to have spent time in a homeless shelter compared with white families (Institute for Children, Poverty, and Homelessness 2012).

Poverty and Income Inequality

The effects of poverty and income inequality are interdependent with racism and sexism in American society. Black women earn less money than most other demographic groups and have higher rates of poverty than black men and women from other races/ethnicities (with the exception of Native American women) (Dumonthier et al. 2017). Despite common negative assumptions that brand all welfare recipients as black, white families outnumber black families among those receiving public assistance in the United States (Sherman et al. 2017). It is well known that living in poverty is strongly associated with poor mental health outcomes, including substance use disorders, major depressive disorder, posttraumatic stress disorder, and anxiety disorders (Wilkinson and Pickett 2009). Poverty is also associated with chronic health conditions such as hypertension, diabetes, and obesity, which are disproportionately high among black women and often co-occur with mental illnesses (Gebreab et al. 2015).

Unemployment, Underemployment, and Job Insecurity

Black women are more likely to participate in the workforce than women from other racial/ethnic groups and are more likely to be the breadwinners in their families. Still, black women face significant job insecurity that comes from high rates of working for minimum wage in positions and jobs that lack important wellness-protecting policies such as paid sick leave, paid family/medical leave, and paid maternity leave (Dumonthier et al. 2017). Often, because of the burden of needing to support their families, black women may take jobs or positions that are far below their qualifications.

The "Crooked Room" and Stereotypes of Black Women

Journalist and political science professor Melissa Harris-Perry, author of *Sister Citizen: Shame, Stereotypes, and Black Women in America,* refers to the unique challenges of black women in the United States as like living in a "crooked room," based on classic studies of the 1970s that involved placing people in a crooked room and asking them to align themselves vertically (Harris-Perry 2011). While some participants recognized they were sitting in a crooked room and contorted themselves to be fully vertical, others aligned themselves in relation to the objects in the room. Harris-Perry (2011) hypothesized that black women often "tilt and bend themselves to fit the distortion" (p. 29) and their behaviors may support stereotypical conceptions of black women. As Harris-Perry succinctly stated, "It can be hard to stand up straight in a crooked room" (p. 29).

The "crooked room" helps us understand why it appears that black women often conform to these stereotypes that we discuss here along with their impact on black women.

Mammy

The stereotype of the "Mammy"—the strong, selfless, caretaking black woman—originated during slavery in the South. Closely tied into this characterization of black women is a focus on being an asexual superwoman who happily puts everyone's needs above her own. One can easily call up numerous depictions of this stereotype in media and entertainment, from the eponymous Mammy in *Gone With the Wind* to recent characterizations like Madea created by actor and filmmaker Tyler Perry.

Jezebel

Another stereotype that originated during slavery is the "Jezebel," an immoral, hypersexual, seductive black woman who lacks self-control and is ruled only by her desires. This stereotype has been used to justify sexual violence against black women and perpetuates a general lack of justice for black women who are victims of violent crimes. Recent popularizations of the Jezebel stereotype include black women depicted in music videos and the character of Leticia Musgrove in *Monster's Ball*, played by Halle Berry. Associated with the stereotype is the "welfare queen," a characterization of black women as having multiple children who must be supported by public assistance programs.

Sapphire

The stereotype of "Sapphire" was popularized in the 1940s and 1950s and was the name of the wife of a character on the *Amos 'n Andy* radio show. The Sapphire stereotype is an image of a domineering, aggressive, emasculating, nagging black woman. The later stereotype of the "angry black woman" arose from the Sapphire stereotype. This stereotype can lead people to disregard or devalue the normal expression of emotions in black women.

"Johnetta" Henry

The authors have taken poetic license with this stereotype, which is a feminized derivation of the syndrome of John Henry. According to the legend, a black man steel-driver sought to prove his prowess by competing against a steam-powered machine used for railroad construction. While John Henry beat the machine, he died with a hammer in his hand. In "Johnetta" Henryism, black women put industriousness into overdrive to excel against all odds, sacrificing their health and well-being. This syndrome is akin to the myth of the Superwoman.

Case Vignettes and Clinical Considerations

The following case vignettes describe common presentations of black women throughout the lifespan in clinical settings replete with intersectional complexity.

These descriptions are composites of aspects of real-life stories of black women whom the authors have encountered in therapeutic work. The names used are fictitious. Discussion of clinical responses to the challenges in each portrayal takes into consideration person-centered, trauma-informed, and culturally at-tuned approaches.

Ms. Allen: College Student

Ms. Allen is a 20-year-old black college student at a predominantly white in-stitution. She is the oldest of six children and the first person in her family to attend college. She feels considerable pressure to succeed. Ms. Allen's father died when she was an infant, and her mother has a history of depression that has been untreated. Having never worked, her mother relied on public assistance to take care of the family, prompting her mother's relatives to call her a "welfare queen," a term that Ms. Allen found embarrassing. Ms. Allen's mother was crit-ical of her darker skin and encouraged her to use bleaching cream on her face, which led to severe skin irritation. The residual scarring made her feel even more ugly and disfigured. Ms. Allen was molested by her uncle throughout her child-hood. She told her mother, who, sadly, did not believe her.

Her anger about her past victimization was reignited when she was sexually assaulted on campus by a white male student. Ms. Allen thought the assault was her fault because she did not respond to him in a more forceful, negative way when he made comments about her body. She did not report the assault because she did not want to bring attention to herself and worried that no one would be-lieve a black girl making an accusation against a white boy. She carried around guilt and shame along with worry about her academic performance. She began losing weight and having trouble with sleep and concentration. She started get-ting failing grades in her classes and began to panic. Ms. Allen felt isolated at school and had not made any friends on campus. She heard about a black stu-dent organization on campus but felt that she did not have time to participate and thought she might not have much in common with the students anyway. She was on the verge of giving up on everything and considered taking a bottle of pills, but instead she decided to see someone at the university counseling center.

Clinical Discussion

Ms. Allen presents with a classic profile of depression with low mood and feel-ings of worthlessness, guilt, and self-blame. Her sexual assault in college layered additional trauma on top of multiple adverse early life experiences, creating a heavy trauma burden that may have contributed to her depression. It would be helpful to measure her depression with a self-report tool such as the Patient Health Questionnaire–9 (PHQ-9), which could quantify the severity of the depression as well as allow for tracking of her progress in treatment over time. If she is willing, she may benefit from antidepressant medication and/or psy-chotherapy using a cognitive-behavioral approach. Exploring her thoughts about how she feels about herself would be important given her familial experiences, including her mother's denigration of her skin color. This is not uncommon in the black community and can lead to physically and psychologically destructive practices.

Processing her experiences with sexual assault is also important, because not being believed can be devastating from an intrapsychic perspective. It is crucial to take a trauma-informed approach to Ms. Allen's sexual abuse, pursuing it gently so as not to re-traumatize her. Another approach, supporting her self-efficacy, is to process some of the "me-too" reports on social media from other women who have experienced sexual harassment and abuse. In reviewing Ms. Allen's options for supports on campus, it is essential to help her create a sense of belonging. The black students' organization could provide a space for engaging with people from similar backgrounds who could relate to her experiences. No matter which courses of action Ms. Allen pursues, her clinician can provide her with a sense of hope that she can overcome depression and sadness related to the circumstances of her life and her past, and that she is capable of thriving academically and socially.

Ms. Bond: Corporate Executive

Ms. Bond is a 40-year-old single black woman with an MBA who has worked in a corporate setting for 15 years and has excelled in her work. She grew up in the Midwest and always did extremely well in school. She wears her hair in a natural style and often proudly dresses in African clothing. Despite her stellar performance and 12-hour workdays, Ms. Bond has not had the opportunity to move up in the company. Time after time, white men and women with lesser qualifications have been given higher positions and salaries. Sometimes, Ms. Bond feels as though she is an imposter and is not as knowledgeable as she works so hard to be. She heard from a coworker that one person in company leadership said she could have a chance at advancement if she changed her hairstyle to a "more professional" look. Ms. Bond saw this as sexual harassment regarding her physical appearance but did not pursue it. She feels exploited by coworkers and supervisors who come to her with their personal problems and treat her as though she were responsible for taking care of them. She has kept her resentment about this inside for fear of letting it out and being labeled an "angry black woman."

Over time, Ms. Bond has begun to develop symptoms of severe anxiety, and one day she passes out on the train on her way to work. Her blood pressure skyrocketed, and she is hospitalized. She is placed on antihypertensive medication and is released with the strong recommendation to cut back on her heavy workload. Ms. Bond decides to seek mental health services to address her lingering anxiety.

Clinical Discussion

A clinician working with Ms. Bond might question if she is actually being discriminated against. This could be a countertransference issue that the clinician may want to explore. The clinician would also want to propose to Ms. Bond that she think about the pros and cons of staying in her job. In doing so, the clinician has an important role in helping Ms. Bond in her decision making and planning her future. Working with Ms. Bond on her feelings of being an imposter would be essential to assist her in owning her accomplishments and excellence despite the external impediments to her advancement. Wearing Afrocentric outfits and hairstyle is an expression of pride in Ms. Bond's identity. Finding a workplace where this is appreciated would also contribute to her well-being. The clinician could encourage Ms. Bond to consider participating in outside activities that bring her joy and relaxation, such as yoga, meditation, mindfulness, physical activity, and music. Pursuing work-life balance and valuing self-identity will help Ms. Bond achieve her goals of success in the workplace.

Mrs. Cole: Hospital Housekeeping Staff Member

Mrs. Cole is a 60-year-old black woman originally from the Deep South whose family migrated to a Northern urban setting in her childhood. She works full-time in a hospital in housekeeping. A high school graduate, she married at age 18 and had four children. Previously she worked as a housekeeper for a white family. Her husband is an alcoholic and has been physically abusive to Mrs. Cole over the years. He often complains that Mrs. Cole is a "know-it-all," needing to be in everyone's business, trying to take charge of everything and constantly nagging him and challenging his manhood (an example of the "Sapphire" stereotype). At one point, he hit her hard, knocking her down and breaking her tooth, which she never got fixed and serves as a constant reminder of her victimization. Despite his violence and continued drinking, she has stayed with him because she takes her marriage vows seriously.

Her husband was diagnosed with cancer of the esophagus, and the weight of caregiving for him has fallen upon her, since her husband's family of origin abandoned him because of his alcoholism. Her youngest son was murdered in his 20s, which was devastating to Mrs. Cole and her family. Her daughter became addicted to heroin and ended up in prison. Because of her work for a white family and taking care of their children in previous years, Mrs. Cole was blamed by her husband's family for making their children "latchkey kids," rendering them vulnerable to getting in trouble. As a result of her daughter's incarceration, Mrs. Cole takes care of her daughter's young children. This has taken a toll on her financially, but she "wouldn't have it any other way" because she could not fathom having her grandchildren placed in foster care.

She is active in her church and is a highly regarded deaconess. The church is an environment in which Mrs. Cole is recognized for her leadership, unlike in the workplace. She is overweight and has diabetes. She is known in the family, at work, and in her neighborhood as a hard worker, a great cook, a relentless volunteer, and a generous, selfless friend. She thinks of her cooking as an expression of love and nurturing to those close to her. Yet her need to use available, low-cost foods often leads her to cook with processed ingredients that are high in fat, carbohydrates, and sodium, and this has contributed to the obesity of her grandchildren. She expresses concerns about frequent sadness, fatigue, and difficulty sleeping. Mrs. Cole prays regularly for the health and safety of her family members and for the Lord to give her strength. When she decided to seek help from a mental health professional, her husband balked at the idea, asking her, "Why would you want to go down there and tell those white folks all of our business and have them tell you you're crazy?"

Clinical Discussion

The case of Mrs. Cole illustrates the excessive hard work identified in "Johnetta" Henryism, with expectations of outsized caregiving and self-sacrifice. Even though she presents with some symptoms of depression, her presentation does not necessarily meet criteria for a diagnosis but, rather, indicates psychological distress. It would be important for the clinician to learn from Mrs. Cole how she understands her situation. The clinician can inquire about what Mrs. Cole thinks has caused her depressed mood and fatigue and about what types of coping she has employed in the past, such as friends, prayer, and church, and how helpful they have been. The clinician could acknowledge her unselfish investment in raising her grandchildren and encourage Mrs. Cole to see how her life of sacrifice, devotion, and giving to others can be balanced with self-care. Exploring with Mrs. Cole about others who could help her with her responsibilities, what things are most important to her, and her short- and long-term goals could help to formulate a plan to reduce her stress and improve her well-being. In promoting a "both-and" approach, the clinician could encourage Mrs. Cole's engagement in religious activity, prayer, and volunteer activities along with mental health services and self-care to achieve a balance that supports her health and well-being.

It would be beneficial for the clinician to give Mrs. Cole a sense that resilience is possible in the face of these personal and family challenges and that coming forward for help would not mean receiving a label but rather is an opportunity for self-exploration and growth with the support of a mental health professional. High rates of voluntarism, civic participation, and social connection are characteristics of black women that may contribute to their resilience and well-being. Clinicians can encourage such activities and participation in support groups that have been helpful to black women experiencing psychological distress, such as Prime Time Sister Circles, created by Drs. Marilyn Gaston and Gayle Porter, and Emotional Emancipation Circles, developed by the Community Healing Network and the Association of Black Psychologists.

Conclusion

In this chapter we reviewed how the checkered past of the United States, with slavery, misogyny, racism, and poverty, has affected black women and their mental health. Black women have endured these negative forces and survived, striving in the face of tremendous odds to raise their children and support their families while holding out hope for the promise of a brighter future. Despite tremendous historical adversity and trauma, black women have collectively demonstrated powerful resilience and a capacity to not only endure but also thrive. This optimistic response to hardship is a cultural imperative reflective of the fact that risk factors are not predictive factors because of protective factors. Regardless of a black woman's psychological and trauma burdens, clinicians can help to mitigate risk factors and determinants of poor mental health by employing cultural humility as well as their understanding of the permutation of psychosocial challenges black women face, as a group and individually. This requires that clinicians join with black women to cultivate protective factors such as strong support systems and resources both within and outside the individual's immediate environment, toward the goal of maximizing the mental health, well-being, and quality of life for themselves, their families, and their communities.

References

Bowleg L: The problem with the phrase women and minorities: intersectionality—an important theoretical framework for public health. Am J Public Health 102(7):1267–1273, 2012 22594719

Broussard PA: Black women's post-slavery silence syndrome: a twenty-first century remnant of slavery, Jim Crow, and systemic racism—who will tell her stories? The Journal of Gender, Race, & Justice 16:373–421, 2013

Carson AE, Anderson E: Prisoners in 2015. Washington, DC, Bureau of Justice Statistics, 2016

Compton MT, Shim RS (eds): The Social Determinants of Mental Health. Arlington, VA, American Psychiatric Publishing, 2015

Dumonthier A, Childers C, Milli J: The Status of Black Women in the United States. Washington DC, Institute for Women's Policy Research, 2017

Felitti VJ, Anda RF, Nordenberg D, et al: Relationship of childhood abuse and household dysfunction to many of the leading causes of death in adults. The Adverse Childhood Experiences (ACE) Study. Am J Prev Med 14(4):245–258, 1998 9635069

Gebreab SY, Diez Roux AV, Brenner AB, et al: The impact of lifecourse socioeconomic position on cardiovascular disease events in African Americans: the Jackson Heart Study. J Am Heart Assoc 4(6 e001553):e001553, 2015 26019130

Harris-Perry MV: Sister Citizen: Shame, Stereotypes, and Black Women in America. New Haven, CT, Yale University Press, 2011

Institute for Children, Poverty, and Homelessness: Intergenerational Disparities Experienced by Homeless Black Families. National Survey Policy Brief. New York, Institute for Children, Poverty, and Homelessness, 2012

Krieger N: Embodying inequality: a review of concepts, measures, and methods for studying health consequences of discrimination. Int J Health Serv 29(2):295–352, 1999 10379455

Krieger N: Discrimination and health inequities. Int J Health Serv 44(4):643–710, 2014 25626224

Moore LD, Elkavich A: Who's using and who's doing time: incarceration, the war on drugs, and public health. Am J Public Health 98(9 suppl):S176–S180, 2008 18687610

The Research and Evaluation Group: Findings From the Philadelphia Urban ACE Survey. Philadelphia, PA, Public Health Management Corporation, 2013

Richie B: Arrested Justice: Black Women, Violence, and America's Prison Nation. New York, NYU Press, 2012

Seng JS, Lopez WD, Sperlich M, et al: Marginalized identities, discrimination burden, and mental health: empirical exploration of an interpersonal-level approach to modeling intersectionality. Soc Sci Med 75(12):2437–2445, 2012 23089613

Sherman A, Shapiro I, Greenstein R: Census data show robust progress across the board in 2016 in income, poverty, and health coverage. Center on Budget and Policy Priorities, September 12, 2017. Available at: https://www.cbpp.org/research/poverty-and-inequality/census-data-show-robust-progress-across-the-board-in-2016-in-income. Accessed December 23, 2017.

Spotlight Team: Boston. Racism. Image. Reality. Boston Globe December 10, 2017

Suglia SF, Chambers E, Sandel MT: Poor housing quality and housing instability, in The Social Determinants of Mental Health. Edited by Compton MT, Shim RS. Arlington, VA, American Psychiatric Publishing, 2015, pp 171–192

Suglia SF, Duarte CS, Sandel MT: Housing quality, housing instability, and maternal mental health. J Urban Health 88(6):1105–1116, 2011 21647798

Tucker J, Lowell C: National Snapshot: Poverty Among Women and Families, 2015. Washington, DC, National Women's Law Center, 2016. Available at: https://nwlc.org/resources/national-snapshot-poverty-among-women-families-2015. Accessed December 23, 2017.

White KJC: Women in the Great Migration. Soc Sci Hist 29(3):413–455, 2005

Wilkinson RG, Pickett K: The Spirit Level: Why Greater Equality Makes Societies Stronger. New York, Bloomsbury Press, 2009, pp 63–72

CHAPTER 11
YOUNG MINORITY FATHERS

Harbingers of Promise for Their Children

Derrick M. Gordon, Ph.D.
David Friedlander, M.A.
Christine Simon, Sc.M.

IN RECENT DECADES, scientific inquiries have documented the positive impact that men and fathers can have on children, families, the mothers of their children, and community outcomes. As this research area has developed, some attention has been paid to adolescent paternity. This attention is an outgrowth of the documented negative effects adolescent paternity has been shown to exert on the development of young men, their partners, and children.

Considering the myriad negative societal outcomes associated with adolescent fatherhood, there are few prevalence data drawn from nationally representative samples on adolescent male paternity. There are a number of challenges associated with limited prevalence data research on adolescent paternity. These include limited awareness and attention to the presence and need of adolescent fathers, biological limitations associated with the fact that males cannot physically be impregnated and carry a fetus to term, and limited interest and strategies specifically focused on the reproductive health needs of men, and specifically young men (Marcell et al. 2011). Estimated rates of adolescent paternity appear to vary by time of data collection and recruitment methodology. There are reports that between 2% and 7% of adolescent males become fathers. More recent analyses by Kiselica and Kiselica (2014a, 2014b) suggest that annually, 180,000 adolescent males will father a child. Other estimates indicate that 9.4% of adolescent males become fathers (Sipsma et al. 2010). While nationally, the rates of adolescent paternity have continued to decline, there are pockets of intransigence in the rates observed.

Pockets Where Adolescent Fatherhood Is Higher

There is evidence that teen fatherhood occurs more often in inner-city neighborhoods where the population is mostly composed of ethnic minority young men. Estimates of teen fatherhood in these settings range from 15% to 20%, and there is some evidence that neighborhoods with greater environmental physical risk factors, such as those found in inner cities, are significantly more predictive of adolescent fatherhood (Sipsma et al. 2010).

A group that is often neglected in discussions and considerations of adolescent paternity is young men involved with child welfare systems. When risk factors associated with adolescent paternity and child welfare involvement are considered, there is significant overlap. This overlap calls for those involved in the delivery of services to these vulnerable young men involved with child welfare systems to consider their reproductive health needs and risks. The challenge associated with this call is the failure by child welfare providers to collect data on the rates at the local, state, and national levels. These social supports often fail to integrate the reproductive health needs and experiences of these young men as they complete case management, discharge planning, and matriculate out of social service systems (Gordon et al. 2011). This experience is challenging and adds to the problems in getting an accurate picture of adolescent paternity.

Although it is difficult to depict accurately the reach of adolescent paternity, there is support for the view that black and Hispanic/Latino young men have disproportionate rates compared with their white counterparts. Support for this perspective is drawn from the higher rates of black and Latino/Hispanic adolescent paternity among samples of early fathers identified and their over-representation in services associated with greater rates of early paternity (e.g., child welfare services, juvenile justice programs). Research suggests that black young men are three to four times more likely to father a child than their same-age, different-race peers. These observations are important, given the risks associated with adolescent paternity and the exacerbation of these risks following the birth of their child. These findings call for more research, intervention development, and policies specifically focused on the needs of this vulnerable group, and greater understanding of the factors associated with adolescent paternity. When the developmental considerations of young men who are fathers are taken into account, paternity status may have important family, physical, mental, educational, juvenile justice, and economic implications at the individual, children, family, and community levels, with negative long-term risks.

Several risk factors predispose young men to fathering a child. The most frequently studied risk factors include family demographic variables, low educational attainment, delinquency, substance use, psychological factors, and physical health risk (e.g., Kiselica and Kiselica 2014a, 2014b). However, longitudinal studies that allow researchers to make causal inferences about these risks are lacking and need to be carried out. Nevertheless, the current associations made between adolescent paternity and its associated risks require some consideration of their presence and impact on adolescent development.

Risk Factors for Adolescent Paternity

Family Demographic Variables

Most adolescent parents come from socioeconomically disadvantaged backgrounds, and recent studies now argue that high rates of poverty among adolescent parents may be in part due to their own childhood experiences of poverty (Berger and Langton 2011; Smeeding et al. 2011). These observations highlight questions about how many of the young men who are fathers are the offspring of teenage parents, are from single-parent homes, or reportedly feel disconnected from their own families (Sipsma et al. 2010). These risks are further compounded when the adolescent's family lacks social support or undergoes numerous transitions in family structure (i.e., parental figures entering and leaving the home, involvement in child welfare system, involvement in criminal justice system). Further complicating the picture are observations from qualitative studies that show adolescent fathers are more likely to report little, poor, or no contact with their own fathers growing up (Kiselica and Kiselica 2014a, 2014b). Clear in the description are the ways that family experiences, structures, and supports affect the paternity risks of young men, especially minority and urban males. What is also evident are the ways that their early paternity signals their risks for poor educational outcomes.

Low Educational Attainment and Employment

Teenage males who experience academic difficulties or drop out of school are more likely to become fathers than their academically successful peers. Low academic competency or being older than expected for grade may result in adolescent paternity. Some studies have found poor school performance to be the single most significant predictor of young fatherhood. Poor academic performance has clear implications for the vocational and employment opportunities of young fathers (Kiselica and Kiselica 2014a, 2014b).

Adolescent fathers are disproportionately likely to be unemployed when compared with their nonfather peers. Adolescent fathers expressed little interest in mental health or substance abuse treatment; they were substantially more interested in obtaining employment or receiving educational-vocational services (Dariotis et al. 2011). When asked, these young men tended to indicate interest in receiving support in getting employment, educational-vocational services, job referrals, vocational education, and job readiness. Because these young men are generally poorly educated, they struggle to find and maintain employment. When they are able to find jobs, they tend to receive very low pay (Alio et al. 2011; Carlson 2016). Some may resort to illegal activities, including drug trafficking, to support themselves or pay child support. Illegal activities are an unstable source of income and carry the obvious risks of arrest and incarceration. The challenges faced when their academic and employment opportunities are limited and their performance is poor can be exacerbated with their engaging in delinquent behaviors.

Delinquency

Research has consistently revealed a link between delinquent behavior (i.e., the commission of criminal acts) and adolescent fatherhood. Unmarried adolescent fathers may be more likely to engage in activities that can lead to incarceration, including substance use (see later discussion). Reports by young fathers indicated histories of jail or prison involvement, recent problems with the law, and probation and parole histories. Furthermore, chronic violent behavior may substantially increase the likelihood of becoming a teen father and the motivations for delinquent acts and adolescent fatherhood may be similar. Adolescent fathers have been linked to gangs and other deviant or aggressive peers (Kiselica and Kiselica 2014a, 2014b). Peer experiences are relevant to young fathers, because developmentally they have been shown to exert significant influence. Adolescent fathers may turn to crime because they lack viable alternatives to support themselves financially (Kiselica and Kiselica 2014a, 2014b). Substance use and drug distribution have been shown to impact the trajectory of young men negatively as they transition to adulthood.

Substance Use

The link between substance use and adolescent fatherhood is well documented. There is also evidence that substance use is associated with other problem behaviors that are known to increase risk for adolescent fatherhood (e.g., disruptive school behavior, delinquency). The risks associated with adolescent paternity and substance use have been shown to be present even after other risk factors, such as aggressive behaviors and sexually transmitted infections, have been taken into account. Compared with their peers, adolescent fathers are more than three times as likely to test positive for drugs, smoke cigarettes, use alcohol, or use hard drugs (Weinman et al. 2002). Despite this frequency, only a small number request substance abuse treatment. Substance use and its relationship to early paternity bring to the fore psychological factors that may also be associated with risks for early paternity.

Psychological Factors

In general, psychological variables have received less scholarly attention as a potential risk for early paternity. Nevertheless, there is evidence that young men are more likely to become fathers if they experience psychological illness, have been victims of sexual or physical abuse, or exhibit early adolescent aggressive behaviors (Kiselica and Kiselica 2014a, 2014b). Childhood aggression links to adolescent risk-taking behaviors, behavioral dysregulation, and antisocial behaviors, which may be a precursor for adolescent paternity. Adolescent fathers have also been shown to have more external loci of control and lower self-esteem than their non-father peers. Other studies have documented anywhere between 25% and 46% of young fathers endorsing "feelings of anger, sadness/depression, nervousness/tension, helplessness, and aggressiveness." Studies also show that compared with childless adolescents, young fathers experience higher levels of stress and psychological distress (e.g., depression, anxiety, guilt, lower life satisfaction), and social isolation, and tend to be less healthy (Berger and Langton 2011; Paschal et al. 2011), putting them at a greater risk of having poor health and mental health outcomes as adults. Despite the fact that these emotional states are identified through screening, only a fraction of the young men request mental health services. Failure to seek appropriate services may be tied to the views that seeking services would indicate weakness or some other outcome not associated with being masculine.

Seeking and receiving appropriate mental health treatment is important for young men at risk for early paternity. Services can lead to positive outcomes that impact their developmental tasks, and research with adult fathers show that men's positive mental health experiences have cascading effects for them, their partners, and their children. While there are links identified between adolescent paternity and the psychological factors described, more research is needed to document how these connections develop and lead to early paternity and, where connections have been established, how interventions can mitigate their effects. Questions are also raised about the physical health consequences of the behaviors that lead to adolescent paternity.

Physical Health Risks

While some attention has been paid to the social and mental health consequences of young fatherhood, less is understood about the physical health impact of young fatherhood. For example, Garfield et al. (2016) found that being a father was associated with an increase in body mass index for men, which is linked to increased risk of obesity and cardiovascular diseases later in life. These health risks are often compounded by racial and ethnic disparities, with men of color experiencing worse health outcomes than their white counterparts later in life. Addressing young minority men's physical health and mental health risks early could prevent adverse health outcomes in adulthood. These recommendations also point to the value that healthful fatherhood practices can add to the experiences of fathers and their children, partners, family, and community. Nowhere is this possibility more promising than through interventions focused on young fathers.

Importance of Addressing the Unique Needs of Adolescent Fathers

While the parenting needs of adolescent fathers have been historically overlooked (Lewin et al. 2015), the growing interest in their role in family life and childrearing presents a unique opportunity for social systems to identify and implement strategies that effectively engage young minority fathers. Despite societal shifts in the perceptions and expectations of fathers' roles in childrearing over the past few decades, society continues to hold negative views of young fathers, particularly young black fathers. Young black fathers are often portrayed as being uncaring, irresponsible, absent, criminal, and violent (Lau Clayton 2016). These broad-brush stereotypes have fueled assumptions about them and have resulted in social systems' approaching adolescent fatherhood from a deficit perspective (Paschal et al. 2011) rather than using a strength-based approach.

Concerns about adverse economic and educational consequences for adolescent parents have been mainly directed toward minority mothers, because they are often seen as the primary, if not sole, caregiver of children. Young fathers, particularly minority fathers, have limited access to, if not complete exclusion from, social systems supports. As a result, a system-wide focus on young mothers overshadows the needs of young fathers and their positive contributions to their children and partners. When fathers are mentioned in the context of understanding their parenting needs, the benefits of building their parenting skills are discussed in the context of improving the lives of mothers and children. Focusing on the unique parenting needs of adolescent fathers can help to lend legitimacy to their role personally, with the mother of their child, their extended family systems, their community, and their broader social systems. It also recognizes the social prescription that such acknowledgment can lend to cementing the "father" identity for these young men and those in their community and beyond.

Adolescent fathers have parent education needs that are not entirely addressed in parenting programs, which often focus on mothers. Young fathers, in particular, need tailored programs that address their unique life position. Most young fathers are simultaneously transitioning into adulthood while also navigating their new role as a parent. Given the varying risks identified as young fathers matriculate into their roles as adults, there is a need for supports that minimize those risks while simultaneously helping these young fathers increase their skills (Paschal et al. 2011). Without proper supports, the cumulative effects of these major life changes can have adverse consequences for young fathers' physical and mental health as well as for their family lives.

Impact on the Transition to Adulthood

Studies show that adolescent fathers' self-confidence and feelings of self-efficacy often overlap with their perceptions of themselves as fathers. Roy and Dyson (2010) noted that despite their experience of past adversity, young fathers aspire to be self-sufficient, in control of their lives, and capable of setting goals for themselves, regardless of whether they have the resources or means to fulfill their goals. Additional studies demonstrate that when fathers feel confident and empowered in their role as men and as fathers, they become more engaged with their children, take on more parenting responsibilities, develop stronger bonds with the children, and prioritize having better relationships with their children's mothers. By helping fathers bridge the gap to adulthood, social systems can help them learn important life skills (e.g., interpersonal communication, planning and goal setting, financial literacy) that they might not otherwise learn (Kiselica and Kiselica 2014a, 2014b). These skills are exceptionally useful for adolescent fathers who are in the child welfare, juvenile justice, or criminal systems, because young fathers in these circumstances have limited contact with their children and fewer resources.

Another positive aspect of young fatherhood is that it can have a stabilizing effect on at-risk fathers (Carlson 2016). Qualitative and quantitative studies on the trajectories of delinquent, criminally involved, and incarcerated adolescent males have documented fatherhood to be a critical turning point in the lives of these adolescent fathers. In several studies, impending fatherhood led many to change their lives and behaviors for the better, so that they could be involved in raising their children (Roy and Dyson 2010; Wilkinson et al. 2013). A few of these studies indicated that while fathers were steadfast in their will to make these necessary life changes, some fathers expressed concern that they would not be able to sustain their new lifestyles, particularly those fathers whose life changes included abstaining from drugs and alcohol. In order to become more effective adults and parents, adolescent fathers need social systems support that will help them address, process, and better manage the complexities of their stressful life events (Lewin et al. 2015). This would help them improve and maintain their physical and mental health while providing them with the tools and skills to become responsible adults and effective parents.

Impact on the Young Children

Similar to adult fathers, adolescent fathers want to be involved and engaged in the upbringing of their children (Paschal et al. 2011). Contrary to popular views about adolescent fathers, findings from some studies (Lau Clayton 2016; Paschal et al. 2011) have highlighted minority fathers' commitment to becoming and remaining involved in their children's lives. Several of these qualitative studies have identified fathers' desire to be "good fathers" and to "be there," meaning emotionally and physically available, for their children as key themes within their study populations (Paschal et al. 2011; Roy and Dyson 2010; Wilkes et al. 2012).

Fathers are important for children, and they are willing to invest their time, support, and limited resources to ensure their children's well-being. Father involvement has been shown to be positively associated with children's health and development across the lifespan. A recent American Academy of Pediatrics report showed that when fathers are involved postpartum, mothers are more likely to initiate breastfeeding earlier and continue it longer than when fathers are not involved (Yogman et al. 2016). Fathers tend to engage in play and caregiving activities differently from mothers, which has positive benefits for children's cognitive, social, and emotional development and school readiness. Early father involvement has been linked to more secure parent-child attachments, higher IQs, and better language development compared to when fathers are absent. For adolescent children, positive father involvement is associated with reduced delinquency and risky behaviors such as substance use, illegal activities, and the onset of sexual activity. These findings are relevant to understanding the impact of nonresidential father involvement on children and adolescent health and behavior.

Fathers also have an important role in sex-role modeling for male and female children. Fathers provide the blueprint for their children's masculine ideals by setting an example for what a man should be. It is important that fathers, particularly young fathers, model positive parenting for their children.

Impact on the Partners of the Young Men

The positive effects of father involvement are not limited to adolescent fathers. Lewin et al. (2015) pointed out in their study on father involvement that their results often did not distinguish between the effects of adolescent fathers and adult fathers and instead grouped data from younger fathers with older fathers (Lewin et al. 2015). However, there are several studies on the impact of adolescent father involvement on adolescent mother outcomes. These studies mainly focus on the benefits of adolescent father involvement for maternal birth outcomes, noting that the role of adolescent fathers during pregnancy is underappreciated (Lewin et al. 2015).

Adolescent fathers provide mothers with multiple forms of social support that have positive implications for maternal health. Adolescent mothers are at a higher risk of experiencing poor birth outcomes, including infant mortality, stillbirths, and birth defects, compared with adult mothers (Alio et al. 2011). For black mothers, the risk of having an adverse birth outcome is much higher than for white mothers. In fact, the infant mortality rate among black mothers is more than twice that of white mothers (Alio et al. 2011). However, fathers' prenatal involvement has been shown to have a protective effect and is associated with better birth outcomes. Additionally, adolescent mothers are at a higher risk of maternal depression, which has been linked to negative consequences for children and adolescents (Lewin et al. 2015). When fathers are involved with their children, not only do adolescent mothers experience lower rates of depressive symptoms, but their children are less affected by their mothers' depression (Lewin et al. 2015).

Adolescent fathers can also be an important source of financial support for adolescent mothers. In the United States, almost half of all children live in poverty or near-poverty, and many of these children live in single-female–headed households (American Academy of Pediatrics Council on Community Pediatrics 2016). Adolescent fathers' financial contributions, though potentially limited, can help offset the cost of living and childrearing for single adolescent mothers and increase the household income for married and cohabiting adolescent mothers (Kiselica and Kiselica 2014a, 2014b). Furthermore, adolescent fathers contribute in-kind support of noncash goods such as food, clothes, and toys. They also can help fix items inside and outside the child's home. Kane et al. (2015) conducted semistructured interviews of 400 low-income nonresidential fathers and found that noncash support made up 25% of children's total support and that children received approximately $60 per month in in-kind goods. The authors also found that a larger proportion of in-kind support came from black fathers and fathers who were underemployed. The authors noted that nonresidential fathers in their study reported that they provided in-kind support to facilitate opportunities to connect with and build bonds with their children and not to compensate for their financial limitations (Kane et al. 2015).

Unfortunately, the nonfinancial ways in which nonresidential minority fathers contribute to the betterment of their children are mitigated based on social systems' overemphasis on fathers' cash support. For many adolescent fathers, spending quality time with their children and being involved in caregiving activities are very meaningful to them. Given the numerous pathways (e.g., social, educational, and psychological) by which fathers can positively influence children's health and development, early father-child interactions may be equally as important to children's overall well-being as financial child support is touted to be, when it was identified as a mechanism for getting at-risk children out of poverty. Social systems should seize the opportunity to invest in adolescent minority fathers by engaging them in services that will help them to be successful adults and responsible parents.

Conclusion

While the national rates of adolescent paternity have consistently declined, there continue to be pockets of significant intransigence: minority individuals (especially black and Latino/Hispanic young men) and those involved in the child welfare and juvenile justice systems. Young minority men are a vulnerable group who experience disparate "system contact." These systems have limited information, interest, and services to support young minority fathers. Early paternity is a marker of risk for physical, mental health, substance use, delinquency, and education outcomes. Fathering may include motivation to learn new skills in preparation for the role, and these skills can position their children for future success.

In this chapter, we identified the potential risks and resources of young minority men who are adolescent fathers and the opportunities for systems to initiate efforts to meet the needs of this vulnerable group. These systems need to attend to the unique developmental, social, and service needs of adolescent fathers as they negotiate their way through these systems. This negotiation begins with attention to and identification of the numbers of young men in their care who are fathers and the resource and risk needs they present. Furthermore, attention to and programming specifically focused on the "identified" risks associated with adolescent paternity should be integrated into any system response to address the unique needs of this vulnerable group. The focus should also include attention and enhancement of the resources and strengths present. Key areas include family, education/vocation, delinquency, substance use, and mental/psychological and physical health. In discussing these areas, we hope to draw attention to the positive effects that intervention can have for the adolescent father, the mother of his child, his child, and the community that they become.

References

Alio AP, Mbah AK, Grunsten RA, et al: Teenage pregnancy and the influence of paternal involvement on fetal outcomes. J Pediatr Adolesc Gynecol 24(6):404–409, 2011 22099734

American Academy of Pediatrics Council on Community Pediatrics: Poverty and child health in the United States. Pediatrics 137(4):55–71, 2016 26962238

Berger LM, Langton C: Young disadvantaged men as fathers. Ann Am Acad Pol Soc Sci 635(1):56–75, 2011 21643452

Carlson DL: Challenges and transformations: childbearing and changes in teens' educational aspirations and expectations. J Youth Stud 19(5):705–724, 2016

Dariotis JK, Pleck JH, Astone NM, et al: Pathways of early fatherhood, marriage, and employment a latent class growth analysis: Demography 48(2):593–623, 2011

Garfield CF, Duncan G, Gutina A, et al: Longitudinal study of body mass index in young males and the transition to fatherhood. Am J Mens Health 10(6):NP158–NP167, 2016 26198724

Gordon DM, Watkins ND, Walling SM, et al: Adolescent fathers involved with child protection: social workers speak. Child Welfare 90(5):95–114, 2011 22533056

Kane JB, Nelson T, Edin K: How much in-kind support do low-income nonresident fathers provide? A mixed-method analysis. J Marriage Fam 77(3):591–611, 2015 26052162

Kiselica AM, Kiselica MS: Improving attitudes, services, and policies regarding adolescent fathers: an affirming rejoinder. Psychol Men Masc 15(3):284–287, 2014a

Kiselica MS, Kiselica AM: The complicated worlds of adolescent fathers: implications for clinical practice, public policy, and research. Psychol Men Masc 15(3):260–274, 2014b

Lau Clayton C: The lives of young fathers: a review of selected evidence. Soc Policy Soc 15(1):129–140, 2016 26740798

Lewin A, Mitchell SJ, Waters D, et al: The protective effects of father involvement for infants of teen mothers with depressive symptoms. Matern Child Health J 19(5):1016–1023, 2015 25102809

Marcell AV, Wibbelsman MC, Seigel WM; Committee on Adolescence: Male adolescent sexual and reproductive health care. Pediatrics Nov 28, 2011; peds.2011-2384; doi: 10.1542/peds.2011-2384

Paschal AM, Lewis-Moss RK, Hsiao T: Perceived fatherhood roles and parenting behaviors among African American teen fathers. J Adolesc Res 26(1):61–83, 2011

Roy KM, Dyson O: Making daddies into fathers: community-based fatherhood programs and the construction of masculinities for low-income African American men. Am J Community Psychol 45(1–2):139–154, 2010 20077133

Sipsma H, Biello KB, Cole-Lewis H, et al: Like father, like son: the intergenerational cycle of adolescent fatherhood. Am J Public Health 100(3):517–524, 2010 20075312

Smeeding TM, Garfinkel I, Mincy RB: Young disadvantaged men: fathers, families, poverty, and policy. Ann Am Acad Pol Soc Sci 635(1):6–21, 2011

Weinman ML, Smith PB, Buzi RS: Young fathers: an analysis of rick behaviors and service needs. Child and Adolescent Social Work Journal 19(6):437–453, 2002

Wilkes L, Mannix J, Jackson D: 'I am going to be a dad': experiences and expectations of adolescent and young adult expectant fathers. J Clin Nurs 21(1–2):180–188, 2012 21645156

Wilkinson DL, Khurana A, Magora A: Intergenerational transmission of fathering among crime-involved urban African American and Latino young men. Spectrum: A Journal on Black Men 2(1):19–45, 2013

Yogman M, Garfield CF; Committee on Psychosocial Aspects of Child and Family Health: Fathers' roles in the care and development of their children: the role of pediatricians. Pediatrics 138(1):e1–e15, 2016 27296867

CHAPTER 12
BLACK ELDERS OF THE TWENTY-FIRST CENTURY

F. M. Baker, M.D., DLFAPA

THE BLACK ELDERLY in 2050 will contain the "baby boomer" birth cohorts (i.e., persons born between 1946 and 1964). The U.S. population will contain a higher percentage of persons age 65 and older, and these elders will be more ethnically diverse than in prior generations (Ortman et al. 2014). Persons age 65 and older will compose 20% of the U.S. population by 2050.

In 2012, some 20.7% of persons age 65 and older were ethnic minorities. This percentage will increase to 39.1% in 2050. In 2050 persons age 85 and older will account for 4.5% of the U.S. population, an increase from 2.5% in 2030. In 2050, some 29.7% of persons age 85 and older will be members of minority groups, compared with 16.3% in 2012. Thus, by 2050, the U.S. population will contain a larger percentage of persons age 65 and older, and these elders will be more culturally and racially diverse (Ortman et al. 2014).

Population projections suggest that in 2050 some 42% of black elders will live in the southern United States. In the 2010 census, 55% of persons who reported their race as black lived in the South, 18% in the Midwest, 17% in the Northeast, and 10% in the West. Some urban-resident black elders decide to "move home" to their parents' home where they grew up in the southern United States, but these elders are moving to southern urban centers, not to rural communities. The move is based on a wish for a slower pace of life, less urban crime, and an opportunity to reconnect with family members.

Black Life Cycle

Neugarten (1979) wrote about the transition and changes characteristic of a given period in the life cycle and noted that they may occur at a different pace for each person. Carter and McGoldrick (1980) described the family life cycle and the joys, tensions, and conflicts that occur as the family moves from its original dyad to a system with one or more children and returns, eventually, to the original dyad—the family life cycle. Levinson (1978) looked in detail at the life of four white, mainly middle-class men and suggested that there are specific tasks that are accomplished at different times in the life cycle. Baker (1987) applied the life cycle concept and the family life cycle concept to black elders of the 1980s.

Historical Events Affecting the Psychosocial Development of Twenty-First-Century Black Elders

Rosow (1978) expanded the cohort concept beyond persons born in a specific year or period who then aged together, to refer to "people about the same age who in a given period have similar experiences that may affect them in the same way." When we are attempting to understand how the black elderly of 2050 will become who they are as elders, it is important to look at their historical and social experiences through their life course that influence the development of their self-image, expectation of society and themselves, and development of coping strategies through their life course.

Childhood

Persons who will be age 65 in 2020 were born in 1955, 1 year after the *Brown v. Board of Education* decision by the U.S. Supreme Court (Tuttle 1999) that overturned the "separate but equal" doctrine. Growing up, these black elders experienced legalized segregation, with separate bathroom facilities, drinking fountains, and schools. If blacks were allowed to patronize a specific store or restaurant, they may have had to access a separate entrance or been required to order food from the back door because the restaurant only seated whites. With the *Brown v. Board of Education* decision, the ending of legalized school segregation was gradually implemented across the nation. Although the U.S. Supreme Court decision was announced in 1954, in many communities, schools were not desegregated until the 1970s. The twenty-first-century black elder would have been a teenager or in his or her 20s before attending school with whites in many communities. In 1967 interracial marriage was legalized by the U.S. Supreme Court decision in the case of *Loving v. Virginia* (Newman 1999), making it legal for blacks and whites to marry and have legitimate sexual relationships.

In December 1955, Ms. Rosa Parks was tired from work and unwilling to give up her bus seat to a white man. For refusing to give up her seat, Ms. Parks was sent to jail, triggering the Montgomery Bus Boycott. Following the decision to continue the initial boycott, the Montgomery Improvement Association was formed, with the Rev. Dr. Martin Luther King Jr. elected as its president. The 13-month mass protest ended with a U.S. Supreme Court decision that segregation on public buses was unconstitutional. The period from 1954 to 1968 is defined as the Civil Rights Movement, led by Dr. King and a number of young black ministers. The Civil Rights Movement focused on ending racial segregation and discrimination against black people and was fought by nonviolent means to secure legal recognition and federal protection of the citizenship rights enumerated in the U.S. Constitution and federal law (Sullivan 1999).

Adolescence and Youth: The First Life Structure

In their 20s, twenty-first-century black elders had the opportunity for the first time of entering colleges that were historically for "whites only." Federal funding was made available through various grants to increase the enrollment of blacks in colleges and professional schools (including medicine and law), resulting in increased opportunities for higher education. The Civil Rights Movement was characterized by acts of nonviolent protest, including sit-ins in segregated lunch counters to open service to blacks as well as marches for voting rights. As a college student, the black elder may have participated in various protests, including the March on Washington in August 1963 where the Rev. Dr. King delivered his famous "I Have a Dream" speech. As a youth, the twenty-first-century black elder was influenced by and became active in a movement demanding equal rights for blacks in the United States and developed a pride from asserting his or her rights as defined by the U.S. Constitution.

Over a period of years, the fabric of American society and the rule of law were called into question. President John F. Kennedy was assassinated in November 1963; Malcolm X was assassinated in February 1965; the Rev. Dr. Martin Luther King Jr. was assassinated in April 1968; and the former attorney general and presidential candidate Robert F. Kennedy was assassinated in June 1968. White leaders who were sympathetic to the goals of the Civil Rights Movement and provided federal support for protestors were killed as well as black leaders who emphasized black pride and excellence through nonviolent action. Anger and frustration in black urban communities erupted in rioting.

Between 1966 and 1975 the Black Power movement emerged. Young black men and women challenged the established black leadership. The leaders of the Black Power movement (Stokely Carmichael and Willie Ricks of the Student Nonviolent Coordinating Committee; Huey Newton and Bobby Seale of the

Black Panther Party) rejected the cooperative attitude toward federal and local governments by the traditional black leaders of the Civil Rights Movement and complained that progress was too slow. The Black Power movement demanded political and economic self-sufficiency for black communities, now.

Although the Rev. Dr. Martin Luther King Jr. won the Nobel Peace Prize in 1964 for his emphasis on nonviolent social change, leaders of the Black Power movement emphasized action and confrontation to achieve improvements for blacks in American society. The Black Power movement was influenced by Malcolm X, who was initially a Black Muslim who advocated separation of black and white persons (Kelly 1999). Studying the Muslim faith, traveling internationally, and making a pilgrimage to Mecca, Malcolm X returned changed by these experiences; he had become alienated from the Black Muslim movement at the time of his death and was developing an international perspective. The twenty-first-century elders began to view themselves as beautiful black people whose heritage began in Africa, resulting in a preference to be described as African American.

Young Adult: An Expanded Focus

In his or her 30s, the twenty-first-century black elder may have benefited from federal funding to increase the number of blacks attending previously all-white colleges and universities and may have become the first person in his or her family to complete a college degree and go on to graduate school. Beginning with their first professional position, black elders of the twenty-first century saw some of their former teenage neighbors caught up in an alternative lifestyle of addiction to heroin or cocaine. Some of their former neighbors were dead from suicide or black-on-black homicide (Griffith and Bell 1989).

Middle Years: Settling Down

By the 1990s the twenty-first-century black elder, now in his or her fourth decade of life, had settled into a career, had probably married, and had a family. Plans for retirement, a new home purchase, and college education for his or her children were made for the future. Medical problems were stable, with employment-related health insurance facilitating payment for doctor visits and medications.

The twenty-first-century black elder may have had to address an unanticipated pregnancy in a child and accept the responsibility of rearing a grandchild while in their 50s. If a child developed a chronic mental illness—for example, schizophrenia—the black elder may have had to provide financial as well as social support for the loved one. At a time of becoming a mentor to younger generations, some twenty-first-century black elders may have found themselves involved in the role of family caregiver. In 2009, at age 54, the twenty-first-century black elder would have seen the election of the first U.S. president of African origin, Barack H. Obama. Going back to the activism of their 20s, the black elder may have been active in the Obama campaign and hoped again for increased societal change. The economic recession of 2007–2009, the most severe since the Great Depression of the 1930s, may have caused the black elder significant concern as his or her retirement savings "disappeared" with lower earnings from the stock market, declining home values, and, in some cases, extensive job losses placing him or her among the unemployed. Plans for retirement and funding college education for children had to be reworked. Concerned about maintaining employment, job stability, and earnings, the black elder may have put on hold seeking a new position with more responsibility and increased income until the economic downturn had resolved.

Late Adult Life: The Elder

The twenty-first-century elder will be age 65 in 2020. Anticipating retirement, the elder may find the impact of medical problems becoming an increasing concern. The black elder may delay retirement because he or she is the caregiver for grandchildren whose parents are addicted or the caregiver for a chronically mentally ill adult child. Facing multiple health problems (see section "Health Concerns of Black Elders" later in this chapter), the twenty-first-century black elder may return to church to seek psychological, spiritual, and social support. The friendship network built through the years is narrowing because of death of friends, particularly of older black male friends, due to multiple medical problems.

In contrast to the black elder of the 1960s, who had limited resources and may have had only Social Security and a small pension from his or her work history, the twenty-first-century black elder may have financial resources beyond Social Security, such as health insurance, a pension or retirement package from work, and a paid mortgage.

Rural Black Elders

Parks (1988) completed detailed interviews with 555 rural elderly black residents in Arkansas, Tennessee, and Mississippi. Among all respondents combined, some 34.8% had 0–4 years of education, 49.1% had completed high school, 10.4% had post–high school or vocational education, 3.9% had 1–3 years of college education, and only 1.8% had postgraduate college education. In this sample, 52.2% described themselves as widowed. Some 3.4% of respondents reported being single/never married and 5.2% described themselves as separated. Fifty-four percent of these rural black elders reported living alone, and 33.3% of the sample reported living with one other person. Only 2.2% of respondents lived with four other persons. Only 349 persons responded to the question of home ownership, and 53.9% (275 of 510) reported that they owned their home outright. Some 64.6% of the sample were retired, and 11.8% were retired on disability. Some 4.2% were employed full-time, and 6.4% were employed part-time. Among the total number of black elders interviewed, 59.2% reported using food stamps to help with meal costs, and 25.4% had had help from an agency or program, with 10.2% having received help from family or friends. Some 55.3% of rural black elders had been receiving food stamps for more than 5 years. Some 18.9% of respondents had seen a doctor at least once in the past 6 months. Arkansans (25.4%) had seen their doctor two or more times in the past 6 months, in contrast to Mississippians, of whom 31.0% had not visited their physician, and 24.0% reported visiting their doctor only once, in the past 6 months (Parks 1988, p. 154). Among rural elderly black residents in Arkansas, some 66.5% said there was not a doctor in their community. Mississippi respondents reported that 34.1% did not have a doctor in their community. In Tennessee, rural elderly black respondents reported that 41.3% did not have a doctor in their community. When religious activity was addressed, two-thirds of rural black elders reported attending church every week, and 51.1% of rural black males indicated that they went to church every week. More than 50% of rural black elders were as active or more active in church than 10 years ago. Some 66.7% of rural black elders had lived all their lives in Tennessee, compared with 26.1% of rural black elders living all their lives in Mississippi. Only 7.2% of rural black elders had spent their entire lives in Arkansas (Parks 1988). The author found that transportation was a major concern for rural black elders, housing was poor, and access to physicians was limited.

Parks's work is one of the few studies that provide information on rural black elders demonstrating that many had less than a high school education and were likely to live alone, to have transportation issues, to have no physician in their community, and to need help with meal costs. These rural black elders remained very involved in their churches and were regular weekly attendees at services. Attempting to screen rural black elders for cognitive impairment and depressive illness will require attention to the data from Parks's study. Selecting the Short Portable Mental Status Questionnaire (SPMSQ) to screen for cognitive impairment (Pfeiffer 1975) and the Center for Epidemiologic Studies–Depression Scale (CES-D) to screen for depression (Baker et al. 1995) would be appropriate. Working with local pastors to set up screenings after Sunday services would facilitate rural black elders' participation, because additional travel would not be required and screening would be sanctioned by their pastor.

Health Concerns of Black Elders

Black elders have had to deal with health issues throughout their lives. The high rates of hypertension among black people beginning in their 20s may be a combination of genetic predisposition, environmental factors, and society pressures from the daily, thousand cuts of microaggressions. The John Henry attitude among some blacks—persevering to accomplish an "impossible" task—may also be a contributory factor.

Poussaint and Alexander (2000) have studied the impact of racial stereotyping resulting in characterization of blacks as happy-go-lucky and less likely to become depressed. These authors pointed out how psychiatric diagnoses were influenced by racial stereotyping, resulting in the misdiagnosis of black patients and their exclusion from mental health facilities, particularly in the southern United States. Although access to healthcare has improved for more blacks today, with employment giving them health insurance coverage and the legislative ending of segregation, not all blacks have access to healthcare and medications, and this is particularly true of rural black residents (Parks 1988) and poor urban residents (Poussaint and Alexander 2000). Poorly treated hypertension over years affects the cardiovascular system and contributes to the impairment of renal function (Bakris 2004).

Diabetes

The rates of obesity among blacks are of concern because of the increased risk for the development of type 2 diabetes. The increased rates of type 2 diabetes in the U.S. population, and particularly among children, have become a public health issue. The combination of hypertension and diabetes increases the risk for the development of end-stage renal disease, which can lead to the need for hemodialysis or renal transplantation (Alebiosu et al. 2003; Bakris 2004).

Leading Causes of Death

The leading causes of death for blacks are heart disease, cancer, stroke, diabetes, and pneumonia or influenza (Sahyoun et al. 2001). Coronary heart disease and stroke account for 24% of excess mortality among black men and 41% of excess mortality among black women. *Excess mortality* refers to the difference in mortality that is observed when comparing blacks and whites. It is defined as the difference between the number of deaths observed in a minority population and the number of deaths that would have occurred in that group if both minority and nonminority groups had the same age- and sex-specific death rates. If one uses the mortality rate observed in whites to calculate mortality in blacks, one finds a predicted death rate. When that mortality rate is compared with the observed black mortality rate, excess deaths are found beyond the predicted mortality rates. The excess mortality among blacks with cancer is attributed to later diagnosis of disease, limited access to treatment, and limited insurance/monies to cover the cost of care. The death rate for all cancers is 30% higher for blacks compared with whites. Although the twenty-first-century cohort of black elders has higher educational attainment and better employment with health benefits compared with earlier generations of black elders, the rates of chronic diseases remain a serious public health concern (Geruso 2012).

Literature from the 1990s documented the increased risk for the development of depression among black elders with multiple medical problems (Bazargan and Hamm-Baugh 1995). It has been established for more than 30 years that persons who experience a left central stroke have a 67% risk of developing a major depressive disorder (Robinson et al. 1984). Recent studies have demonstrated that early treatment of depression improves recovery from stroke (Robinson and Jorge 2016).

Mental Health Concerns of Black Elders

In the preceding sections we have looked at the social and psychological factors affecting black elders during their life course, as well as their physical health concerns. Mental health issues do not occur in a vacuum, so it is important to establish the reality of life for the black elderly.

The presence of chronic medical problems such as hypertension and diabetes increases the risks for cardiovascular disease and impairment of renal function (Bakris 2004). Since the 1990s research has shown that chronic medical problems increase the risk for the development of depressive illness (Bazargan and Hamm-Baugh 1995). As noted earlier, individuals who have had a left central stroke have a 67% increased risk of developing a major depressive disorder (Robinson and Jorge 2016).

Depression

In a study of 1,022 black urban-resident elders, depression was greatest among elderly black persons who reported kidney, vision, and/or circulatory problems (Bazargan and Hamm-Baugh 1995). Among these New Orleans, Louisiana, black elders, factors associated with depression included financial difficulties, more stressful life events, lower self-perceptions, less support from friends, and less instrumental support (Bazargan and Hamm-Baugh 1995).

Cognitive Impairment

Black elders are more at risk for cognitive impairment from multiple causes, including multiple medical problems, the prescription of multiple medications, and psychosocial stressors involving finances and family concerns. Because of a long history of hypertension beginning in their 20s, black elders in their 60s and older are at increased risk to develop vascular dementia (Heyman et al. 1991). As they age, black elders enter cohorts that are at an increased risk of developing a major neurocognitive disorder of the Alzheimer's type (Heyman et al. 1991). Thus, black elders are at an increased risk of having more than one type of dementing illness as they age.

Older black Americans may attempt to save the cost of an office visit and the prescribed 1 month of medication by accepting "a few pills" from a friend or neighbor who has the same symptoms as the elder. Unfortunately, this new medication may trigger a drug-drug interaction with one or more of the multiple medications that the black elder takes daily. The new onset of "dementia" within a few days should be a flag for the elder's family that something has changed and that a thorough evaluation is indicated. If the black elder is getting his or her medication from more than one pharmacy, there is not one pharmacist monitoring the elder's multiple prescriptions, increasing the risk for undetected drug-drug interactions.

Another factor affecting the cognitive function of older black Americans is the possible history of alcohol use. If the black elder drank heavily and regularly in his or her third, fourth, and fifth decades of life, the black elder is at an increased risk for an alcohol-related neurocognitive disorder. The relationship between alcohol dependence and the development of depression has also been established. Recent research conducted by Yale University and the University of Pennsylvania found a genetic link for the comorbidity of alcohol dependence and depression in the 4,653 black participants and no association among the 3,169 white participants (Zhou et al. 2017). The identified genetic locus was rs139438618 of the semaphorin 3A gene (*SEMA3A* [OMIM603961]). Future research may lead to medications created specifically for persons with this genotype to address their risk for both alcohol dependence and depression.

Chronic Mental Illness

Black elders with chronic mental illness (diagnoses of schizophrenia or bipolar disorder made during their 20s or 30s) can reach their sixth decade of life. Psychosocial rehabilitation programs help these persons with chronic mental illness to stay in treatment and to get and to take their prescribed medications for physical and mental illnesses; they also provide a psychosocial structure that facilitates their growth and development (Bachrach 1992). These psychosocial rehabilitation programs are crucial for chronically mentally ill black elders, for their survival as well as for their quality of life.

In 2018 the U.S. Congress intends to draft legislation that will make changes in the Affordable Care Act. Changes in the tax codes are also being discussed. Depending on the changes made, the funding from Medicaid that supports elderly residents in nursing homes, as well as funding for the psychosocial rehabilitation programs serving the chronically mentally ill, may be decreased or cut. Management of these elders without these funding sources would have a significant impact on already stressed community mental health centers, community-based clinics, local hospitals, and the families of these elders. If this does occur, the mental health and health care systems may become further strained as these black elderly persons seek needed physical and mental healthcare.

Substance Abuse Epidemic

Another factor affecting the mental health of older black Americans is the substance abuse epidemic. Some older black Americans have become the caregivers of grandchildren and great-grandchildren because the parents of these children are addicted to heroin or cocaine and are no longer able to care for the children. Older black Americans may become caregivers for young children at a time in their lives when they expected to be getting visits from their grandchildren, not to be raising them. Children are very important to black elders, who will sacrifice to help their younger family members. Using data from the National Survey of Families and Households, Fuller-Thomson et al. (1997) found that women, recently bereaved parents, and African Americans were twice as likely to become caregiving grandparents.

In a study of grandmothers caring for grandchildren whose parents were crack cocaine addicts (Minkler et al. 1992), the authors found that the grandparents tended to minimize their own health problems and symptoms. Thus, friends and the healthcare team of a black elder will need to monitor the elder closely for a decline in his or her baseline health and function. The elder may exhibit increasing confusion from fatigue and sleep deprivation. Dealing with the additional stresses of being a caregiver, the black elder is at increased risk to experience a decline in his or her physical health and is at risk to develop symptoms of depression.

Suicide

Higher rates of suicide were observed among black youth ages 25–29 for the period from 1981 to 2002, with a rate of 41.05 per 100,000. The age-specific suicide rate for black women age 65 and older was 4.5 per 100,000 following a lower suicide rate across the life cycle. The age-specific rates for older black men were lower at age 65 (25 per 100,000) and increased with age. For ages 70–74, a rate of 30 per 100,000 was noted, and for ages 80–84, a rate of 33 per 100,000 was observed. Thus, for black men there was a bimodal distribution, with the observed rates of suicide increasing in youth (ages 25–29) and in old age (ages 65–84) (Joe 2006). Risks factors identified for suicide among blacks include mental disorders, substance abuse, poor social support, family dysfunction, and access to firearms. Using an age-period-cohort analysis, Joe (2006) found that the age-adjusted suicide mortality rates increased for males from 1981 to 1989, remained flat from 1990 to 1993, and then declined sharply. Among black females, the trends rose from 1983 and 1988 and began to decline in 1989, reaching an all-time low in 2002. The author suggested that the peak rate of suicide among younger blacks in the early 1990s followed by a decline reflected the height of deindustrialization, a period effect.

One must recognize that among the black elderly of 2050 will be men who have spent their youth through middle years incarcerated and are attempting to build their first life structure as an elder. More likely single, with limitations on employment because of their incarceration, these elders will face financial pressures and housing concerns with minimal social supports because members of their family of origin may have died due to multiple medical problems or community violence. These elders are at increased risk for depression. Involvement in church or the Nation of Islam may provide the resources and social support that these elders need to prevent a downward spiral into substance abuse and suicidal behavior. Further research is needed to better understand factors contributing to the higher rates of suicide among older black men.

Faith: A Psychosocial Mediator

The role of faith as an important mediator of psychosocial stresses for black elders needs to be recognized. Younger cohorts of black persons are less involved in formal religion, and the congregations of established churches—for example, Baptists, Methodists, and Presbyterians—are aging (Gentzler 2008). Black elders may participate in Bible study groups and may be members of a prayer chain. These groups aid the black elderly in deepening their understanding of scripture as well as provide a social support network for these elders. The black church can be a financial aid for the black elderly as well. Pastoral counseling can be an important resource for the black elders attempting to balance the care of grandchildren or a mentally ill adult child and keeping themselves physically and mentally well.

Conclusion

The black elderly of 2050 will make up a larger proportion of the U.S. population age 65 and older and will be better educated, with a broader range of employment options compared to prior cohorts of black elders. Entering their late adult years with multiple medical problems, urban-resident black elders are at risk of developing depression related to multiple chronic medical problems and/or related to the stresses of becoming caregivers for an adult child with chronic mental illness (e.g., schizophrenia) or addiction, as well as of becoming the caregiver for their grandchildren. The black elder is also at risk for cognitive

impairment due to a stroke or earlier alcohol use or undetected drug-drug interactions, as well as, with age, an increased risk of developing a major neurocognitive disorder due to Alzheimer's disease.

Coping strategies developed during their young adult years as activists in the
Civil Rights Movement and the Black Power movement can facilitate these elders' adjustment to the changing daily schedule with retirement from work and
living on a fixed retirement income. Strategies used to adjust because of the economic downturn of the 2006–2009 period were used by these elders, again, to
stretch their income in their eighth decade of life. Screenings for the presence of
cognitive impairment and depression should be done in their doctor's office and/or
through a church-based health fair.

Rural-resident black elders will have fewer resources with limited access to
physicians who live in their communities, limited transportation options, and
poorer quality of housing. The strong faith of rural-resident elders provides them
with the support of their church family, who may serve as an "extended family"
for the rural elder with multiple medical problems. With limited medical care,
the early diagnosis of mental disorders (depression, dementia, delirium, drug-
related psychotic disorder) is less likely to happen, resulting in hospitalization.
Lower educational level will require the use of appropriate screening instruments for cognitive impairment (i.e., SPMSQ) and depression (i.e., CES-D).
If the U.S. Congress acts to change the Affordable Care Act, the resulting legislation may further limit the resources available to these rural black elders.

Utilizing appropriate screening instruments, initiating public health initiatives such as screening clinics at the local church after Sunday services, and establishing joint initiatives between churches and local health departments can
facilitate the early identification and treatment of mental disorders among the
rural black elderly of 2050. The development of creative mental health resources
within the psychosocial spheres of these elders would be the most effective intervention to facilitate the health and mental health of the black elders of 2050.

References

Alebiosu CO, Odusan O, Jaiyesimi A: Morbidity in relation to stage of diabetic nephropa-
     thy in type-2 diabetic patients. J Natl Med Assoc 95(11):1042–1047, 2003 14651370
Bachrach LL: Psychosocial rehabilitation and psychiatry in the care of long-term pa-
     tients. Am J Psychiatry 149(11):1455–1463, 1992 1415813
Baker FM: The Afro-American life cycle: success, failure, and mental health. J Natl
     Med Assoc 79(6):625–633, 1987 3302279
Baker FM, Velli SA, Friedman J, et al: Screening tests for depression in older black vs.
     white patients. Am J Geriatr Psychiatry 3(1):43–51, 1995 28530957
Bakris GL: The importance of blood pressure control in the patient with diabetes. Am
     J Med 116 (suppl 5A):30S–38S, 2004 15019861

Bazargan M, Hamm-Baugh VP: The relationship between chronic illness and depression in a community of urban black elderly persons. J Gerontol B Psychol Sci Soc Sci 50(2):S119–S127, 1995 7757840

Carter EA, McGoldrick M: The Family Life Cycle: A Framework for Family Therapy. New York, Gardner Press, 1980

Fuller-Thomson E, Minkler M, Driver D: A profile of grandparents raising grandchildren in the United States. Gerontologist 37(3):406–411, 1997 9203764

Gentzler RH: Aging and Ministry in the 21st Century: An Inquiry Approach. Nashville, TN, Discipleship Resources Distribution Center, 2008

Geruso M: Black-white disparities in life expectancy: how much can the standard SES variables explain? Demography 49(2):553–574, 2012 22287272

Griffith EE, Bell CC: Recent trends in suicide and homicide among blacks. JAMA 262(16):2265–2269, 1989 2677427

Heyman A, Fillenbaum G, Prosnitz B, et al: Estimated prevalence of dementia among elderly black and white community residents. Arch Neurol 48(6):594–598, 1991 2039381

Joe S: Explaining changes in the patterns of black suicide in the United States from 1981 to 2002: an age, cohort, and period analysis. J Black Psychol 32(3):262–284, 2006 19759855

Kelly R: Malcolm X, in Africana: The Encyclopedia of the African and African American Experience. Edited by Appiah KA, Gates HL Jr. New York, Basic Civitas Books, 1999, pp 1233–1236

Levinson DJ: The Seasons of a Man's Life. New York, Knopf, 1978

Minkler M, Roe KM, Price M: The physical and emotional health of grandmothers raising grandchildren in the crack cocaine epidemic. Gerontologist 32(6):752–761, 1992 1478493

Neugarten BL: Time, age, and the life cycle. Am J Psychiatry 136:887–894, 1979

Newman R: Miscegenation, in Africana: The Encyclopedia of the African And African American Experience. Edited by Appiah KA, Gates HL Jr. New York, Basic Civitas Books, 1999, pp 1320

Ortman JM, Velkoff VA, Hogan H: An Aging Nation: The Older Population in the United States. Population Estimates and Projections. Washington, DC, U.S. Census Bureau, 2014

Parks AG: Black Elderly in Rural America. Bristol IN, Wyndham Hall Press, 1988

Pfeiffer E: A short portable mental status questionnaire for the assessment of organic brain deficit in elderly patients. J Am Geriatr Soc 23(10):433–441, 1975 1159263

Poussaint AF, Alexander A: "Boy, you must be crazy," in Lay My Burden Down: Suicide and the Mental Health Crisis Among African-Americans. Boston, MA, Beacon Press, 2000, pp 65–83

Robinson RG, Jorge RE: Post-stroke depression: a review. Am J Psychiatry 173(3):221–231, 2016 26684921

Robinson RG, Kubos KL, Starr LB, et al: Mood disorders in stroke patients: importance of location of lesion. Brain 107 (Pt 1):81–93, 1984 6697163

Rosow I: What is a cohort and why? Hum Dev 21:65–75, 1978

Sahyoun NR, Lentzner H, Hoyert D, et al: Trends in causes of death among the elderly. Aging Trends, No 1. Hyattsville, MD, National Center for Health Statistics, 2001

Sullivan P: Civil Rights Movement, in Africana: The Encyclopedia of the African and African American Experience. Edited by Appiah KA, Gates Jr. HL. New York, Basic Civitas Books, 1999, pp 446–455

Tuttle K: Brown v. Board of Education, in Africana: The Encyclopedia of the African and African American Experience. Edited by Appiah KA, Gates HL Jr. New York, Basic Civitas Books, 1999, pp 321–322

Zhou H, Polimanti R, Yang B-Z, et al: Genetic risks variants associated with comorbid alcohol dependence and major depression. JAMA Psychiatry 74(12):1234–1241, 2017 29071344

CHAPTER 13
BLACK LESBIAN, GAY, BISEXUAL, TRANSGENDER, AND QUEER IDENTITIES AND MENTAL HEALTH

Kenneth B. Ashley, M.D., FACLP, DFAPA

Lorraine E. Lothwell, M.D., FAPA

IN 2013 it was estimated that slightly more than 1 million black adults in the United States (3.7%) identified as lesbian, gay, bisexual, or transgender (LGBT); by comparison, 3.5% of the U.S. population identifies as lesbian, gay, or bisexual and 0.3% identifies as transgender (Kastanis and Gates 2013). Although there is limited literature on mental health issues in the black lesbian, gay, bisexual, transgender, and queer (LGBTQ) population, there is a growing body of scientific research. In this chapter, we cover some of the basic findings on black LGBTQ mental health.

Given the issues and complexities involved in attempting to assess individuals with multiple identities, more recent studies have used an intersectional approach to address how antiblack racism, heterosexism, antihomosexual bias and homophobia, homonegativity, misogyny, gender bias, biphobia, transphobia, social class, and privilege significantly and simultaneously affect the lived experience of black LGBTQ people.

Studies have indicated that lesbian, gay, and bisexual (LGB) individuals, overall, have a higher prevalence of anxiety, mood, and substance use disorders and suicide attempts than do heterosexuals. When prevalence was examined by race, it was found that relative to whites, black LGB individuals had lower prevalence of any anxiety, mood, or substance use disorder, or any disorder, but a higher prevalence of serious suicide attempts. Serious suicide attempts occurred at a younger age and were thought to coincide with the coming-out period. As a result, the higher rate of serious suicide attempts was related to higher social disapproval of an LGB identity (Meyer et al. 2008).

It has been recognized that black LGBTQ persons are less likely to share their sexuality with members of the black community. This has been identified as one of the ways to maintain ties to the black community, which is a source of support and appears to play a role in the development of resilience (Choi et al. 2011; Moradi et al. 2010).

One of the ongoing debates is whether, compared with other racial/ethnic groups, the black community is more biased against the LGBTQ community. The issue is as complex and as diverse as the black community. Some of the significant characteristics of the black community that play a role in the perception are faith-based traditions, community unity, black male masculinity, and gender bias. It is important to recognize that individuals are often accepting of their LGBTQ family and friends, and there is evidence of increasing acceptance and support (Hill 2013).

Findings also indicate sources of resilience in the black LGBT community that have defied the expectation of greater mental illness in the community related to the multiple minority identities based on the minority stress model (Barnes and Meyer 2012; Meyer 2003, 2010; Moradi et al. 2010). It is important that the factors involved in developing this resilience be explored further because they have a role in the development of interventions to promote improved outcomes.

Terminology

It will be useful to familiarize the reader with some of the basic terminology in the literature.

- **Sex:** A term that refers to the male or female division of a species and takes into account the sum of biological and anatomical differences (e.g., male, female, intersex).
- **Gender:** A set of characteristics, behavioral differences, and social and cultural distinctions divided into a binary between men and women. *Sex* and *gender* are not interchangeable terms.
- **Sexual orientation:** Individuals' inner feelings of who they are attracted to physically and emotionally, in relation to their own gender identity.
- **Gender identity:** Individuals' sense of their own gender: "Do I feel male, female, androgynous, or genderqueer?"

- **Gay:** Men who are primarily or exclusively attracted to other men and have, or desire to have, emotional and sexual relationships primarily or exclusively with other men.
- **Men who have sex with men (MSM):** Male persons who engage in sexual activity with members of the same sex, regardless of how they identify themselves. Many such men do not sexually identify as gay, homosexual, or bisexual.
- **Same gender loving:** A description coined by activist Cleo Manago for homosexuals and bisexuals in the African American community.
- **Lesbian:** Women who are primarily or exclusively attracted to other women and have, or desire to have, emotional and sexual relationships primarily or exclusively with other women.
- **Bisexual:** Men and women who are attracted to both men and women, although their attraction may be stronger to one particular gender. Bisexuals may have emotional and sexual relationships with any gender. Some individuals who have sex with individuals of different genders may still describe themselves as gay, lesbian, or heterosexual; may use another label altogether; or may prefer not to label themselves at all.
- **Sexual and gender minority (SGM)/Gender diverse and sexual minority:** Terms that aim at inclusion that are growing in acceptance including those who identify as lesbian, gay, bisexual, transgender, queer, or intersex.
- **Intersex:** General term used for a variety of conditions in which a person is born with or develops a reproductive or sexual anatomy that does not seem to fit the typical definitions of female or male.
- **Heterosexual:** Persons who are primarily or exclusively attracted to persons of the opposite gender and have, or desire to have, emotional and sexual relationships primarily or exclusively with persons of the opposite gender.
- **Transgender:** The term *transgender* has been defined in many different ways, and the definition is evolving. It is generally viewed as an umbrella term that comprises anyone who does not conform to traditional gender norms. This includes the following:

1. Those who identify and/or express their gender as opposite the sex they were assigned at birth.
2. Those who define their gender as outside the binary construct of exclusively male or female, including those who identify with having a fluid or changeable gender identity, those who prefer not to define themselves by any gender, those who feel their gender comprises both male and female elements, and those who feel gender cannot be restricted to just the two categories of male and female. Some people will use different labels for this, such as gender nonconforming (GNC), genderqueer, or queer.

- **Nonbinary:** See the second definition under *transgender.*
- **Cisgender:** People who identify and/or express their gender in congruence with the sex they were assigned at birth.
- **Heterosexism:** Institutionalized belief system that naturalizes and idealizes heterosexuality and dismisses or ignores LGB subjectivity (Morin and Garfinkle 1978).
- **Homonegativity:** Negative attitudes toward homosexuals.
- **Externalized homophobia (antihomosexual bias):** An irrational fear and hatred toward LGB people (Weinberg 1972).
- **Internalized homophobia:** Self-loathing that LGB people feel for themselves (Weinberg 1972).
- **Biphobia:** An irrational fear and hatred that people feel toward bisexual people.
- **Transphobia:** An irrational fear and hatred that people feel toward transgender people.

Intersectionality

Intersectionality is the theory that social identities; related systems of oppression, domination, or discrimination; and multiple group identities intersect to create a whole that is different from the component identities. Multiple aspects of identity continuously and simultaneously interact and impact an individual's experience. Data that indicate that LGB black individuals are less likely to openly identify their sexual orientation have been replicated in a number of studies (Choi et al. 2011; Moradi et al. 2010). However, black LGB individuals manage their LGBT identities utilizing social support from family and friends essentially in the same manner as whites. They reported that both their racial identity and their sexual identity are important (Meyer 2010).

Youth

The literature has consistently found that LGBT youth have elevated rates of suicidality (ideation, attempts, completed) when compared with their heterosexual peers. A study using data from the 2005 and 2007 Youth Risk Behavior Surveys confirmed these findings among sexual minority youth ages 13–18 years. As well as identifying increased feelings of sadness in these youth, the study also found disparities in mental health and suicidality based on sexes and race/ethnicity. Young women scored higher on sadness, suicidal ideation, suicide plan, and self-harm. Rates of suicide attempts were the same across sexes. Young men had increased prevalence for being treated for suicide attempts. Blacks, relative to whites, had a decreased prevalence of suicidal ideation, self-harm, and suicide plan but increased suicide attempts for male youth. Findings indicate that blacks tend to have a more negative view of suicide, which acts as a buffer against the stigma of being a sexual minority (Bostwick et al. 2014b).

Elders

LGBT elders have a host of issues to deal with: heterosexism in the aged community, ageism in the LGBT community, racism in the LGBT community, and heterosexism in the black community. The sexuality of older adults is often not discussed because of the perception that they are no longer sexual individuals. When the provider does not broach the subject, the patient typically is not given the opportunity to disclose issues of sexuality or sexual orientation, and the message is sent that discussion of the topic is not welcome. Also, as a result of heterosexism, there may be a presumption of heterosexuality based on the patient's history of heterosexual marriage and/or children. This may also decrease the likelihood of disclosure of sexual minority status.

LGBT older adults have often faced discrimination and victimization attributed to their sexual and/or gender identities. In one study (Kim et al. 2017), such discrimination (covert or overt actions that prevent LGBT individuals from social, economic, housing, and political opportunities) and victimization (intentional physical, verbal, or psychological abuse) were important predictors of poorer physical and psychological health–related quality of life. Compared with Hispanics and non-Hispanic whites, African Americans had higher rates of lifetime LGBT-related discrimination; however, African Americans did not have higher rates of lifetime LGBT-related victimization or day-to-day discrimination.

This study suggested that a positive sense of identity is an important protective factor associated with health-related quality of life that may help to support resilience and self-worth. It was also determined that the increased spiritual resources (defined as individual-level understanding of spirituality as opposed to participation in or affiliation with formal religious activity) found in the African American and Hispanic participants in the study were significantly associated with better psychological health-related quality of life (Kim et al. 2017) and, as has been shown in other studies, likely act as a protective resource.

Bisexuals

There is limited research on bisexual adults. Much of the literature does not identify bisexuals separately from gay men and lesbian women. In general, the studies that have looked at bisexuals have found that they often have worse mental health than heterosexual and gay men and lesbians. There is also evidence that bisexuals experience stigma and discrimination in a manner qualitatively different from that experienced by lesbians and gay men. Bisexuals often experience biphobia from both the heterosexual and the homosexual communities. Bisexuals are often met with discrimination, rejection, and exclusion from a community where acceptance is expected. There can be a lack of connectedness to the LGBT community, and bisexuals can also find themselves defending their identity as authentic (Bostwick et al. 2014a). Patients should self-identify their sexual orientation, regardless of sexual behavior and/or desire. Issues that arise in treatment related to identity should be explored.

Transgender and Gender-Nonconforming Individuals

Gender dysphoria is a term used to describe incongruency between individuals' gender identity and their physical or assigned gender, resulting in psychological distress and discomfort with their physical appearance. This distress often worsens at the time of puberty with the development of secondary sex characteristics.

Historically, mental health providers were "gatekeepers" in the transitioning process. Their input and evaluation were required for individuals seeking treatment of gender dysphoria via medical transition with hormone therapy, surgery, or both. Currently, only informed consent is required for hormone therapy. Guidelines on the role of mental health professionals in the process of medical transition for adults vary, with some *recommending* a presurgical mental health evaluation (Hembree et al. 2017), whereas others *require* such an evaluation (World Professional Association for Transgender Health 2011). It is understood that mental healthcare should be available to individuals before, during, and after transitioning. Providers are expected to be able to distinguish gender dysphoria from other psychiatric or psychological problems and should be familiar with the economic, social, and psychological stress associated with transitioning.

Over the course of their lifetimes, transgender and gender-nonconforming individuals are exposed to a great deal of mistreatment and discrimination, including verbal harassment and physical violence, related to their expressed gender identity. It is important for providers to be aware that this includes reports of discrimination experienced in healthcare settings. Among the research looking at the experiences of transgender individuals, most studies are based on male-to-female transgender populations. In one of the few studies of transgender men (individuals whose sex was assigned female at birth), approximately 40% reported having experienced verbal harassment, denial of equal treatment, or physical assault in a doctor's office or hospital setting. Study participants reported experiencing increased anxiety associated with seeking gynecological care and being refused care altogether from some healthcare providers (Shires and Jaffee 2015).

The 2015 U.S. Transgender Survey, with 27,715 respondents age 18 and older, documented the impact of high rates of stigma and discrimination on transgender individuals (James et al. 2016). In the survey, 33% of respondents reported having had at least one negative experience while seeking medical care, and 23% reported that they avoided seeking medical treatment out of fear of being mistreated. Nearly 40% reported having attempted suicide at some point within their lifetime, and 39% reported having experienced severe psychological distress in the month prior to completing the survey. This is almost nine times the attempted suicide rate in the general U.S. population. When asked about their experiences in grades K–12, 54% of respondents reported experiencing verbal harassment, 24% reported being the victim of physical violence, 13% reported being subjected to sexual assault, and 17% reported having to leave their school as a result of these harmful conditions. In adulthood, 30% reported experiencing some form of mistreatment, ranging from verbal harassment, to being fired for being transgender, and to even physical and sexual assault in the workplace. The survey also noted higher rates of stressors for transgender people of color (black, Latinx [a gender-neutral, gender-inclusive word vs. *Latino/a*], American Indian, and multiracial). They were three times as likely to be living in poverty and four times as likely to be unemployed.

Mental health providers can advocate for their transgender patients to prevent stigma and discrimination in healthcare settings. For example, we can work to change the erasure of patients' transgender identities in medical records, hospital policies, and procedures and insurance billing and coding when providing care, including medically necessary transition-related care. We can also improve the experiences of patients and decrease stigma in medical settings by training providers to understand the healthcare needs of transgender individuals.

HIV/AIDS

In 2015, African Americans accounted for 45% of new HIV diagnoses, with almost 60% occurring in MSM (Centers for Disease Control and Prevention 2016). Rates of HIV infection are also significantly increased among transgender women. In the 2015 U.S. Transgender Survey (James et al. 2016), the overall rate of HIV infection was five times as great as in the general U.S. population (1.4% vs. 0.3%), and for black transgender women the rate of HIV infection was 19%.

Despite these staggering numbers, recent rates of new diagnoses either are falling or have stabilized among many demographics, including black MSM. It is important to be aware of HIV risk behaviors in all patients, but when working with black MSM and transgender women, it is essential that providers discuss HIV. Issues that should be discussed include testing, linkage to care, and prevention. People who are diagnosed early and maintained in treatment with an undetectable HIV viral load have a normal life expectancy and do not transmit the virus. Safer behaviors include pre-exposure prophylaxis (referred to as PrEP), which is taking a medication that is almost 90% effective in preventing the acquisition of HIV in MSM, and postexposure prophylaxis (PEP), which is taking a 30-day regimen of medication to prevent acquisition of HIV after a potential exposure (Spinner et al. 2016).

Substance Use

A recent study comparing substance use across various intersecting identities found that for black sexual minority men, the rates of substance use were similar to those for black heterosexual men and less than those for white sexual minority men. Significantly, black sexual minority women had a rate of substance use four times that of black heterosexual women and twice that of white sexual minority women (Mereish and Bradford 2014)

Studies indicate higher prevalence of cigarette smoking in LGB individuals compared with heterosexuals. Rates were most elevated for bisexuals, particularly bisexual women (Fallin et al. 2015). Cigarette smoking is associated with a host of medical conditions, causing increased morbidity and mortality.

Clinicians should assess substance use with all patients. Providers should note the disparities in rates of substance use in black sexual minority women and appropriately assess and treat. Clinicians should also assess cigarette smoking and provide information and treatment for smoking cessation.

Resilience

There has been a question as to whether LGB people of color are exposed to higher levels of heterosexist stigma with negative consequences (risk) or are more resistant to this stigma (resilience). The minority stress model posits that as LGBT persons experience increased stress (prejudice events, expectations of rejection, hiding and concealing, internalized homophobia), they experience an increase in mental health problems (Meyer 2003), but more recent literature favors resilience.

For black LGB persons, strategies developed to cope with racism may serve as a source of resilience. Such strategies include confronting prejudice, developing supportive networks, practicing active self-acceptance, managing and reducing exposure to stigmatization and prejudice by being flexible in self-presentation and disclosure, and having a personal relationship with God or connection with faith and a religious community (Barnes and Meyer 2012; Choi et al. 2011; Follins et al. 2014; Meyer et al. 2008; Moradi et al. 2010). Black lesbians reported the following qualities as necessary for resilience: strong, positive racial group membership identity (black friends and family, other black LGB people, black religious communities); racial and religious socialization; and culturally specific coping skills (see strategies discussed earlier in this section).

Recently, black gay men, bisexual men, and MSM have most often had their psychological health assessed in the context of HIV risk behavior (Follins et al. 2014). Nonetheless, resilience was associated with a strong sense of racial group membership, integration of multiple identities, and a personal connection to spirituality. Black transgender individuals (it should be noted that few transmen are included in this research literature) noted family support and acceptance, as well as being connected to their racial community, as being important for the development of resilience.

Religion and Spirituality

The church has been significant in the black community, offering a refuge from the racism of the majority culture. The church also provides support and meaning. It appears to play a role in the development of the resilience that is seen in the black LGBT population, but there are conflicting data (Follins et al. 2014). For black LGBT individuals, participation in nonaffirming religious settings was related to internalized homophobia (Barnes and Meyer 2012). Internalized homophobia predicted depressive symptoms and less psychological well-being; however, participation in nonaffirming religious settings was not related to adverse mental health outcomes. It has been theorized that the support provided by the church counters the deleterious effects of the nonaffirming environment (Barnes and Meyer 2012).

As has been noted, some aspect of resilience may appear related to connection to the black community and faith traditions. One strategy to maintain these supports has been to selectively share sexual identity and orientation. However, it is important that clinicians not rush to recommend that patients come out; rather, the issue needs to be explored, addressing thoughts about the coming-out process and the potential risks and benefits.

Clinicians working with black LGBT patients need to be aware of the religious background of their patients and the role it plays in their lives. Patients' exposures to nonaffirming and homophobic religious environments should be explored, as well as how the patients have responded to the strain that engagement in these environments may have caused them. Although many black LGBT individuals abandon nonaffirming religious settings, finding affirming settings or avoiding religious settings altogether, many maintain their connection with nonaffirming and homophobic religious situations. In the latter circumstance, clinicians need to understand the positive effects and reasons for continued affiliation and, as appropriate, sensitively explore potential alternative religious settings for the patient.

Discussion

Just as there is no monolithic black community, the black LGBT community is also diverse. However, black LGBT persons share the lived experience of having multiple stigmatized racial, sexual, and gender identities. Although there is some work assessing the mental health of black LGBT persons, much work remains to be done. The literature is particularly sparse on transgender men, nonurban populations, bisexually identified men and women separate from gay men and lesbian women, and those younger than 18 years. Although the impact of HIV on black MSM cannot be overstated, studies also need to be done on the mental health issues in this community that do not focus on HIV. More research is necessary to determine risk factors for mental illness, resources for resilience, and effective interventions. That research should be done using an intersectional approach to appreciate the various roles of the multiple identities.

Clinicians need to be aware of some significant issues and the health disparities in black LGBT patients to be able to address them, whether they be gender dysphoria in transgender persons, HIV in black MSM, or substance use in black sexual minority women. Mental healthcare providers should be aware of the discrimination black LGBTQ individuals may experience—racism in the majority LGBTQ community and bias against sexual minorities in the black community—and the role these experiences may have on the lives of their patients.

Studies have shown that, contrary to what the minority stress model would have predicted, black LGBTQ persons have generally lower rates of mental illness relative to the white LGBTQ community. Various sources of resilience have been proposed, most often identifying the role of spirituality or religion and a connection with the black community (e.g., family, social network). The clinician should be aware of what psychosocial supports exist for their patient and work to strengthen them when present or attempt to create them when absent.

Black LGBTQ people are also generally less likely to be open about their sexual minority status in many situations, including with providers. In most cases, it does not appear to decrease their acceptance of this status but functions as a way to maintain connection with the black community. Clinicians should provide an open, safe, and nonjudgmental space where patients may feel comfortable sharing all aspects of their identity. One can provide visual clues for LGBTQ patients through the use of inclusive brochures and educational materials as well as inclusive forms. Clinicians should also be aware of local resources for their black LGBTQ patients and understand some of the potential issues and limitations with majority culture LGBTQ resources as well as with resources in the black sexual majority community.

Resources

AGLP (Association of LGBTQ Psychiatrists): www.aglp.org

American Medical Association: https://www.ama-assn.org/delivering-care/physician-resources-lgbtq-inclusive-practice

American Psychiatry Association: www.psychiatry.org

American Psychological Association, Resources Related to LGBT Psychology: www.apadivisions.org/division-44/resources

Center for Black Equity: http://centerforblackequity.org

DBGM: http://dbgm.org/about-dbgm

GLMA (Health Professionals Advancing LGBT Equality): www.glma.org

National LGBT Health Education Center: www.lgbthealtheducation.org

References

Barnes DM, Meyer IH: Religious affiliation, internalized homophobia, and mental health in lesbians, gay men, and bisexuals. Am J Orthopsychiatry 82(4):505–515, 2012 23039348

Bostwick WB, Boyd CJ, Hughes TL, et al: Discrimination and mental health among lesbian, gay, and bisexual adults in the United States. Am J Orthopsychiatry 84(1):35–45, 2014a 24826824

Bostwick WB, Meyer I, Aranda F, et al: Mental health and suicidality among racially/ethnically diverse sexual minority youths. Am J Public Health 104(6):1129–1136, 2014b 24825217

Centers for Disease Control and Prevention: HIV Among African Americans. Atlanta, GA, Centers for Disease Control and Prevention, 2016. Available at: www.cdc.gov/hiv/group/racialethnic/africanamericans/index.html. Accessed December 10, 2017.

Choi KH, Han CS, Paul J, et al: Strategies for managing racism and homophobia among U.S. ethnic and racial minority men who have sex with men. AIDS Educ Prev 23(2):145–158, 2011 21517663

Fallin A, Goodin A, Lee YO, et al: Smoking characteristics among lesbian, gay, and bisexual adults. Prev Med 74:123–130, 2015 25485860

Follins LD, Walker JJ, Lewis MK: Resilience in black lesbian, gay, bisexual, and transgender individuals: a critical review of the literature. J Gay Lesbian Ment Health 18(2):190–212, 2014

Hembree WC, Cohen-Kettenis PT, Gooren L, et al: Endocrine treatment of gender-dysphoric/gender-incongruent persons: an Endocrine Society clinical practice guideline. J Clin Endocrinol Metab 102(11):3869–3903, 2017 28945902

Hill MJ: J Gay Lesbian Ment Health 17(2):208–214, 2013

James SE, Herman JL, Rankin S, et al: The Report of the 2015 U.S. Transgender Survey. Washington, DC, National Center for Transgender Equality, 2016

Kastanis A, Gates GJ: LGBT African-Americans and African-American Same-Sex Couples. Los Angeles, CA, Williams Institute, UCLA School of Law, 2013. Available at: http://williamsinstitute.law.ucla.edu/wp-content/uploads/Census-AFAMER-Oct-2013.pdf. Accessed December 10, 2017.

Kim H-J, Jen S, Fredriksen-Goldsen KI: Race/ethnicity and health-related quality of life among LGBT older adults. Gerontologist 57 (suppl 1):S30–S39, 2017 28087793

Mereish EH, Bradford JB: Intersecting identities and substance use problems: sexual orientation, gender, race, and lifetime substance use problems. J Stud Alcohol Drugs 75(1):179–188, 2014 24411810

Meyer IH: Prejudice, social stress, and mental health in lesbian, gay, and bisexual populations: conceptual issues and research evidence. Psychol Bull 129(5):674–697, 2003 12956539

Meyer IH: Identity, stress, and resilience in lesbians, gay men, and bisexuals of color. Couns Psychol 38(3):38, 2010 24347674

Meyer IH, Dietrich J, Schwartz S: Lifetime prevalence of mental disorders and suicide attempts in diverse lesbian, gay, and bisexual populations. Am J Public Health 98(6):1004–1006, 2008 17901444

Moradi B, Wiseman MC, DeBlaere C, et al: LGB of color and white individuals' perceptions of heterosexist stigma, internalized homophobia, and outness: comparisons of levels and links. Couns Psychol 38(3):397–424, 2010

Morin S, Garfinkle E: Male homophobia. J Soc Issues 34:29–47, 1978

Shires DA, Jaffee K: Factors associated with health care discrimination experiences among a national sample of female-to-male transgender individuals. Health Soc Work 40(2):134–141, 2015 26027422

Spinner CD, Boesecke C, Zink A, et al: HIV pre-exposure prophylaxis (PrEP): a review of current knowledge of oral systemic HIV PrEP in humans. Infection 44(2):151–158, 2016 26471511

Weinberg G: Society and the Healthy Homosexual. New York, Anchor Books, 1972

World Professional Association for Transgender Health: Standards of Care for the Health of Transsexual, Transgender, and Gender Nonconforming People, Version 7. Minneapolis, MN, World Professional Association for Transgender Health, 2011. Available at: https://s3.amazonaws.com/amo_hub_content/Association140/files/Standards%20of%20Care%20V7%20-%202011%20WPATH%20(2)(1).pdf. Accessed December 15, 2017.

CHAPTER 14
ADULT ATTENTION-DEFICIT/HYPERACTIVITY DISORDER IN AFRICAN AMERICAN POPULATIONS

Patricia A. Newton, M.D., M.P.H., M.A.

ATTENTION-DEFICIT/HYPERACTIVITY DISORDER (ADHD) is often unrecognized and underdiagnosed in adult populations. ADHD has been estimated to have an overall prevalence of roughly 4.4% in adults over the age of 18 in the United States and 7% overall in children (Kessler et al. 2006; see also Ginsberg et al. 2014; National Center for Health Statistics 1994). Rates for children diagnosed with ADHD are, in general, higher overall than for adults in all ethnic and racial categories (8.9% non-Hispanic African American children; 6.3% Hispanic children; and 11.5% in non-Hispanic white children) (Pastor et al. 2015b). However, these same studies show an increase in the rate of diagnosis among children from an overall prevalence of 7.0% in 1997–1999 to 10.2% in 2012–2014 (Pastor et al. 2015a). Also, during the same period, prevalence increased among non-Hispanic white children from 8.4% to 12.5%, among non-Hispanic African American children from 5.5% to 9.6%, and among Hispanic children from 3.8% to 6.4% (Pastor et al. 2015a). Prevalence rates for ADHD in African American adults have been variable, with no consensus reported that can be considered reliable despite the fact that overall diagnoses have been reported to have increased over the last decade at a rate of 6.2% (Kessler et al. 2006).

Several factors contribute to the lack of recognition of the disorder in this population: presence of comorbid conditions such as alcohol and substance use disorders, affective disorders, anxiety disorders, and posttraumatic stress disorder and historical trauma; implicit bias among healthcare providers; cultural factors; and general disparities relative to the healthcare delivery system (Suite et al. 2007). Social stigma regarding mental health treatment among African Americans, coupled with fear and distrust of psychiatry, also contributes to the failure to seek treatment. A major reason for this lack of trust and underutilization of mental health services by African Americans can be directly traced to a history of racism in medical research and diagnosis (Suite et al. 2007).

Misdiagnoses in African American populations can be problematic (American Psychiatric Association 2013), and inadequate knowledge about ADHD and its manifestations in adults also weighs heavily in the scheme of things relative to recognition, diagnosis, and treatment among this population group (American Psychiatric Association 2013). Because of the serious social, legal, and healthcare consequences created by the misdiagnosis and underdiagnosis of the disorder in African Americans, clinical and cultural competence in assessment and treatment of ADHD in adult populations are essential to improving the overall quality of life in affected individuals.

Effects of ADHD on Quality of Life

In a series of focus groups in Europe and North America (sponsored by Shire Pharmaceuticals), adults with ADHD reported inattention, impulse-control problems, irritability, and forgetfulness as contributors to difficulty in interpersonal relationships and misunderstandings. The average focus group size was seven participants (range, three to nine participants), with a mean age of 36 years. Participants were asked questions based on a script/guide designed for the focus group based on a literature review and feedback on prior experience from expert clinicians from each country. The guide was designed to elicit commentary from participants in several areas, including how they were diagnosed, their childhood experiences of ADHD, and social, physiological, and physical functioning in their daily lives (Brod et al. 2012).

Research indicates that adults with ADHD may have had disrupted education earlier in life. A study of 500 adults (age > 18 years) with self-reported ADHD, who were compared with 501 healthy control subjects, found that the adults with ADHD were less likely to have achieved a college degree (19% vs. 26%; $P < 0.01$) (Biederman et al. 2006). Reasons for this included an inability to handle large workloads, inattention, disorganization, difficulty following instructions, and making careless errors (Biederman et al. 2006). Adults with ADHD have been noted to experience work-related difficulties that have an impact on their reputations and productivity and lead to high job turnover and frequent unemployment (Biederman et al. 2006; Brod et al. 2012; Shifrin et al. 2010).

Several studies (Barkley et al. 2002; Brod et al. 2012; Lichtenstein and Larsson 2013; Piñeiro-Dieguez et al. 2016; Sørensen et al. 2017) have indicated that adults with ADHD, compared with persons without ADHD, have a higher incidence of criminality and arrests, aggressive reckless driving, traffic violations, suspension of driving licenses, and substance use disorders. A U.S. study comprehensively evaluated driving in 105 adults with ADHD (ages 17–28 years) and 64 community control adults in five domains of driving ability using a battery of executive function tasks. Compared with community control subjects, adults with ADHD were associated with more traffic violation tickets verified by self-reports and Department of Motor Vehicle records (Piñeiro-Dieguez et al. 2016). In a series of European and North American focus groups (sponsored by Shire Pharmaceuticals), some adults with ADHD reported aggressive or reckless driving often accompanied by anger directed at the other driver (Brod et al. 2012).

ADHD and Medical Comorbidity

Adults and children diagnosed with ADHD may also have symptoms that meet criteria for other psychiatric diagnoses (Kessler et al. 2006; Torgersen et al. 2006). Data analyzed from the National Comorbidity Survey Replication demonstrated that ADHD in adults was associated with other psychiatric disorders: mood disorders (odds ratio [OR]=5), anxiety disorders of all types (OR=3.7), and any substance abuse (use) disorder (OR=3.0) (Jain et al. 2017; Kessler et al. 2006; Torgersen et al. 2006).

Adults with ADHD have an increased risk of having comorbid medical illnesses such as sleep disorders, asthma, migraine headaches, and obesity. The management and outcomes in patients with chronic medical illness are impacted greatly in patients with ADHD. Careful lifestyle changes and medication management (e.g., hypertension, diabetes) (Nigg 2013) are essential in this population and have profound health consequences. As Jain et al. (2017) note, "When the high overall comorbidity rate of ADHD with other psychiatric disorders is considered in light of the low rate of ADHD diagnosis in adults, it could be speculated that the underdiagnosis and therefore lack of treatment in many adults with ADHD may be partially the result of misdiagnosis of ADHD as a different and often comorbid disorder" (p. e4). This becomes a critical clinical outcome issue, especially in African American patients, who have a disproportionate prevalence of hypertension, diabetes, obesity, and associated healthcare disparities and underdiagnosis of ADHD (Nigg 2013; Shifrin et al. 2010; U.S. Department of Health and Human Services 1989).

TABLE 14–1. ADHD community survey

Question	Yes	No	Unsure
Have you ever heard of ADHD?	550 (100%)	0	0
Does anyone in your family have ADHD?	231 (42%)	264 (48%)	55 (10%)
Do all children diagnosed with ADHD eventually grow out of it?	440 (80%)	88 (16%)	22 (4%)
In adult populations, do you see ADHD?	110 (20%)	385 (70%)	55 (10%)
Is there any association between ADHD and substance abuse?	110 (20%)	275 (50%)	165 (30%)

Note.   *N*=550; females: 330; males: 220. Age range: 19–87 years; median age: 46 years.
Source.   Unpublished results based on survey at Mondawmin Mall in Baltimore, Maryland.

ADHD and Community Awareness

The serious effects that ADHD has on the well-being of African American adults and on their overall quality of life frequently go undiagnosed and therefore untreated. There is an apparent need to have a better understanding of the impact that the disorder has on this group. In September 2016, the author conducted a public opinion survey among African Americans in Baltimore, Maryland. The survey was completed over a period of 10 days at a local mall in the inner city. Mondawmin Mall is a heavily traversed shopping center located in a residential area that is predominantly inhabited (82%) by African Americans. A brief survey (Table 14–1) was conducted of African Americans shopping at the mall. A total of 550 persons (ages 19–87 years) were questioned regarding their knowledge of ADHD. The participants (60% female; 40% male) who agreed to participate in the survey had heard of ADHD as a diagnosis in children. Less than half (42%) of the respondents had family members who had been diagnosed with ADHD, and a small percentage (10%) had no idea if a family member had ever been diagnosed with the disorder. Seventy percent of respondents felt that ADHD was not a disorder of adults and, for the most part, believed that children grew out of the disorder (80%) once they reached adulthood.

Eighty percent of those interviewed had either no idea whether there was an association of ADHD with alcoholism, substance use disorders, or other psychiatric conditions or felt there was no such association. Interestingly, the small percentage (20%) of individuals who had heard of ADHD in adults and who believed that it was associated with other mental conditions as well as alcoholism and substance use disorders were all female (Table 14–2).

TABLE 14–2. ADHD community survey attitudes by gender

Question	Females	Males	Both genders
Has anyone in your family been diagnosed with ADHD?	Yes (42%)	No (48%)	(10%) (Unsure)
Do all children diagnosed with ADHD eventually grow out of it?	No (16%)	Yes (80%)	(4%) (Unsure)
In adult populations, do you see ADHD?	Yes (20%)	No (70%)	(10%) (Unsure)
Is there any association between ADHD and substance abuse?	Yes (20%)	No (50%)	(30%) (Unsure)

Note. N=550; females: 330; males: 220. Age range: 19–87 years; median age: 46 years.
Source. Unpublished results based on survey at Mondawmin Mall in Baltimore, Maryland.

As a result of this brief survey, the author wondered whether the results might reflect the knowledge base of the greater African American community in the city (and perhaps in the nation as a whole). The findings were discussed with key leaders of Black Psychiatrists of America (BPA) in terms of these findings' relevance to the overall mental health and well-being of the African American community. As a result, BPA decided on a national road show both to educate healthcare providers serving African American populations and to improve the general knowledge regarding ADHD in the African American community across the United States.

The BPA adult ADHD program is entitled "Get a Check-Up from the Neck-Up" and has two phased tiers:

1. *Phase I:* Educating primary care physicians and adolescent medicine physicians and reeducating adult psychiatrists about ADHD in adult populations. (Nurse practitioners and physician assistants are also encouraged to acquire knowledge about adult ADHD as well in this educational outreach effort.)
2. *Phase II:* Enhancing community awareness of ADHD in adult populations through a partnership with the faith-based community. BPA has a cooperative agreement with the Samuel DeWitt Proctor Conference, an interfaith United Nations nongovernmental organization composed of seminarians and practicing clergy from across the nation targeting African American communities and disenfranchised groups globally.

These phased tiers are thought to be essential in eliminating basic gaps in knowledge about those at the greatest risk of being underdiagnosed and receiving inadequate treatment of the disorder by healthcare providers. Eliminating those gaps will also enhance both provider and public awareness of the association of ADHD with other health comorbidities that affect patient outcomes in the African American community. Likewise, improving the general knowledge base on ADHD in adult populations may alleviate quality-of-life problems that often plague this group, such as substance use disorders, interpersonal conflicts, and legal matters, while increasing the numbers of those adults who had been unknowingly affected who seek and receive adequate treatment. This would mitigate some of the adverse outcomes associated with the disorder that have continued to affect the African American community in adverse ways.

In 2017, BPA was awarded an educational grant from Shire Pharmaceuticals to initiate Phase I of this project. From August 2017 through January 2018, BPA continued its national road show to educate healthcare providers about ADHD in adult populations. Five cities with large African American populations were targeted: Nashville, Tennessee; Atlanta, Georgia; Oakland, California; Detroit, Michigan; and Houston, Texas. Family medicine and adolescent medicine physicians, as well as adult psychiatrists, were in attendance. Physician extenders, including nurse practitioners and physician assistants, were also present. The preliminary results of the provider educational phase have been positive in terms of acquisition of new knowledge and enhanced awareness of the problem in adult patients. The BPA is seeking additional funding to extend Phase I activities in 2018 and 2019 to reach other cities where providers treat large African American populations.

BPA has also initiated a cooperative agreement with a large faith-based association that is interdenominational and serves the African American community nationwide to begin Phase II of the project. Funding for Phase II is in the planning stages but with the intent that a national education campaign targeting the larger African American community can begin in the last quarter of 2018 as well. It is anticipated that this program will expand knowledge to both providers who treat African Americans and consumers of healthcare in African American communities. Evaluations of the overall effectiveness of the "Get a Check-Up from the Neck-Up" program designed to fill the treatment gaps associated with adult ADHD are being conducted throughout the entirety of the project. The results of these evaluations are serving as a guide for program expansion and improved healthcare and social quality of life outcomes.

Conclusion and Future Considerations

Adult ADHD is a health condition that is underdiagnosed and undertreated in the African American community. Healthcare providers as well as the public have clear knowledge gaps in providing and receiving adequate services to this population group. The lack of awareness in the general African American community regarding ADHD in adult populations is highly correlated with social, legal, and personal challenges and difficulties being faced by this group here in the United States. The failure of the healthcare system in general and mental healthcare providers in particular in recognizing the implications of this disorder in adults has a great impact on the general well-being of affected individuals. This represents a major gap in effective diagnosis and treatment in physical as well as emotional health.

The distrust, fear, and racism that have been experienced by African Americans relative to the healthcare system also serve to create challenges in terms of providing adequate treatment to adults affected with ADHD (Suite et al. 2007). The high correlation of education, work, social, and legal dysfunction with the disorder in adult populations cannot be overstated. The impact of ADHD on African Americans caught in the downward spiral created by this condition relative to successful attainment of positive life goals cannot be ignored. Serious questions come to mind concerning the comorbidities associated with ADHD in adult populations.

There is a clear and urgent need to educate law enforcement officials, courts, and probation officers about the devastating effect of ADHD in adult populations. Such efforts can lead to improved diagnosis and treatment outcomes. Treatment should be made available to offenders; this may prevent future legal violations and actions against them. In addition, substance use and abuse counselors require reeducation regarding the impact of ADHD in adults and the high correlation of ADHD with relapse, which complicates treatment recovery.

Recognizing and treating adult ADHD is just the tip of the iceberg relative to healing the African American community, but it is a major step in the right direction toward improving the quality of life and personal and professional competency and minimizing legal as well as societal conflicts that plague a large segment of this community.

The BPA, as it approaches its fiftieth year of existence in 2019, is committed to improving the lives of African American patient populations through the recognition and treatment of a disorder that has far too long plagued the social fabric of this community. The public health implications are significant. In terms of costs and morbidity to the entire nation, ADHD in adults should not be disregarded or marginalized any longer.

References

American Psychiatric Association: Diagnostic and Statistical Manual of Mental Disorders, 5th Edition. Arlington, VA, American Psychiatric Association, 2013

Barkley RA, Murphy KR, Dupaul GI, et al: Driving in young adults with attention deficit hyperactivity disorder: knowledge, performance, adverse outcomes, and the role of executive functioning. J Int Neuropsychol Soc 8(5):655–672, 2002 12164675

Biederman J, Faraone SV, Spencer TJ, et al: Functional impairments in adults with self-reports of diagnosed ADHD: a controlled study of 1001 adults in the community. J Clin Psychiatry 67(4):524–540, 2006 16669717

Brod M, Pohlman B, Lasser R, et al: Comparison of the burden of illness for adults with ADHD across seven countries: a qualitative study. Health Qual Life Outcomes 10:47, 2012 22583562

Ginsberg Y, Quintero J, Anand E, et al: Underdiagnosis of attention-deficit/hyperactivity disorder in adult patients: a review of the literature. Prim Care Companion CNS Disord 16(3):e1–e8, 2014 25317367

Jain R, Jain S, Montano CB: Addressing diagnosis and treatment gaps in adults with attention-deficit/hyperactivity disorder. Prim Care Companion CNS Disord 19(5):e1–e9, 2017 28906602

Kessler RC, Adler L, Barkley R, et al: The prevalence and correlates of adult ADHD in the United States: results from the National Comorbidity Survey Replication. Am J Psychiatry 163(4):716–723, 2006 16585449

Lichtenstein P, Larsson H: Medication for attention deficit-hyperactivity disorder and criminality (letter). N Engl J Med 368(8):776, 2013 23425178

National Center for Health Statistics: Current estimates from the National Health Interview Survey, 1992 (Vital and Health Statistics, Series 10, No 189). Hyattsville, MD, National Center for Health Statistics, 1994

Nigg JT: Attention-deficit/hyperactivity disorder and adverse health outcomes. Clin Psychol Rev 33(2):215–228, 2013 23298633

Pastor PN, Duran C, Reuben C: QuickStats: Percentage of children and adolescents aged 5–17 years with diagnosed attention-deficit/hyperactivity disorder (ADHD), by race and Hispanic ethnicity—National Health Interview Survey, United States 1997–2014. MMWR Morbid Mortal Weekly Rep (MMWR) 64(33):925. August 26, 2015a

Pastor PN, Reuben CA, Duran CR, Hawkins LD: Association between diagnosed ADHD and selected characteristics among children aged 4–17 years: United States, 2011–2013. NCHS DataBrief No 201. Hyattsville, MD, National Center for Health Statistics, May 2015b

Piñeiro-Dieguez B, Balanzá-Martínez V, García-García P, et al: Psychiatry comorbidity at the time of diagnosis in adults with ADHD: the CAT study. J Atten Disord 20(12):1066–1075, 2016 24464326

Shifrin JG, Proctor BE, Prevatt FF: Work performance differences between college students with and without ADHD. J Atten Disord 13(5):489–496, 2010 19474462

Sørensen L, Sonuga-Barke E, Eichele H, et al: Suboptimal decision making by children with ADHD in the face of risk: poor risk adjustment and delay aversion rather than general proneness to taking risks. Neuropsychology 31(2):119–128, 2017 27267090

Suite DH, La Bril R, Primm A, et al: Beyond misdiagnosis, misunderstanding and mistrust: relevance of the historical perspective in the medical and mental health treatment of people of color. J Natl Med Assoc 99(8):879–885, 2007 17722664

Torgersen T, Gjervan B, Rasmussen K: ADHD in adults: a study of clinical characteristics, impairment and comorbidity. Nord J Psychiatry 60(1):38–43, 2006 16500798

U.S. Department of Health and Human Services: Report of the Secretary's Task Force on Black and Minority Health, Vol 1: Executive Summary (DHHS Publ No 241-80-841/05306). Washington, DC, U.S. Department of Health and Human Services, 1989

CHAPTER 15
PSYCHOTHERAPY WITH AFRICAN AMERICANS AND PEOPLE OF AFRICAN DESCENT

Anderson J. Franklin, Ph.D.

PSYCHOTHERAPY IS ONE MAJOR intervention for treating general life stressors and mental health disorders, but there is less access to and utilization of psychotherapy by blacks than in the general population. There are a number of reasons for this disparity in access and utilization in spite of decades of efforts and leadership by black psychiatrists, psychologists, and other allied mental health providers to advocate for cultural competency in training and practices. In this chapter I discuss some factors in psychotherapy with African Americans and people of African descent to shed light on the challenges that remain to provide psychotherapy as effective interventions for the community.[1] I first place access to and utilization of mental health interventions within the larger framework of health and mental health disparities for African Americans in this country. After a discussion of the tensions between the black community's and professionals' curative knowledge and mental health practices, I explore factors—both systemic and experiential—that

---

[1]In this chapter, I use the terms *blacks, African Americans,* and *people of African descent* interchangeably.

shape black peoples' orientation to and engagement of psychotherapy and other mental health services. The chapter concludes with a discussion of the orientation, assumptions, and expectations of psychotherapy practices and process.

Psychotherapy is one of the current behavioral health procedures in the treatment of mental health disorders. It is interactive, with both verbal and nonverbal communication between patient and therapist. There can be different procedural approaches and goals to change or modify behavior. Common procedures include insight-oriented, cognitive-behavioral, and manualized empirically supported treatments as well as supportive therapy and drug management. Psychotherapy is commonly utilized to manage an array of general life stressors that have created dysfunctions in adjustment and adaptation to everyday life and overall psychological well-being. Psychotherapy is also viewed within a generic framework, encompassing an array of orientations and treatments. It can be provided exclusively for an individual, as well as within group, couples, or family therapies. Treatment can be in-hospital or outpatient. For the purposes of this chapter, the discussion of psychotherapy is based on services received in various outpatient facilities such as private offices, community mental health centers, or any other social service facilities that provide therapeutic interventions. For African Americans and people of African descent, as for the average person, psychotherapy is another way to acquire healing.

Summary of Black Mental Health: Some Indicators and Rates

To discuss psychotherapy as a mental health intervention for blacks in treating disorders, maladaptive behavior, and psychological well-being in general, it must also be viewed within the larger framework of health and mental health disparities for African Americans in the country. Moreover, we must think of psychotherapy as an intervention for mental health distress potentially available to the average black citizen. Rates of utilization, however, are less than needs. This is in part because utilization is tied to the structural inequities impacting the black community.

There are many inequities and disparities for blacks across economic, health, and social demographic indicators (Williams and Wyatt 2015; see also Chapter 24, "Racism and Mental Health," in this book). Blacks have the lowest median family income compared with other racial groups (DeNavas-Walt and Proctor 2014). Regarding health disparities, blacks have higher rates of hypertension and heart attacks than whites and most other ethnic groups. There is nonequivalence across socioeconomic levels, wherein blacks at the same levels of education as whites make less income, have less purchasing power, and have less wealth (Williams et al. 2016). Even poor blacks are poorer than poor whites. The consequences of disparities are many. One mental health disparity of interest is the lower rates of depression among blacks compared with whites, even after potential stressors, such as vigilant anticipatory coping (LaVeist et al. 2014), which is a form of alertness about things to come such as racial microaggressions (Sue et al. 2008), are taken into account. The disparities in health and mental health are persistent structural barriers to opportunities for the black community, which contextualize the life narratives for black patients entering psychotherapy. Disparities are also manifested in the manner in which black people are referred to, engage in, and benefit from conventional mental health interventions, and psychotherapy specifically. Having less access to and lower quality of healthcare and mental health services for many generations of black history required black people to find alternatives to compensate for inadequate care. Such self-reliance yielded community conventional wisdom and practices about health and mental health treatments to promote healing and maintain the well-being of individuals and the community at large.

Tensions Between the Black Community's and Professionals' Curative Knowledge and Mental Health Practices: Disconnect and Overlap

Black people are no strangers to practices of healing. We have created and utilized curative interventions for maintaining health, ameliorating mental health illnesses, and fixing everyday problems for generations. Psychotherapy is just another curative practice for black people. Conventional beliefs about illness and a legacy of home remedies compete with professional practices in the treatment of health and mental health problems. Embracing indigenous health practices is not different from many other ethnic and cultural populations' approach to health and mental health illness. In the absence of adequate health services and treatment, we create our own conventional wisdom and solutions about care. A case in point is the black community's traditional reliance on the church and religion. For an array of personal, health, family, or mental health distress, such as bereavement, blacks connected to the church will seek help from their pastor first, and their family physician next, before engaging psychiatrists or psychologists (Chatters et al. 2011). This help-seeking behavior, of course, like any other research inquiry into behavioral outcomes, has far more levels of complexity and unknown variables. However, it is important for the clinical practitioner to be aware of such complexity in one phase of a therapeutic process when conceptualizing cases—that is, why are black patients seeking help?

Therefore, to situate psychotherapy as a health practice within the black community, we must consider how it is viewed within the help-seeking beliefs and schema of the community.

Psychotherapy as Social Construction

The perception of psychotherapy is a product of social construction. In other words, both actors—people in the black community as well as members of our professional society—interpret and attach meaning to behavior considered normal, deviant, or resilient and therefore act from their points of reference. As psychiatrists and psychologists, we construct our orientation to diagnosis and treatments, such as best practices and empirically supported treatments. Persons who emerge as our patients often have a lay diagnostic and treatment system that is a parallel process to our protocols for determining what is wrong with them and how to fix it. African Americans rely on their family and community to guide understanding about psychological well-being and employ conventional wisdom and "best practices" for dealing with it, such as praying and putting into the hands of God the healing of someone who has had a "nervous breakdown."

I convey this cautiously because we professionals often quickly dismiss home-grown conventional wisdom as ineffective indigenous "folk medicine" nonsense. However, an overly dismissive attitude prohibits understanding of the biopsychosocial context of black people's conventional wisdom, much less lay curative practices. From my experiences with black patients in psychotherapy, irrespective of education or income level, "old folks' wisdom" and lay practices have currency in the belief system undergirding health and help-seeking behavior. The black elderly still hold on to the stigma associated with mental illness and psychotherapeutic interventions (Sirey et al. 2014). What determines utilization includes both beliefs about lay "folk medicine" practices and whatever else has worked in the experiences of family and friends in treating personal problems, which might include family success with psychotherapy, religion, or both. Therefore, successful psychotherapy for black people in part is dependent on the person's attitudes and beliefs about mental health determinants and appropriate interventions (Obasi and Leong 2009), plus what we as providers deliver in the form of trained knowledge about mental health determinants and related interventions.

Psychotherapy's Responsiveness to Population Diversity

An important element in effectiveness of psychotherapy with black people is knowledge of the diversity that exists among peoples of African descent. There are third-generation African American descendants of slaves, Africans, West Indians of different nationalities, and other persons in the United States from throughout the African diaspora (e.g., Canada, United Kingdom, Brazil) who are lumped under the generic label of *black* or *African American*. Moreover, there are intermarriages and other interrelationships among blacks from these distinctive populations within the African diaspora that add to interpersonal dynamics and personal narratives.

Other very important intrapsychic stratifications often not considered in the effectiveness of psychotherapy are variations in the degree of acceptance and adoption of black racial and ethnic identity among individual black people (Chae et al. 2011). Blacks raised in a predominantly black community are socialized in a more homogeneous ethnic environment, shaping them to likely be more black-identified than blacks raised in a predominantly white community with little black racial socialization. However, such identification also depends on the racial socialization practices of the family. These factors represent a salient research question. The point is that there are stratification complexities within the black community and among black people that are important. We as psychiatrists, psychologists, and allied service providers need to be aware of and knowledgeable about these complexities to augment effectiveness of interventions with black patients. The complex economic and psychosocial stratifications that make up the diverse black populations are a challenge to researchers' and practitioners' aspirations for more parsimonious protocols for diagnosis and treatments of behavior disorders.

Engagement and Utilization of Psychotherapy: Why and Why Not

Therapist and patient each bring to psychotherapy their implicit biases and expectations about the purpose of engaging in it (van Ryn et al. 2011). Guided by our theoretical orientation and practices, we as professionals can have criteria for "good" or "suitable" patients for treatment that are not always informed by evidence-based practices. I believe it is important for therapists to recognize our own assumptions and biases about patient behavior in the framework of diagnosis and psychotherapy (Trierweiler et al. 2006). Our training and place of work also help to shape our orientation to expectations. That is, if we are working in a hospital or community mental health center, that neighborhood location and workplace attributes of our setting determine parameters of our professional behavior, just as private practice has its own unique conditions governing practice behavior. I mention these different workplace contexts for psychotherapy in recognition that just as emergency departments are often the primary source of health treatment and experiences for blacks, and therefore contextualize health services for black people, so too are public community mental health centers and social service agencies. They are the frequent points of engagement by black patients for psychiatric and psychotherapy interventions that shape experiences of this modality of care as well as cultivate the help-seeking and utilization beliefs of black people.

One profound example of this early conditioning of beliefs is how black boys are often introduced to counseling and psychotherapeutic forms of interventions during their school years from referrals for behavior problems or emotional regulation related to attention-deficit/hyperactivity disorder. The preponderance of black boys identified with school behavior problems and sanctioned or dispelled disproportionately from school in contrast to the general school population pulls the therapeutic workforce into what Michelle Alexander (2012) refers to as the "school-to-prison pipeline" reality. These experiences of black boys' public school mental health referrals, plus the help-seeking narratives they generate, socialize these youths' gender attitudes toward therapeutic interventions in particular.

Role of Referral Process in Contextualizing Psychotherapy by Shaping Experiences

Another systemic factor that shapes black peoples' orientation to psychotherapy and other mental health services is the constraint of access. Health insurance costs, benefits, and patients' ability to pay determine setting and manner of access to psychotherapy. Therefore, we must understand that the general black patient population's experiences of psychotherapy, as well as our profession's capacity to put the best foot forward in delivery of high-quality services, are held captive by these health cost realities of the community. Poor black families and persons with no health insurance are at the mercy of public aid and whatever psychotherapy services come with it, if at all. Therefore, this constituency within the black community brings a distinctive view of psychotherapy and its effectiveness. They contribute another story line to the black community's narrative and conventional wisdom about mental health services and treatment.

Black people are more often coming into psychotherapy because of being referred by an organization, such as schools, work, family courts, or trusted persons (e.g., minister or friend) who advise them to seek treatment (Chatters et al. 2011). Needs of children frequently govern black parents' use of psychotherapy and mental health services. Some patients are mandated to treatment because of custody or family disputes, child/wife/partner abuse, or substance abuse, for example. A preponderance of young black males come to us from the criminal justice system (Alexander 2012). These types of referral circumstances are another factor that shape and determine health beliefs, help-seeking behavior, and utilization of psychotherapy by the black general population.

Blacks who engage in psychotherapy in private practice constitute a distinct population within our community. They can afford the costs through insurance and level of income. The millennial and contemporary generation of black middle class will seek out private practice for help with personal distress, particularly issues related to partner/marital relationship problems or those of a child. Black millennials are part of a generation that has been exposed to the contemporary era of lessening stigma to seek psychotherapy and utilizing mental health services.

Role of Race in Psychotherapy and the Significance of Asking for a Black Therapist

Augmenting the quality of psychotherapy for black people is behind the common request to be seen by a black psychiatrist or psychologist (Earl et al. 2011). The frequency of this type of request speaks to the assumptions of black patients that there are shared experiences and knowledge of black people's lives, lived and/or intuited by black mental health service providers. There is a belief that attributes of the black therapist can facilitate therapeutic bonds and promote cultural efficacious interventions. This ethnic-cultural connection is important to the success of joining and bonding during the initial session with black patients as well as to reducing early termination of treatment. Either implicit or explicit in requests for a black therapist by black people is the quest for racial identity alignment between black patient and black therapist about genuine understanding of real black life matters.

This "racial identity alignment" between black patients and black therapist is often a miscalculation by agencies believing that to match race of therapist to race of patient is sufficient in fulfilling specific requests by black patients for a black psychiatrist or psychologist for medications or psychotherapy. Do not misunderstand the caution; there are benefits in fulfilling this request. Nevertheless, such matching is done predominantly to placate the black patient, rather than from an informed or empirical knowledge about how it is value added to psychotherapy effectiveness for black patients (Cabral and Smith 2011). In spite of these caveats, the caution is that skin color alone does not ensure therapeutic alliance or effectiveness. Again, just as "not all black people are alike," "not all black psychiatrists and psychologists are like black people." We too are a product of our personal life experiences and family racial socialization as well as our formal training. How we reconcile and integrate these personal attributes into our professional identity are factors that impact our provider effectiveness with black patients in psychotherapy.

Gender and Poverty as Factors in Psychotherapy

Another trend in the utilization of psychotherapy for blacks is that females use it more than males. This disparity is not that different from trends in the general population. Poor black families do not receive much psychotherapy or adequate quality assurance of best practices. In addition, the lesser number of black males utilizing psychotherapy does present challenges to meeting the broad scope of needs for the general black population. Gender disparities have implications for the well-being of relationships, family functioning, and community leadership.

Black males and black females have parallel but distinct life experiences, as well as particular needs for psychotherapeutic interventions. Franklin (2004) raised some of these life distinctions through his discussion of how racial stereotypes in the public domain about black males create navigational obstacles in life that shape development of intrapsychic structures and personal self-concepts manifested by an "invisibility syndrome." The invisibility syndrome is cultivated by the dominance of public stereotypes about black men that obscure the genuine person, eclipse life opportunities, and force a counternarrative to public presumptions about black males in order to protect psychological well-being. Some of this narrative is embedded in the contemporary Black Lives Matter movement to raise public awareness of inequitable police treatment of black males by the justice system (Alexander 2012).

This systemic generational dilemma of strained interactions between police authorities and black males foreshadows the complexity of power dynamics in the therapist–black male patient relationship. As one black male patient who was a successful professional and businessman conveyed in therapy, "It's hard for folks to see me as something other than the athlete I was." The significance of this statement lies in its pinpointing of a psychosocial legacy over generations that speaks to everyday stressors for black people that test identity, resilience, and psychological well-being (Jones 1997). Racism and experiences of discrimination have been shown to be stressors that put the health and mental health of black people at risk (Williams et al. 2016). Consequently, just considering the gender factor of black males in the larger schema of societal interactions should increase vigilance for manifest racial stereotypes within the therapeutic context. This should be as much a question for patient characteristics research as it is a concern about best practices in psychotherapy regarding effectiveness.

Psychotherapy Practices and Process: Orientation, Assumptions, and Expectations

The promotion of cultural competency training in professional development has improved awareness of some characteristics of black people as prospective patients. The differentiation within the community of African descent is multifaceted and presents a challenge to the average mental health provider to acquire sophistication in his or her awareness, knowledge, and skills. Such levels of sophistication in cultural competency are what inform the dynamics in therapist–black patient interactions. For example, when the average person thinks of psychotherapy, it is often in the public domain's conception of it as "talk therapy." Some embellish that thinking with the belief we can "read their minds," which forms some black patients' initial skepticism of psychotherapy. Like the general public, black patients come with preconceptions about the practices of psychiatry and psychotherapy. Few are sophisticated about the theoretical and practice orientations that distinguish our schools of theory and approaches to treatment. Like the average person, few black people genuinely know the differences between psychoanalytic, psychodynamic, cognitive-behavioral, dialectical behavioral, and empirically supported treatment or, in general, evidence-based practices, much less accompanying pharmacological treatments (see Chapter 16, "Biological Therapies and Black Patients"). Certainly, we do not expect patients to know how we utilize DSM-5 or ICD-11 diagnostic classification systems (American Psychiatric Association 2013; World Health Organization 2018) and their organizing of mental health assessment and diagnosis. Moreover, few patients consider how theoretical orientation to psychotherapy is a way in which we as psychiatrists, psychologists, and mental health providers conceptualize their presenting and underlying problems to formulate and to guide our interpretations of their behavior and to determine therapeutic interventions. People often are just coming in to simply talk over their problems and get a solution.

In past decades the advocacy for evidence-based practices and empirically supported treatments has introduced another form of therapeutic intervention that the black community is no less informed about than the general population. This domain of interventions is guided by an integration of research evidence, clinical expertise, and patient characteristics. Both psychiatry (https://psychiatryonline.org/guidelines) and psychology (https://www.div12.org/psychological-treatments/) provide information on empirically supported treatments and best practices. The growing utilization of and advocacy for this modality for best practices has merit. However, there are shortcomings for both the therapist and the black patient. Let's consider the three legs of integrated support for evidence-based practices: research evidence, clinical expertise, and patient characteristics. When the research evidence is considered, there remains significant underrepresentation of black patients in clinical trials in empirically supported treatments. Clinical expertise presumes experiences in diagnosis of disorders and evolved knowledge from patient contact. For black patients, given their average standard of living as well as inequities in health care, clinical expertise of the professional through patient contact is acquired most often in less quality-assured settings and/or circumstances than other, more privileged groups. Finally, there are deficiencies in knowledge about characteristics of black patients wherein the cultural and biopsychosocial determinants of psychological well-being are not fully understood (Whaley and Davis 2007).

Nevertheless, in spite of continuing challenges to achieve effectiveness of psychotherapy and evidence-based practices, there has been considerable progress in knowledge, sophistication, and best practices over the past decades. The receptivity by black patients to our best practices in psychotherapy remains determined by an initial alignment with their conventional assumptions and expectations about how their problems are going to be solved by us, the providers. This alignment is another factor in the equation determining early termination from treatment. There is also, however, a vein of "healthy cultural suspicion" of healthcare providers (Boyd-Franklin 2003). Clearly, the Tuskegee experiment is the quintessential example of compromised trust in healthcare for the black community, but long before that horrific experiment was disclosed, the black community had many personal experiences during other periods of history with mistreatment within the health and mental healthcare system that helped form skepticism and mistrust about equitable care for the black community. In spite of misgivings, black people, when in personal distress, like most of the general public, invest confidence that our formal training truly has provided us with diagnostic proficiency and clinical competency. Trust is an important element of psychotherapy, and it must be cultivated.

Conclusion: Reflections and Observations

Psychotherapy is an important and significant intervention in mental health treatment for black people. Access to and utilization of psychotherapy are a function of how psychotherapy is perceived as a credible curative intervention. Health disparities mirror the continued second-class citizenship of the black community and the persistence of discrimination and racism. The supposition of second-class citizenship by the black community is reinforced by the underrepresentation of blacks in psychotherapy research and clinical trials for empirically supported treatments. There is a need for greater inclusion and sophistication in sampling and recognizing demographic and health variables (e.g., intragroup ethnic variation and socioeconomic status) in highly differentiated and stratified black populations within the African diaspora. Psychiatrists and psychologists need to sustain and continue to advance cultural competency in their professional training and for the broad mental health workforce. It is paramount that there be social policy that allows affordable access to psychotherapy and mental health services. The perception of psychotherapy by black people remains tied to the legacy of health and mental health treatment, as well as experiences of mental healthcare in the community. Black people will utilize psychotherapy if it has curative relevancy to their well-being, is affordable, and is delivered with cultural competency.

References

Alexander M: The New Jim Crow: Mass Incarceration in the Age of Colorblindness, Revised Edition. New York, The New Press, 2012

American Psychiatric Association: Diagnostic and Statistical Manual of Mental Disorders, 5th Edition. Arlington, VA, American Psychiatric Association, 2013

Boyd-Franklin N: Black Families in Therapy: Understanding the African American Experience, 2nd Edition. New York, Guilford, 2003

Cabral RR, Smith TB: Racial/ethnic matching of clients and therapists in mental health services: a meta-analytic review of preferences, perceptions, and outcomes. J Couns Psychol 58(4):537–554, 2011 21875181

Chae DH, Lincoln KD, Jackson JS: Discrimination, attribution, and racial group identification: implications for psychological distress among Black Americans in the National Survey of American Life (2001–2003). Am J Orthopsychiatry 81(4):498–506, 2011 21977935

Chatters LM, Mattis JS, Woodward AT, et al: Use of ministers for a serious personal problem among African Americans: findings from the National Survey of American Life. Am J Orthopsychiatry 81(1):118–127, 2011 21219283

DeNavas-Walt C, Proctor BD: Income and poverty in the United States: 2013 (Current Population Reports Series). Suitland, MD, U.S. Census Bureau, 2014. Available at: https://www.census.gov/content/dam/Census/library/publications/2014/demo/p60-249.pdf. Accessed December 11, 2017.

Earl TR, Alegría M, Mendieta F, et al: "Just be straight with me": an exploration of black patient experiences in initial mental health encounters. Am J Orthopsychiatry 81(4):519–525, 2011 21977937

Franklin AJ: From Brotherhood to Manhood: How Black Men Rescue Their Relationships and Dreams From the Invisibility Syndrome. New York, Wiley, 2004

Jones JM: Prejudice and Racism, 2nd Edition. New York, McGraw-Hill, 1997

LaVeist TA, Thorpe RJ Jr, Pierre G, et al: The relationships among vigilant coping style, race, and depression. J Soc Issues 70(2):241–255, 2014 24954953

Obasi EM, Leong FTL: Psychological distress, acculturation, and mental health-seeking attitudes among people of African descent in the United States: a preliminary investigation. J Couns Psychol 56(2):227–238, 2009

Sirey JA, Franklin AJ, McKenzie SE, et al: Race, stigma, and mental health referrals among clients of aging services who screened positive for depression. Psychiatr Serv 65(4):537–540, 2014 24687104

Sue DW, Capodilupo CM, Holder AMB: Racial microaggressions in the life experience of black Americans. Prof Psychol Res Pr 39(3):329–336, 2008

Trierweiler SJ, Neighbors HW, Munday C, et al: Differences in patterns of symptom attribution in diagnosing schizophrenia between African American and non-African American clinicians. Am J Orthopsychiatry 76(2):154–160, 2006 16719633

van Ryn M, Burgess DJ, Dovidio JF, et al: The impact of racism on clinician cognition, behavior, and clinical decision making. Du Bois Rev 8(1):199–218, 2011 24761152

Whaley AL, Davis KE: Cultural competence and evidence-based practice in mental health services: a complementary perspective. Am Psychol 62(6):563–574, 2007 17874897

Williams DR, Wyatt R: Racial bias in health care and health: challenges and opportunities. JAMA 314(6):555–556, 2015 26262792

Williams DR, Priest N, Anderson NB: Understanding associations among race, socioeconomic status, and health: patterns and prospects. Health Psychol 35(4):407–411, 2016 27018733

World Health Organization: International Statistical Classification of Diseases and Related Health Problems, 11th Revision. Geneva, World Health Organization, 2018

CHAPTER 16
BIOLOGICAL THERAPIES AND BLACK PATIENTS

William B. Lawson, M.D., Ph.D., DLFAPA

IN THEIR CHAPTER "Black Psychiatric Researchers" published in *Black Psychiatrists and American Psychiatry* in 1999, Drs. Baker and Grady-Weliky noted the dearth of either part- or full-time researchers (Baker and Grady-Weliky 1999; see also Ozarin 2002). The good news is that there were African Americans who spent much of their time doing academic research, but the bad news is that there were not many. Moreover, the numbers unfortunately reflected the paucity of both African Americans in academic careers and those who were able to become funded researchers in the medical field, irrespective of discipline. At the time they were preparing their chapter, Drs. Baker and Gray-Weliky found that only 4% of African American psychiatrists were pursuing academic careers (Baker and Grady-Weliky 1999). Moreover, African American psychiatrists spent much of their time addressing the large clinical demands of their patients, who often had limited access to services, in programs that had a predominantly teaching or clinical mission or provided services to individuals who were reluctant to participate in medical research.

Unfortunately, many of these barriers to research careers continue. The numbers of African Americans going into medicine have changed little over the past two decades and may have declined for African American males. Surveys of minority medical students still show a strong reluctance of these students to go into academic medicine (Mervis 2016). Of those who go into academic medicine, many physicians of color often end up primarily doing administrative work, providing teaching, or doing clinical work. African Americans disproportionately provide services in low-income communities or have academic positions at smaller institutions that often lack a track record, culture, or mentorship for research (Primm and Lawson 2010).

Evidence that African Americans are less likely to be involved primarily in research is provided by examining submissions and funding from the National Institutes of Health, the primary funder for those in research careers. African Americans are far less likely to receive funding: only 15% had complete submissions, and only 1.9% were funded (Ginther et al. 2011). The primary award for research support, the R01 grant, is rarely obtained. The problem begins early and continues through their medical career. In general, most life science majors do not earn biomedical doctoral or medical doctor degrees, most medical doctors will not enter academia, and most academics will never apply for an R01 grant, much less obtain one.

Impact of African American Researchers

The first African American psychiatrist was Dr. Solomon Carter Fuller (1872–1953; Ozarin 2002). Kraepelin's clinic and laboratory at the Royal Psychiatric Hospital at the University of Munich in 1903 offered new opportunities for clinical and pathological studies of the brain. When Alzheimer joined the facility, he selected five foreign visiting students as his graduate research assistants, and one was an American, Dr. Fuller. Dr. Fuller performed groundbreaking research on the physical changes that take place in the brains of Alzheimer's patients. He reported that "[t]he plaques were the deposits in brain tissue of a chemical substance resulting from pathological metabolism of nervous elements" (Fuller 1911, p. 150). In a later paper he used the term "amyloid." He also helped correctly diagnose and train others to correctly diagnose the side effects of syphilis to prevent black war veterans from getting misdiagnosed, discharged, and ineligible for military benefits. He later helped train other African American psychiatrists (Ozarin 2002).

Another groundbreaking researcher was Dr. Chester Middlebrook Pierce (1927–2016), who also made substantial contributions to psychiatry outside of research that are well documented by Dr. Ezra Griffith in his excellent book *Race and Excellence* (Griffith 1999). Dr. Pierce began his work in Antarctica studying soldiers in extreme environments. That experience served him well when he later worked for NASA helping to bring American and Russian cultures together on the International Space Station. He was elected to the Institute of Medicine at the National Academy of Sciences for his career achievements. He later helped found Black Psychiatrists of America (BPA), developed a global psychiatry program at Harvard, and promoted international conferences involving people of African ancestry in the diaspora that helped to promote research on the African continent. Moreover, he had an enormous impact on race relations in multiple institutions.

The Need for African American Researchers

The contributions of these investigators show the kind of impact that African Americans can have on the field as a whole. Clearly, there is a greater need for African American researchers than ever before. Moreover, Drs. Fuller and Pierce have shown that African American researchers can have a disproportionate impact on the field, especially in addressing misconceptions by providers, people with lived experiences, and policy makers. In addition, the need for researchers of color emerges from the need for investigators who have an unbiased view, appreciate people of color as fellow human beings, and can to some extent understand their life experiences irrespective of the emotional distance required for objectivity. Such a perspective has often not been seen in the United States. The perspective of mental life of African Americans can readily be traced to the history of the understanding of mental health in the time of American slavery, when diagnoses of mental illness were overwhelmingly dominated by racism and the perceived inferiority of African Americans (Primm and Lawson 2010). Mental disorders thought to be peculiar to enslaved men and women included *drapetomania* and *dysaesthesia aethiopis,* the former referring to the tendency to run away from slave owners and the latter described as "a form of madness manifest by 'rascality' and 'disrespect for the master's property' that was to be 'cured' by extensive whipping" (Metzl 2009). During and after slavery, African Americans were thought not to require the same mental health services.

African Americans were structurally and ideologically segregated from the rest of American health. Treatment often was not provided to African Americans; unmanageable individuals were often incarcerated. Later, as services were deemed necessary, African Americans were treated in mental hospitals exclusively devoted to them, or they were segregated to separate wards or buildings. Even at the turn of the twentieth century, a leading academic psychiatrist claimed that "Negroes" were "psychologically unfit" for freedom (Metzl 2009). The belief that slavery or later racial segregation was necessary for the mental health of African Americans persisted well into the twentieth century. Similar beliefs continue to influence the diagnosis and treatment of African Americans (Primm and Lawson 2010).

The Need for Information

The Problem of Diagnosis

Throughout the twentieth century medical professionals commonly believed that if African Americans had mental disorders at all, they were much more likely to be diagnosed with disorders with more pessimistic outcomes such as psychosis and schizophrenia and rarely diagnosed with disorders with more optimistic prognoses such as affective disorders, including depression and bipolar disorder (Adebimpe 1981). Epidemiological studies were absent, and the field depended on clinical observations by practitioners, who were often influenced by the larger context of pervasive structural racism, even those who were trying to be well meaning. Since African Americans were thought to have a limited or no mental life, affective disorders such as depression were thought to be uncommon and even rare. Mental disorders such as schizophrenia and paranoia were believed to be the predominant disorders. Psychotherapy was often felt to be unnecessary, and treatment consisted of confinement or medication when it became available. Drs. Billy Jones and Carl Bell, among other African American psychiatrists, documented that affective disorders indeed occurred among African Americans and that the underdiagnosis of these disorders contributed to the disparities in care seen in African Americans (Primm and Lawson 2010). Dr. Victor Adebimpe, a well-regarded African American psychiatrist in both clinical care and research, helped to show that misdiagnosis was pervasive, occurred in spite of objective evidence to the contrary, and had a significant impact on patient care (Adebimpe 1981).

The validity and reliability of psychiatric diagnosing improved over the years with various refinements of DSM. Racial differences in psychiatric disorders were seldom found in large epidemiological studies, in which more objective, structured instruments were used, but overdiagnosing of schizophrenia and underdiagnosing of bipolar disorder and depression continued in clinical settings. The search to find diagnostically valid instruments and the drive to improve the diagnostic system were due in part to the impact of the findings of these researchers. Moreover, the persistence of biased clinical judgments despite evidence to the contrary helped to galvanize the development of professional activism in the 1960s and 1970s. BPA was founded in 1969 to address racial and ethnic issues that mainstream psychiatric organizations were not prioritizing, with Dr. Chester Pierce serving as the group's first president. The issue of racism in psychiatry was a key point of discussion at the 1969 annual meeting of the American Psychiatric Association (APA). Members, including Drs. J. Alfred Cannon, James P. Comer, Chester Pierce, James Ralph, and Charles Wilkinson, led a protest insisting that the APA not only grant to its African American members all the rights and privileges of full membership but, more importantly, take immediate steps to improve the mental healthcare of African Americans in the United States. The APA responded positively, by appointing African American psychiatrists as observer-consultants to its councils, boards, and task forces (Pierce 1970). The APA in later years made active efforts to ensure that the clinical base for DSM, the diagnostic system sanctioned by the APA, had strong ethnic representation in its field trials and clinical deliberations. Moreover, initiatives such as a cultural formulation were developed and had an impact on both National Institute of Mental Health (NIMH) research and the guidelines for the use of DSM-III, DSM-IV, and DSM-5 (American Psychiatric Association 1980, 1994, 2013).

With the emergence of more objective assessments possible with biomarkers and the emergence of genomics, valid diagnostic systems are essential for progress to be made in utilizing these technologies in the clinical setting. During my tenure as chair at Howard University, we participated in a multi-site study to address racial differences in diagnosing affective disorders and found that overdiagnosing of schizophrenia persisted for African Americans despite multiple approaches to reduce racial bias. African Americans with affective psychosis were overdiagnosed with schizophrenia despite the use of experts as multistage face-to-face reviewers and the use of transcripts (Gara et al. 2012). Clearly, there is a need to conduct additional research in this area and to aggressively promote minority participation in such studies.

Psychiatric Genetics

In recent years there have been substantial advances in the neurosciences. Failure to address biases and misconceptions can limit the translation to clinical care and acceptance of these approaches. Moreover, there remains a paucity of data about African Americans' mental disorders and health, in both the psychosocial and the biological underpinnings. Racial and ethnic minorities are often not included in psychological, biological marker, or treatment studies. When race is indicated, less than 1% of studies include African Americans. With a few exceptions, blacks or African Americans are also underrepresented in genetic studies of psychiatric disorders. Non-Hispanic whites have typically composed 90% or more of samples in U.S.-based family history studies, adoption and/or twin studies, and genetic linkage studies. On the other hand, non-Hispanic blacks, who made up approximately 11%–13% of the U.S. population between 1980 and 2006, have made up 0% to less than 5% of the sample in such studies. Furthermore, among blacks, there are no within-group formal family history studies of major depression (Murphy and Thompson 2009). Yet genetic studies will become important in showing diagnostic boundaries in psychiatry and in determining the best treatment modalities. Also, genetic differences have been found for bipolar disorder in whites and African Americans, suggesting different ancestry contributions to the disorder (Smith et al. 2009). Moreover gene-environment interactions may be especially relevant for African Americans given the importance of past traumatic events, such as slavery and early life traumatic events.

Psychopharmacology

The supplement to the 1999 Surgeon General report on mental health, *Mental Health: Culture, Race, and Ethnicity*, documented racial and ethnic disparities in care but it also emphasized the lack of participation of African Americans in pharmaceutical trials, especially since evidence continues to emerge about ethnic differences in basic pharmacology that may necessitate different dosing (Office of the Surgeon General et al. 2001). I have previously reported the results of a literature review that showed ethnic disparities in psychopharmacotherapy (Lawson 1986). More recently, Dr. Annelle Primm, former director of the Office of Minority and National Affairs at the APA, reviewed this literature along with me and found that many of these disparities still persist (Lawson 1986; Primm and Lawson 2010). African Americans are more likely to get antipsychotic medication irrespective of diagnosis; to get higher doses of medication; to be given medication alone rather than psychotherapy or psychotherapy plus medication; and to get older medications, which may have more side effects and as a result may lead to less adherence to medication or discontinuation of treatment earlier. Dr. David Henderson, chair of psychiatry at Boston University and an internationally known schizophrenia researcher, found evidence that clozapine, an antipsychotic that may be more effective for psychosis than any other medication, may have more metabolic side effects for African Americans (Henderson et al. 2015). Dr. Rahn Bailey, former president of the National Medical Association and chair of psychiatry at Wake Forest University, has done extensive work involving clinical trials, as has Dr. Napoleon Higgins, who is in private practice.

African Americans may in fact require different dosing. African Americans tend to be slower metabolizers of antidepressants and antipsychotics, which would lead to lower dose requirements. However, African Americans receive either the same or higher dosing, suggesting that provider preference and misconceptions rather than patient needs may be determining treatment (Primm and Lawson 2010). Such considerations should be given to other psychotropic medications as well. Dr. Samuel Okpaku, president of BPA, was one of the first using in vitro research to show that African Americans metabolize lithium differently. It was subsequently shown that these differences have an impact on clinical dosing of lithium in African Americans.

While the importance of participation of people of color in these studies continues to be shown, some investigators claim that participants of color cannot be found, often because of a lack of knowledge, social contacts, or awareness of how to reach out to people of color (Primm and Lawson 2010). African American investigators have consistently met their goals in recruitment for clinical trials and included African Americans in studies.

Research Participation

Barriers

Multiple studies have shown that African Americans are often reluctant to participate in clinical trials or other research studies (Primm and Lawson 2010).

Yet there is a need for increased population diversity in clinical trials (Mervis 2016). Historical mistreatment, including the Tuskegee syphilis study, does not encourage research participation (Roy 1995). Dr. Evaristus Nwulia, a professor at Howard University and internationally known for research in the genetics of psychiatric disorders, found that even the African American volunteers in a psychiatric genetic study had concerns about how the data would be used (Nwulia et al. 2011). Furthermore, lack of information about research and about mental disorders further contributes to lack of participation (Murphy and Thompson 2009). Yet other research shows that African Americans will participate as often as other groups when given the opportunity, despite fears that research may be harmful. As we showed earlier, African American investigators are also important in increasing participation.

Solutions

African American psychiatrists also encourage research in areas that strongly impact our communities, especially in areas that often do not generate interest in general psychiatry. Moreover, African American patients often seek treatment outside of specialized mental health centers and in settings where research is not encouraged or is rarely done. U.S. jails and prisons hold a disproportionate number of individuals with substance abuse and mental health issues (Office of the Surgeon General et al. 2001). In addition, racial and ethnic minorities, in particular African Americans, are overrepresented in the criminal justice system (Thompson et al. 2016). There is further evidence of racial disparities in mental health treatment among incarcerated populations; persons of color are less likely than white inmates to receive treatment (Thompson et al. 2016). These intersections of race, mental health, and criminal justice provide additional avenues for research to address the needs of African Americans. In many communities the criminal justice system often serves or houses more mentally ill individuals, particularly African Americans, than the mental health system (Office of the Surgeon General et al. 2001). This type of research could also focus on police encounters, access to care, research on mental health services for populations in the criminal justice system, and mental health treatment for formerly incarcerated individuals. Psychiatrists such as Dr. Donald Williams, former chair of the department at Michigan State University, and Dr. Rahn Bailey have contributed to research in such settings. The correctional setting, especially with parolees, has been important for myself and Dr. Tanya Alim, an associate professor at Howard University, to address issues of drug abuse, recidivism, and AIDS.

Violence has had a significant impact on the African American community but has faced strong headwinds as a subject for research. National legislation has been instituted to limit research on gun violence. Nevertheless, Dr. Carl Bell has continued to promote violence as a public health issue and has conducted groundbreaking research (Bell 2017). Primary care settings are where African Americans overwhelmingly seek mental health services (Office of the Surgeon General et al. 2001). Dr. Tanya Alim and Dr. Glenda Wrenn, at Morehouse School of Medicine, have done high-quality psychiatric research in these settings (Alim et al. 2006). Moreover, there is limited research involving the church, despite the relevance of the church to the African American community (Primm and Lawson 2010). The church often is a key site to address mental health needs (see Chapter 17 in this book). Dr. Sidney Hankerson has carried out quantitative studies involving church members.

Substance abuse has emerged as an important area of research for psychiatry. Problems such as alcoholism served as important areas of research by psychiatrists such as Dr. Bankole Johnson, chair at the University of Maryland, and Dr. Deborah Deas, who is now dean of the University of California, Riverside School of Medicine. Dr. Alim and I have carried out multiple studies involving opiate and cocaine users in the Washington, D.C., area (Mbaba et al. 2018). Cocaine has long been a concern in the African American community, and its association with violence, and opiate use has become a key area of concern because of its association with AIDS and hepatitis C and its association in recent years with substantially increased mortality.

Child psychiatry has often not encouraged research. Yet numerous African American psychiatrists have made key contributions, including Dr. Jeanne Spurlock, who mentored many individuals as chair at Meharry Medical College and as deputy medical director at the APA, and Dr. Gale Mattox, as chair at Morehouse School of Medicine Department of Psychiatry: both encouraged African American participation in clinical trials. The late Dr. Harry Wright, who was a well-regarded teacher and clinician, played a key role in identifying the putative gene for autism, and Dr. Deas did extensive research with adolescent substance abusers.

At the other end of the age continuum, the elderly have not received their share of research. In recent years, as life expectancy has improved, it has become increasingly clear that there are vast areas of inquiry that need to be researched in African Americans. Dr. Fran Baker has made her career studying African American elders and has made substantial contributions to an understudied area (Baker and Grady-Weliky 1999).

Research Support: Solutions

As noted, ensuring adequate research funding and having a culture that supports research are crucial. Federal funding has been particularly difficult to gain for researchers despite multiple programs directed to support minorities (Mervis 2016). One outcome of the African American psychiatrists' confrontation with the APA in 1969 was the advocacy by the APA for an Office of Minority

Affairs at NIMH and later at other institutes. Also, there have been ongoing efforts to get African Americans on study committees. A particularly useful program was the minority supplement program, later the diversity supplement program, in which an individual could be funded to work with a funded investigator. One fruitful effort was to get a section chief in the intramural program, the federally supported research component that develops research activities within the national institutes, rather than to fund investigators with extramural grants, to support projects by independent investigators at other institutions such as colleges and universities. Dr. Jean Cadet, an established substance abuse and AIDS researcher, became the first African American psychiatry chief at the National Institute on Drug Abuse (NIDA) and as such was very influential in determining the direction of NIDA research.

A key avenue to securing research funding has been forming a partnership with an individual or organization with existing funding. An area where such partnerships have been successful are historically black colleges and universities (HBCUs). HBCUs served as early sites to address racial disparities in care for mental illness and also to educate the community. Founded shortly after the end of the Civil War, both Howard University and Meharry Medical College provided training for African American clinicians, including psychiatrists and other mental health workers. Both institutions were often considered ahead of their time in promoting community mental health care for African Americans. In 1957, Dr. E.Y. Williams started the department of psychiatry at Howard University College of Medicine. The department included a biopsychosocial model of African American patients that addressed such issues as racism and discrimination. Shortly after, Dr. Lloyd Elam founded the department of psychiatry at Meharry Medical College, which also addressed the impact of racism on mental health. Both departments had faculty who were actively involved in their local communities and offered services to the indigent at a time when many mental health services were absent in African American communities. However, both institutions often had difficulty promoting research because of their clinical and teaching missions. The HBCU medical schools were not able to get R01 and other grant support until recently. Dr. Bailey was able to develop a clinical trial program at Meharry, Dr. Mattox encouraged clinical trials at Morehouse on HIV, and I initially was able to do the same at Howard. Charles R. Drew University of Medicine and Science, through its strong AIDS research with Dr. Eric Bing, a partnership that we had with the intramural program at NIMH, and the partnership of Morehouse with NIMH, led to most of the medical school HBCUs eventually getting R01 and other grants. The HBCUs continue to be important because of their role in training future investigators, their relationship with our community, and their historical commitment to the underserved. The Department of Veterans Affairs/Veterans Health Administration represents another key opportunity, because African Americans are overrepresented in the system. It also has its own research infrastructure. During the

Clinton administration, the Veterans Administration system, through a presidential executive order, was asked to partner with HBCUs on research. That partnership is ongoing and has been effective in promoting research activity and encouraging investigators. The Congressional Black Caucus Veterans Braintrust, of which I am a member, plays a major role in facilitating this program.

We noted that pharmaceutical industry support can be crucial for funding in the absence of federal funding. Unfortunately, in recent years industry support, especially for studies involving central nervous system (CNS) drugs, has been extremely competitive as more companies have shifted their support to studies involving drugs for other, less-costly disease states. However, psychiatrists have gained leadership positions in the industry, and this may have long-term gains. Dr. Freda Lewis-Hall, an African American psychiatrist who is the executive vice president and chief medical officer for Pfizer, the largest pharmaceutical company in the world, has been a strong advocate for CNS clinical trials and community participation. Dr. William Carson is president and chief executive officer of pharmaceutical development and commercialization for Otsuka America. He has played a strong role in including African American investigators and patients in clinical trials, supporting programs of interest to the communities we serve, and developing products relevant to our community needs.

Conclusion

While black psychiatrists who are primarily researchers are only a minority among minorities, they have played a key role in reducing mental health misinformation for patients and served as their patients' advocates in directing the direction of research to their needs. Moreover, they have clearly influenced policy. Their findings are leading to better treatments and access to treatment. Yet barriers still remain, and the numbers remain small. We are now seeing emerging leadership in research funders. The awareness of the problem and the creativity of committed individuals beckon to a bright future.

References

Adebimpe VR: Overview: white norms and psychiatric diagnosis of black patients. Am J Psychiatry 138(3):279–285, 1981 7008631

Alim TN, Graves E, Mellman TA, et al: Trauma exposure, posttraumatic stress disorder and depression in an African-American primary care population. J Natl Med Assoc 98(10):1630–1636, 2006 17052054

American Psychiatric Association: Diagnostic and Statistical Manual of Mental Disorders, 3rd Edition. Washington, DC, American Psychiatric Association, 1980

American Psychiatric Association: Diagnostic and Statistical Manual of Mental Disorders, 4th Edition. Washington, DC, American Psychiatric Association, 1994

American Psychiatric Association: Diagnostic and Statistical Manual of Mental Disorders, 5th Edition. Arlington, VA, American Psychiatric Association, 2013

Baker FM, Grady-Weliky TA: Black psychiatric researchers, in Black Psychiatrists and American Psychiatrists. Edited by Spurlock J. Washington, DC, American Psychiatric Press, 1999, pp 141–152

Bell CC: Lessons learned from 50 years of violence prevention activities in the African American community. J Natl Med Assoc 109(4):224–237, 2017 29173929

Fuller SC: A study of the miliary plaques found in brains of the aged. American Journal of Insanity 28(2), 1911

Gara MA, Vega WA, Arndt S, et al: Influence of patient race and ethnicity on clinical assessment in patients with affective disorders. Arch Gen Psychiatry 69(6):593–600, 2012 22309972

Ginther DK, Schaffer WT, Schnell J, et al: Race, ethnicity, and NIH research awards. Science 333(6045):1015–1019, 2011 21852498

Griffith EEH: Race and Excellence: My Dialogue With Chester Pierce. Iowa City, University of Iowa Press, 1999

Henderson DC, Vincenzi B, Andrea NV, et al: Pathophysiological mechanisms of increased cardiometabolic risk in people with schizophrenia and other severe mental illnesses. Lancet Psychiatry 2(5):452–464, 2015 26360288

Lawson WB: Racial and ethnic factors in psychiatric research. Hosp Community Psychiatry 37(1):50–54, 1986 2867967

Mbaba M, Brown SE, Wooditch A, et al: Prevalence, diagnosis, and treatment rates of mood disorders among opioid users under criminal justice supervision. Subst Use Misuse 15:1–10, 2018 29333954

Mervis J: Mentoring's moment. Science 353(6303):980–982, 2016 27701098

Metzl J: The Protest Psychosis: How Schizophrenia Became a Black Disease. Boston, MA, Beacon Press, 2009

Murphy E, Thompson A: An exploration of attitudes among black Americans towards psychiatric genetic research. Psychiatry 72(2):177–194, 2009 19614555

Nwulia EA, Hipolito MM, Aamir S, et al: Ethnic disparities in the perception of ethical risks from psychiatric genetic studies. Am J Med Genet B Neuropsychiatr Genet 156B(5):569–580, 2011 21595007

Office of the Surgeon General, Center for Mental Health Services, National Institute of Mental Health: Mental Health: Culture, Race, and Ethnicity. A Supplement to Mental Health: A Report of the Surgeon General. Rockville, MD, Substance Abuse and Mental Health Services Administration, 2001

Ozarin E: Solomon Carter Fuller: first black psychiatrist. Psychiatric News, September 6, 2002. Available at: https://psychnews.psychiatryonline.org/doi/full/10.1176%2Fpn.37.17.0019. Assessed October 1, 2017.

Pierce CM: Black psychiatry one year after Miami. J Natl Med Assoc 62(6):471–473, 1970 5493608

Primm AB, Lawson WB: African Americans, in Disparities in Psychiatric Care: Clinical and Cross-Cultural Perspectives. Edited by Ruiz P, Primm A. Baltimore, MD, Lippincott Williams & Wilkins, 2010, pp 19–29

Roy B: The Tuskegee Syphilis Experiment: biotechnology and the administrative state. J Natl Med Assoc 87(1):56–67, 1995 7869408

Smith EN, Bloss CS, Badner JA, et al: Genome-wide association study of bipolar disorder in European American and African American individuals. Mol Psychiatry 14(8):755–763, 2009 19488044

Thompson M, Newell S, Carlson MJ: Race and access to mental health and substance abuse treatment in the criminal justice system. J Offender Rehabil 55(2):69–94, 2016

CHAPTER 17
THE BLACK CHURCH AND MENTAL HEALTH

Sidney H. Hankerson, M.D., M.B.A.
Eunice C. Wong, Ph.D.
Kenneth Polite, Ph.D.

ACCORDING TO THE PEW FORUM on Religion and Public Life's most recent demographic study of the religious landscape in the United States, African Americans report the greatest degree of religious belief among all the racial-ethnic groups across the United States (Pew Research Center 2015). Specifically, 97% of all African Americans reported belief in God, with 83% reporting belief in God with absolute certainty, and 75% of African Americans reported religion was very important in their lives, compared with 53% of people in the general population. Moreover, 83% of African Americans reported that they attended religious services, compared with 69% of the general U.S. population, with 47% attending at least once a week versus 36% of the general population. These data, along with African Americans' reliance on extended family members and friends (i.e., informal support systems) when faced with psychiatric problems, suggest that black churches are excellent portals for reaching African Americans to implement mental health interventions.

Despite high rates of religious attendance and importance, African Americans underutilize professional mental health services relative to their white counterparts (Hankerson et al. 2011). Factors that contribute to these racial treatment disparities include distrust of providers, limited access to care, financial constraints, high attrition rates, and the stigma of mental illness (Hankerson et al. 2015). African Americans who do seek professional treatment are more likely to receive lower-quality care and are significantly less likely to receive guideline-concordant care (González et al. 2010). Given the enormous individual and societal costs associated with mental disorders (Murray and Lopez 1997), exploring the role of African American faith-based organizations is an essential component of black mental health.

Thus, in this chapter, we have two overarching objectives. First, we briefly review the origins of the black church and examine its role in mental health service provision. Second, we provide case examples of how two black churches in Los Angeles are addressing the mental health needs of their congregants and surrounding community.

Brief History of the Black Church

The term *black church* is classically defined as the collection of seven major historically black denominations of the Christian faith in the United States (Lincoln and Mamiya 1990): African Methodist Episcopal (AME) Church; African Methodist Episcopal Zion (AMEZ) Church; the Christian Methodist Episcopal Church; the National Baptist Convention USA. Inc. (NBA); the National Baptist Convention of America (NBCA); the Progressive National Baptist Convention (PNBC); and the Church of God in Christ (COGIC). These dominations encompass approximately 65,000–75,000 churches in the United States, with an estimated membership between 20 and 24 million. Roughly 80% of all African American Christians are projected to belong to one of these seven denominations (Lincoln and Mamiya 1990).

Following the Union's victory in the Civil War, the black church emerged as the spiritual, cultural, economic, and political hub of African American communities. Black churches had multiple roles. A primary goal of the church was to provide spiritual and emotional catharsis for people of African descent who endured the harrowing experience of the transatlantic slave trade, the brutality of slavery, and the humiliation of being initially defined by the U.S. Constitution as "three-fifths" human (Lincoln and Mamiya 1990). This catharsis would often take place through energetic singing and dancing, passionate call and response between preacher and audience, and loud shouting by congregants (Griffith and Mathewson 1981). Another role of the black church was to promote the economic development of African American communities. Churches initiated the creation of schools, insurance companies, banks, and housing developments in black neighborhoods. The central objective of the black church, however, was the personal conversion of the individual member to become a follower of Jesus Christ. The Afro-Christian conversion experience, however, took on a unique transcendent quality that was strongly influenced by African culture. Numerous aspects of black culture, including music, art, and language, have religious undertones. Throughout its history, the black church has focused simultaneously on personal conversion and social/racial equity (Lincoln and Mamiya 1990).

Perhaps the most recognized illustration of the black church's involvement in promoting social justice is its role in the Civil Rights Movement of the 1950s and 1960s. Renowned figures of the movement, including the Rev. Dr. Martin Luther King Jr., Rev. Ralph Abernathy, Rev. Joseph Lowery, and Rev. Jesse Jackson, first established themselves as leaders in African American churches. Churches functioned as operational hubs for numerous aspects of the movement, from the organized bus boycotts to community gatherings to promote higher wages for laborers. The theology of black churches in the Civil Rights Movement focused on freedom and equality. Indeed, Congressman John Lewis described the moral shape of the Civil Rights Movement as "nothing less than the Christian concept of the Kingdom of God on earth" and as a "redemptive society" that addresses social divisions (Marsh 2005, p. 3).

Those opposed to racial integration also recognized the centrality of the black church in the Civil Rights Movement. Consequently, numerous churches in the South were bombed throughout the struggle for racial equality. Perhaps the most infamous bombing occurred at the 16th Street Baptist Church in Birmingham, Alabama. On Sunday morning, September 15, 1963, a bomb tore through the basement of the church, killing 4 young girls and injuring 22 others. This tragedy proved to be a turning point that led to the passage of the landmark Civil Rights Act of 1964. For a more in-depth exploration of the historical role of the black church, we refer readers to classic texts by Lincoln and Mamiya (1990) and Taylor et al. (2004) and the more recent volume by Charles Marsh (2005).

The Black Church and Mental Health Service Provision

The black church has a long history of addressing the health concerns of its members. "Health ministry" committees have evolved to become formal groups of church leaders and lay members who focus on health education and service provision for congregants (Williams et al. 2014). Church-based health promotion (CBHP), the central task of health ministries, is designed to provide measurable benefits to individuals through education, screening, and treatment. Programs involving CBHP have focused on numerous medical conditions among African Americans, including diabetes, cancer, obesity, cardiovascular disease, and HIV/AIDS (DeHaven et al. 2004). As such, CBHP has received growing attention as a way to provide culturally sensitive community-based health programs (Campbell et al. 2007). Importantly, a meticulous review of faith-based programs concluded that such programs are effective at improving health outcomes for participants (DeHaven et al. 2004).

Despite the potential of CBHP to address mental health problems, the current literature on church-based programs for mental disorders among African Americans is sparse. Hankerson and Weissman (2012) conducted a systematic review of articles to identify African American church–based studies published in scholarly journals between January 1, 1980, and December 31, 2009. Inclusion criteria were as follows: studies were conducted in a church; the primary objective involved assessment, perceptions and attitudes, education, prevention, group support, or treatment for DSM-IV (American Psychiatric Association 1994) mental disorders or their correlates; the number of participants was reported; qualitative or quantitative data were reported; and African Americans were the target population. Of 1,451 studies identified, only eight met the inclusion criteria (Hankerson and Weissman 2012). Five studies focused on substance-related disorders, six were designed to assess the effects of a specific intervention, and six targeted adults. One study focused on depression, and it was limited by a small sample size of seven participants. Thus, there is an emerging opportunity for black churches to provide concrete mental health services.

Clergy as Mental Health Providers

Clergy have an invaluable role in the U.S. mental healthcare delivery system. Findings from the National Comorbidity Survey, a nationally representative general population survey of 8,098 adults in the United States, showed that a higher percentage of people sought help for mental disorders from clergy (25%) compared with psychiatrists (16.7%) or general medical doctors (16.7%) (Wang et al. 2003). Clergy provide the only source of mental health care for many low-income patients (Molock et al. 2008). Clergy encounter a diverse range of psychological issues, including death and dying, anxiety, marital problems, substance use, and depression (Moran et al. 2005).

African American clergy in particular are the primary source of mental healthcare for socioeconomically diverse black adults and are trusted "gatekeepers" for referrals to mental health specialists. In one study, approximately 50% of African Americans utilizing only one source of mental healthcare sought help from clergy providers (Neighbors et al. 1998). A detailed analysis of African American clergy in a large city revealed that clergy averaged more than 6 hours of counseling work per week and often addressed serious problems similar to those seen by secular mental health professionals (Young et al. 2003).

Case Examples

We now describe how two churches in California are addressing the mental health needs of their congregants and surrounding community. These examples are by no means representative of all black churches, which we have described above as a heterogeneous group of institutions. However, our case examples highlight two innovative faith-based efforts to increase access to mental health care among African Americans.

Faithful Central Bible Church

The Faithful Central Bible Church (FCBC) was founded as Faithful Central Missionary Baptist Church in 1936 with a membership of 18 people. FCBC is located in Inglewood, California, a municipality adjacent to Los Angeles. It currently serves more than 5,000 congregants, most of whom are African American. Bishop Kenneth C. Ulmer is the senior pastor and is a nationally recognized preacher and educator.

Champion Counseling Center

Bishop Ulmer's generous support helped make the Champion Counseling Center (CCC) a reality. CCC is a faith-based community mental health center affiliated with FCBC. While many CCC clients are Christian, one does not have to be a Christian or a member of Faithful Central to receive services. The mission of CCC is to serve both the community and the church. The CCC website describes the agency as follows:

> The Champion Counseling Center (CCC) provides educational and counseling services to meet the needs of children, teens, adults, couples, and families. Our trained staff and professional counselors offer the application of sound psychological practices within the context of a therapeutic environment. Trained in the integration of Theology and Psychology, we utilize proven, researched psychological and educational techniques that provide real-world solutions to the problems clients face. Our interventions are culturally sensitive and individually tailored to help individuals, groups, and families reach their full potential. (Faithful Central Bible Church 2018)

History of Champion Counseling Center

In the spring of 2003, one of the pastors at FCBC approached Kenneth Polite, Ph.D., about mental health referrals to meet the psychological needs of a FCBC congregant. Dr. Polite, who is both an ordained minister and a licensed clinical psychologist, was an active member at FCBC. Dr. Polite discussed ways to address the mental health needs of the broader FCBC congregation with his psychological assistant, Erica Holmes, Ph.D. They decided that Dr. Holmes would begin seeing clients in the church's lay counseling center (defunct) under Dr. Polite's supervision. This arrangement, in which Dr. Holmes saw clients and Dr. Polite provided clinical supervision, lasted for nearly 2 years.

Organizationally, CCC was designed to have two major divisions: lay services and professional services. Two lay-run services already existed: premarital education classes and lay counseling sessions. The lay premarital education classes were run by the Marriage Mentors Ministry. These classes were actively serving the congregants of FCBC and members of other churches in greater Los Angeles. The lay counseling ministry, referred to as "the Encouragers," had become inactive and needed to be revived. The Encouragers provide prayer and support over the course of 10 sessions.

The professional services division had to be built from the ground up. The guiding psychologists decided that psychological and educational services would be offered for all age groups and most psychiatric diagnoses, with the exception of severe and persistent mental illness (e.g., schizophrenia). People identified as having severe mental illness received referrals to community mental health clinics and were not eligible for psychological treatment at CCC.

Dr. Holmes spearheaded the development of a training manual that outlined policies and procedures for running a counseling center. CCC developed training agreements with a broad group of universities that train psychologists and/or marriage and family therapists, including the following: Azusa Pacific University; Biola University/Rosemead School of Psychology; Alliant International University/California School of Professional Psychology; Pepperdine University; California State University, Dominguez Hills; and California State University, Northridge. The trainees from these institutions provide the majority of professional services offered under the direct supervision of Drs. Holmes and Polite.

How Champion Counseling Center Operates

CCC is housed in the church's three-story office building and occupies approximately 3,500 square feet of space. CCC has nine consulting rooms, two group rooms, a seminar room that seats 50 people, a waiting room, a file room, and an administrative office. In 2016, the staff, trainees, and volunteers of CCC provided more than 6,000 hours of service to the church and the community.

When a client calls for service at CCC, he or she is placed on an intake log and later given a telephone interview by one or more of the trainees. The interview results are reviewed by one of the supervising psychologists, and two initial determinations are made. First, it is determined if the case is appropriate to be seen in the counseling center. If the case does not meet the criteria, the caller is provided with three referrals. Those cases deemed appropriate for CCC are assigned to a clinician. Second, a determination is made about which clinician at CCC will provide care for this particular client. The training needs of supervisees, clinical severity of the case, and clients' and clinicians' schedules are all considered in this second determination.

West Angeles Church of God in Christ

West Angeles Church of God in Christ (COGIC) was founded by C.E. Church Sr. in 1943 inside a small storefront on Vermont Avenue in the heart of Los

Angeles. Under the leadership of Bishop Charles E. Blake Sr., West Angeles's current pastor, the church has grown exponentially, with a present-day membership of more than 22,000 congregants. The church has been recognized as one of the fastest-growing churches in the nation, with extensive ministry and outreach services. West Angeles is deeply involved not only in providing for the spiritual life of its people but also in providing more than 80 programs for the psychological, social, and economic enhancement of the community.

West Angeles Counseling Center

The West Angeles Counseling Center, a ministry of West Angeles COGIC, was established more than 20 years ago and provides specialized classes, workshops, support groups, and client sessions conducted by peer, pastoral, professional, and crisis intervention counselors. The Counseling Center recognizes the trichotomy of man and provides services that consider aspects of the spirit, soul, and body. The mission of the Counseling Center is to be innovative in its purpose, and its purpose is to help "heal the hurting." Healing is facilitated by providing counseling and by empowering individuals to make rational and healthy life choices for a more abundant life. Empowerment comes through spiritual and relational education, cognitive redirection, coping skills, and emotional management, which enable individuals to work through the contradictions between wholeness and dysfunctional behavior. The Counseling Center utilizes an integrated treatment model that combines traditional psychological approaches, systems theory, and spiritual interventions. The Counseling Center has opened its doors to countless numbers in the community as well as to those who have traveled long distances to seek its services. The Counseling Center is currently under the directorship of Ms. Paula Litt.

Since the Counseling Center is colocated with West Angeles Church, additional partnerships have been established as a result of ongoing referrals to the various internal and external programs. Referrals have been made to Weight Watchers; Women, Infants, and Children (WIC); Maternal Support Services; West Central Department of Mental Health; Kaiser Permanente; area universities; community mental health and healthcare providers; community-based organizations; law enforcement agencies; and other faith-based entities. Organizationally, collaboration is a hallmark of the West Angeles Church, as the Counseling Center was established as a result of Bishop Blake's desire to integrate psychological approaches with spiritual interventions, coupled with an outcry from church members and community leaders to help families with overwhelming mental health needs. While examples of West Angeles's collaborative efforts are numerous, a few follow to highlight the efforts of the Counseling Center.

United by a mission to improve health outcomes through the development of sustainable infrastructure, client education, and new research, today West

Angeles continues its trend through various collaborations such as the Faith-Based Mental Health and Substance Abuse (FMHSA) Collaborative. The primary goal of the FMHSA Collaborative has been to advocate, develop, and implement regional collaborative programs to improve the health access and health outcomes faced by the West Angeles congregants and residents of the greater Los Angeles communities. The Counseling Center works with more than 175 churches (crossing denominational walls), community-based organizations, and other government agencies to empower their communities. West Angeles is committed to strengthening smaller churches and to being an agent of change within their own communities utilizing faith-based approaches.

Given the current economic climate and overwhelming demands on the local church, the FMHSA Collaborative continues to target the coordination and replication of faith-based models and approaches to reduce duplication of services and to ensure a focused approach to addressing critical healthcare needs. The model initially used by the FMHSA Collaborative was the Link Project, which highlighted faith-based models throughout Los Angeles County that could be easily replicated in other areas of need. The initial focus of the project was to provide comprehensive services to those who had been diagnosed with HIV/AIDS, cardiovascular disease, diabetes, or hypertension or who had an ongoing chronic disease that was being poorly managed. The project's goals were to improve health outcomes for patients in Los Angeles County; strengthen the collaborations of the faith-based communities with local healthcare providers; and, based on the lessons learned and assessment results, produce and distribute a generalizable model of care for implementing the SAVE model within the African American faith-based community.

West Angeles COGIC/RAND Partnership

In 2007, West Angeles COGIC participated in a community-based participatory research project, funded by the California Endowment, for purposes of planning and designing a "one stop" shop that would address mild-to-moderate depression and substance abuse for a South Central Los Angeles African American community (Wong et al. 2011). One of the major goals of the grant was to build a collaborative network between community and academic partners with the purpose of improving care for depression and substance abuse services to the Los Angeles African American community. A leadership group, along with community members representing diverse perspectives, was assembled and regularly convened to develop a plan to address the goals of the grant. The founding partners who largely composed the leadership group included West Angeles, the Los Angeles Ecumenical Congress, Kaiser Watts Counseling and Learning Center, Los Angeles County Department of Mental Health, Healthy African American Families, RAND, and University of California, Los Angeles. The project ended with a feedback roundtable report to the community, which occurred in October 2008. Since then West Angeles (Paula Litt) and RAND (Eunice Wong) have continued to meet regularly to expand on a mutual interest in growing the capacity of faith-based organizations to serve the mental health needs of the Los Angeles African American community.

Conclusion

The black church is a heterogeneous group of institutions that have historically served the spiritual, social, economic, and political needs of its members. Multiple elements of the black church are woven into the fabric of African American culture. African American religious congregations have the most extensive involvement in the delivery of social service programs, including counseling (Blank et al. 2002). Moreover, findings indicate that black religious congregations may be more willing and ready to engage in collaborative efforts with mental health providers (Young et al. 2003). Church-based health programs specifically geared toward mental disorders among African Americans, however, are at a fledgling stage of development. On the basis of our brief literature review and case reports, we have identified lessons learned and suggest areas of future development.

Pastoral support for faith-based mental health services can go a long way toward destigmatizing psychological services. At both FCBC and West Angeles COGIC, the lead pastor provided unwavering support toward the implementation and expansion of mental health services. Importantly, pastors can earmark funds specifically for CBHP, which can help to overcome a major hurdle to starting new initiatives. Recruiting the lead pastor as a local "champion" in support of health programs has been cited as a key factor in successfully establishing and sustaining these initiatives in black churches (Campbell et al. 2007).

Engaging clergy in CBHP for mental disorders, in addition to their role as program champions, leverages their trusted role as counselors and gatekeepers for referrals to mental health specialists. In the United States, more people contact clergy for mental health problems than psychiatrists, psychologists, or general medical practitioners (Wang et al. 2003). However, clergy may be underprepared to accurately assess common mental disorders (Moran et al. 2005). To address this limitation, efforts should be made to improve clergy's knowledge about common mental disorders. This can be done on at least two fronts. First, introductory-level pastoral counseling could be a required course for all seminary students. Second, research could be conducted to test the feasibility of training clergy in evidence-based mental health interventions. One such initiative is to train clergy in Mental Health First Aid, a public education program designed to teach people the signs and symptoms of common mental health problems and promote help seeking.

Both churches in our case examples—Faithful Central Bible Church and West Angeles Church of God in Christ—also benefited from leveraging the professional expertise of their own members. Both are classified as megachurches, defined as having more than 2,000 people attend Sunday services (Bopp and Webb 2012). Given the financial resources and vocational diversity of members at megachurches, these institutions appear particularly well suited to implement or expand CBHP for mental health problems. Asking church members who have professional or personal experience with mental health problems to participate in CBHP initiatives can build momentum for program rollout. Future studies could identify characteristics of church congregants that work with CBHP. This information could help other congregations identify congregants who are best suited to replicate mental health programs at their institutions.

In conclusion, increasing mental healthcare among African Americans is a complex issue for which there is no single solution. We argue that the black church can play a central role in mental health service provision, but the current literature on CBHP for mental disorders is extremely limited. We have highlighted how two innovative megachurches in Los Angeles are addressing the mental health needs of their congregations and surrounding communities. Additional work, especially that which utilizes participatory approaches, is needed to explore opportunities and limitations of church-based mental healthcare for African Americans.

References

American Psychiatric Association: Diagnostic and Statistical Manual of Mental Disorders, 4th Edition. Washington, DC, American Psychiatric Association, 1994

Blank MB, Mahmood M, Fox JC, et al: Alternative mental health services: the role of the black church in the South. Am J Public Health 92(10):1668–1672, 2002 12356619

Bopp M, Webb B: Health promotion in megachurches: an untapped resource with megareach? Health Promot Pract 13(5):679–686, 2012 22491133

Campbell MK, Hudson MA, Resnicow K, et al: Church-based health promotion interventions: evidence and lessons learned. Annu Rev Public Health 28:213–234, 2007 17155879

DeHaven MJ, Hunler IB, Wilder L, et al: Health programs in faith-based organizations: are they effective? Am J Public Health 94(6):1030–1036, 2004 15249311

Faithful Central Bible Church: Champion Counseling Center. Available at: https://www.faithfulcentral.com/ccc. Accessed March 16, 2018.

González HM, Vega WA, Williams DR, et al: Depression care in the United States: too little for too few. Arch Gen Psychiatry 67(1):37–46, 2010 20048221

Griffith EE, Mathewson MA: Communitas and charisma in a black church service. J Natl Med Assoc 73(11):1023–1027, 1981 7310918

Hankerson SH, Weissman MM: Church-based health programs for mental disorders among African Americans: a review. Psychiatr Serv 63(3):243–249, 2012 22388529

Hankerson SH, Fenton MC, Geier TJ, et al: Racial differences in symptoms, comorbidity, and treatment for major depressive disorder among black and white adults. J Natl Med Assoc 103(7):576–584, 2011 21999032

Hankerson SH, Suite D, Bailey RK: Treatment disparities among African American men with depression: implications for clinical practice. J Health Care Poor Underserved 26(1):21–34, 2015 25702724

Lincoln CE, Mamiya LH: The Black Church in the African American Experience. Durham, NC, Duke University Press, 1990

Marsh C: The Beloved Community: How Faith Shapes Social Justice, From the Civil Rights Movement to Today. New York, Basic Books, 2005

Molock SD, Matlin S, Barksdale C, et al: Developing suicide prevention programs for African American youth in African American churches. Suicide Life Threat Behav 38(3):323–333, 2008 18611131

Moran M, Flannelly KJ, Weaver AJ, et al: A study of pastoral care, referral, and consultation practices among clergy in four settings in the New York City area. Pastoral Psychol 53(3):255–266, 2005

Murray CJ, Lopez AD: Alternative projections of mortality and disability by cause 1990–2020: Global Burden of Disease Study. Lancet 349(9064):1498–1504, 1997 9167458

Neighbors HW, Musick MA, Williams DR: The African American minister as a source of help for serious personal crises: bridge or barrier to mental health care? Health Educ Behav 25(6):759–777, 1998 9813746

Pew Research Center: America's Changing Religious Landscape, May 12, 2015. Available at: http://www.pewforum.org/2015/05/12/americas-changing-religious-landscape/. Accessed December 2017.

Taylor RJ, Chatters LM, Levin J: Religion in the Lives of African Americans: Social, Psychological, and Health Perspectives. Thousand Oaks, CA, Sage, 2004

Wang PS, Berglund PA, Kessler RC: Patterns and correlates of contacting clergy for mental disorders in the United States. Health Serv Res 38(2):647–673, 2003 12785566

Williams L, Gorman R, Hankerson S: Implementing a mental health ministry committee in faith-based organizations: the Promoting Emotional Wellness and Spirituality Program. Soc Work Health Care 53(4):414–434, 2014 24717187

Wong EC, Chung B, Stover G, et al: Addressing unmet mental health and substance abuse needs: a partnered planning effort between grassroots community agencies, faith-based organizations, service providers, and academic institutions. Ethn Dis 21(3 suppl l):S1–107-13, 2011 22352088

Young JL, Griffith EE, Williams DR: The integral role of pastoral counseling by African-American clergy in community mental health. Psychiatr Serv 54(5):688–692, 2003 12719499

PART III

Training of Black Mental Health Care Providers

CHAPTER 18
PSYCHIATRIC TRAINING AND BLACK MENTAL HEALTH

Iverson Bell Jr., M.D.
Anthony P.S. Guerrero, M.D.
Jyotsna S. Ranga, M.D.

THE PRACTICE OF PSYCHIATRY has always intersected with the need to understand cultural and social norms. The practitioner views the patient from the perspective of his or her own culture and environment and must try to understand and empathize with the patient's own background. Also, the patient must feel comfortable discussing issues with the psychiatrist and feel understood. Success in treatment depends on understanding this interaction. These differing perspectives and understanding must be part of the process of training to become a psychiatrist.

The inherent stress that comes with being a member of a minority with the history of slavery and ongoing racism is widely acknowledged and well studied. A number of studies indicate, however, that the black American minority has apparent rates of mental illness similar to those of the majority (white) Americans when one considers the overall prevalence of mental health conditions (Regier et al. 1984). Other studies show that in virtually every field of medicine, black patients as a group have worse treatment outcomes (Tweedy 2015).

Trust of the doctors may be part of the reason for these conflicting statements. As Tweedy (2015) noted, "Black patients, compared with those of other races, tend to be far less trusting of physicians and their medical advice, and as a rule, black patients are more likely to feel comfortable with black doctors. Studies have shown that they are more likely to seek them out for treatment, and to report higher satisfaction with their care" (p. 1). Spurlock (1982) described the need to promote psychiatric training directed at a better understanding of blacks and the transference-countertransference patterns that impact the service provided to them. She noted that "a curriculum that is culturally relevant for black trainees and patients should be considered relevant for all trainees and patients and be integrated into general psychiatric residency training programs" (p. 163). She recounted numerous prior attempts to develop a model curriculum specifically designed to train residents to treat black Americans. They include Sharpley's presentation at the Solomon Fuller Roundtable Conference in 1977, published as "Treatment Issues: Foreign Medical Graduates and Black Patient Populations" (Sharpley 1977); a special session at the 1977 American Psychiatric Association Annual Meeting; and a training conference sponsored by Black Psychiatrists of America for black psychiatry residents and postresidency psychiatrists in 1980. Others (Jones et al. 1970; Kramer 1973) have written about the deficiencies in traditional residency training programs.

In short, we can all be more effective practitioners when all of the cultural/ racial stressors are considered. Practicing psychiatry from a cross-cultural perspective can address the physical and mental health needs of minority individuals and the needs of the community. Disparities in healthcare between communities become more visible and are more appropriately addressed when differences in culture are considered. The skill to understand and use cross-cultural psychiatry can be taught to resident trainees and practicing psychiatrists, though it is not clear if there is a best method to teach this.

From Culture-Bound Syndromes to Cultural Formulation Interviews

Psychiatric thought has always been influenced by the social norms of the times. Benjamin Rush, the psychiatrist, was also an abolitionist and a signatory of the Declaration of Independence. From his perspective, black Americans suffered from "Negritude," a "disease of pigmentation similar to leprosy and with proper treatment, blacks could be cured and become white" (Butterfield 1951; Rush 1799). Other terms that were later used to describe the behavior of Africans and black American slaves were *drapetomania* and *dysaesthesia aethiopis* (Cartwright 1851). These so-called mental illnesses were said to be common to slaves and led to running away and "lack of work ethic." The treatments for these mental diseases were "whipping and prayer." This intentional blindness to the effects of slavery and the slave trade was self-serving and clearly not therapeutic. Later, psychiatrist Emil Kraepelin and neurologist Sigmund Freud noted cultural differences in presentation of mental illnesses. Dr. E.D. Wittkower began studying transcultural psychiatry to formalize the study of cross-cultural distinctions. He established "transcultural psychiatry" as a distinct discipline in 1955 (Wittkower 1964).

Subsequently, DSM-IV included and described "culture-bound syndromes" (American Psychiatric Association 1994). The more than two dozen "syndromes" in this list were thought to be specific to certain cultures, but there were often similarities in the symptoms of these syndromes. Kleinman noted that approximately 90% of DSM-IV categories were found in and were "culture-bound" to North America and Western Europe. The term *culture-bound syndrome*, however, was primarily applied to cultures outside of Euro-American society (Kleinman 1977). It appears that non-Euro-American cultures, and the psychopathology in those cultures, have been viewed as separate and distinct from the "normal." The designation of "culture-bound" was more likely to be applied to these other cultures.

The DSM-5 (American Psychiatric Association 2013) cultural issues subgroup reviewed culture-bound syndromes by looking at similar symptoms across cultural lines and attempted to standardize diagnoses. Dr. Anthony Guerrero, the former child and adolescent psychiatry training director at the University of Hawai'i, stated that "what the DSM-5 does not explicitly cover is the depth that a culture should be assessed outside the immediate patient/family. Clinicians often rely on the DSM-5 cultural formulation to cover and hopefully hardwire a lot of these points, however."

Challenges in Teaching Cross-Cultural Psychiatry

Different model curricula have been designed to teach transcultural (or cross-cultural) psychiatry. Seminars, readings, lectures, and interactive experiences are usually included. In this chapter we consider the methods and perspectives of two training programs in examining how the field of cross-cultural psychiatry can be examined and effectively taught. We also review how education has evolved to address these issues and the challenges for lifelong learning and maintenance of certification.

Dr. Guerrero advocates for a training curriculum that includes discussion, experiential sharing, and, to the degree of comfort of trainees, personal reflections. Although he works in a specific cultural environment, he understands that there is still a need for a dedicated effort to examine the role of culture and apply the tools available (e.g., DSM-5 Cultural Formulation Interview) to optimize patient care. An effective curriculum blends the history of a cultural group with the psychiatric knowledge of the group to reduce health disparities and inequities

(McDermott and Andrade 2011). To address health and mental health disparities, we must have an adequate and diverse workforce. This means developing a
curriculum that incorporates culture, diversity, and disparities reduction with
basic psychiatric knowledge. Psychiatric educators have a responsibility to ensure
that all trainees have opportunities to learn best practices in treating underserved
and underrepresented patients. They must also ensure that the future healthcare workforce includes students from underrepresented groups who have access
to academic and career development support.

Many training programs in the United States are multicultural, with training directors and residents from cultures that are not the majority. Dr. Guerrero
contends that in any multicultural setting, especially one where a particular
ethnocultural group has endured forced migration (slavery or other human trafficking) or colonization, one must understand the principles of integration, assimilation, marginalization, and separation. He suggests that certain questions
need to be considered:

- To what degree are languages other than English spoken in the community?
- What is the typical language spoken within the family, by whom, and in
  what settings (both inside and outside the home)?

In black communities one would also need to review what the methods of
communication are, how they might be different than expected, and how distress
is communicated. Cultures are not monolithic. A psychiatrist may be familiar
with interactions and communication in a northern black community, for example, but the physician must be aware that there are also differences in northern
black communities. Because of the different routes of post–Civil War migration, many modes of interactions and social values have migrated as well.

Model Curricula

Dr. Guerrero reports that as a nonindigenous voluntary immigrant entrusted with
leading a psychiatry department in a publicly supported medical school in Hawai'i,
he makes a special effort to ensure that teaching and research efforts address disparities affecting Native Hawaiians. He shares perspectives on acculturation and
biculturalism based on personal experiences in Hawai'i's "stew pot" (McDermott
and Andrade 2011). Although his curriculum was not designed specifically to
treat black patients, he proposes it as one model for a cross-cultural training curriculum and notes it addresses a number of issues in the design that must be considered regardless of the cultural identity of the population served:

- How should one address cultural differences?
- How does one establish sensitivity to different cultures?

- What methods may be used in comparing backgrounds, cross-cultural experiences, and social experiences?
- What are the individual and family experiences and values of the cultural group?
- How does one explore race/color feelings?

He also identifies some of the specific challenges and opportunities in teaching in a multicultural environment:

- The importance of asking about cultural identification rather than making assumptions based on appearance (especially since many people describe themselves as "multiracial")
- The need to consider and teach about the dynamics of cultural interfaces (e.g., integration vs. assimilation, marginalization, separation)
- The need to assess the "outside" culture in addition to the patient's/family's culture; the importance of learning the history of the patient's culture
- Most importantly, even though it is tempting to view the multiethnic "stew pot" as a level playing field, that there are genuine health disparities that must be addressed

Another one of the authors of this chapter, Dr. Jyotsna Ranga, has a different perspective and method of educating about cross-cultural psychiatry. Dr. Ranga is the training director for the Child and Adolescent Psychiatry Program at the University of Tennessee Health Science Center in Memphis (UTHSC). She sees the necessity of teaching "cultural humility" as an empathic method of understanding other cultures. Hook et al. (2013) conceptualize cultural humility as the "ability to maintain an interpersonal stance that is 'other-oriented' (or open to the other) in relation to aspects of cultural identity that are most important to the [person]."

Over the past decade, patient centeredness and cultural competence have gained much attention in healthcare delivery. In comparing patient centeredness and cultural competency, Saha et al. (2008) concluded that although these two concepts are different in terms of origins, histories, and foci, many of their core features are the same, and each approach results in improving the quality of healthcare not only for the individual patients but also for communities and population groups. It is critical to include these concepts in residency training to enhance residents' and fellows' confidence and comfort in interacting with patients from diverse cultural backgrounds.

UTHSC has an interesting cultural mix among residents. Demographically, Memphis is 63% black, 29% white, 6% Latino, and 1% Asian. The total resident demographics at UTHSC (Table 18–1) differ considerably from those of the local population, as they do at many universities and training programs (Hall 2017).

TABLE 18-1. Demographics of UTHSC residency programs

Race/Gender	Number	Percentage
American Indian/Alaskan	5	< 1%
Asian	153	18%
Black/African American	56	6%
Hispanic	4	< 1%
Native Hawaiian/Pacific Islander	1	< 1%
White/Not Hispanic	601	73%
Gender		
Female	336	59%
Male	484	41%

Note. UTHSC = University of Tennessee Health Science Center, Memphis.
Source. Graduate Medical Education statistics, October 2017.

The psychiatry training program is small. The demographics do vary from one year to another because of the small number, but the percentages of white and Asian residents still vary from the percentages in the local population (Table 18–2).

Given this diversity, it is essential in our medical education milieu to focus on cultural humility for improving the quality of patient care provided. The goal is to enhance cultural humility (in the fellows), and one must start with the understanding of where we may be on this journey. Dr. Ranga states, "We understand that moving along this trajectory of increasing cultural sensitivity requires a multipronged approach including series of seminars, videos, discussions about patient care experiences, and reflection and self-assessment" (J. Ranga, personal communication, December 8, 2017).

One of the first steps in improving the cultural humility among trainees is to encourage reflection on one's own cultural identity. Dr. Ranga shares her personal journey with the fellows during didactic sessions focused on cultural competency and humility. She states that being an Indian Brahmin woman who grew up in Austria and then returned to India to live with her grandparents to study medicine gave her one set of perspectives. She then journeyed back to Germany, where she developed her interest in psychiatry that led her to the University of Missouri to pursue her training. She continues, "I discuss my ethnic identity as well as linguistic ability, being proficient in accented English. Since many of our trainees are from other countries, I discuss how it may be important to think of the local cultural semantics as we speak with patients" (J. Ranga, personal communication, December 8, 2017).

TABLE 18-2. Demographics of UTHSC psychiatry residents

Race/Gender	Number	Percentage
Asian	2	14%
Black/African American	4	29%
White/Not Hispanic	8	57%
Gender		
Female	8	57%
Male	6	43%

Note. UTHSC = University of Tennessee Health Science Center, Memphis.
Source. UTHSC Psychiatry Program 2017.

The trainees are encouraged to develop their own narratives and share with others in a group didactic session. The fellows are encouraged to provide some pictures and a timeline of their path to this point in their career. They take the Harvard Implicit Association Test (IAT; Greenwald et al. 1998) so that they may become familiar with their blind spots. They also discuss and use the DSM-5 Cultural Formulation Interview (CFI; American Psychiatric Association 2013) to factor in the following points as they assess each patient:

1. Cultural identity of the patient using multiple factors such as ethnicity, languages spoken, occupation, religion, and spirituality
2. Cultural conceptualization of the illness and understanding of how the patient, family, and community view or process mental illness, and the role of stigma and bias in seeking care and managing illness
3. Role of culture in the presenting symptoms or issues: understanding this aspect on a case-by-case basis, using the patient story and matching it with any themes that have been explored
4. An understanding of psychosocial stressors and resilience that may impact the outcome
5. Reflection on transference and countertransference between patient, their family, and clinician that may be culturally influenced, including discussion of clinician bias as well as the bias of the institution, community, and society

To encourage cultural fluency, each fellow is assigned a patient to administer the CFI and then asked to present the cultural formulation in detail to his or her peers. The fellows understand that within the constraints of practice they may not be able to do the detailed CFI with every patient; however, if they can crystallize and incorporate the above five points in their overall formulation of the patient, their understanding of the case will be more complete. Fellows are encouraged to write a biopsychosocial, developmental, and cultural formulation on each of their patients. A succinct narrative that encapsulates the patient's life is then incorporated in each patient note, which will be referred to during subsequent patient visits to remain mindful of the unique complexities of each individual.

As part of the overall professional identity development, the fellows discuss well-being in detail and the role of mindfulness in promoting self-care. Mindfulness has also been discussed as playing an important role in reducing implicit bias (Lueke and Gibson 2015). In that study, participants listened to either a mindfulness or a control audio before completing the race and age IATs. Mindfulness meditation caused an increased awareness and a decrease in implicit race and age bias. Therefore, encouraging a "pause and thought" is very important for all trainees, and it may improve our blind spots. As Stephen Covey paraphrased Viktor Frankl in the eloquent statement, "Between stimulus and response there is a space. And in that space, is our power to choose our response. In our response, is our growth and freedom" (Covey et al. 1994, p. 59).

Both methods of addressing cultural differences help the psychiatrist to have a more complete understanding and aid communication between doctor and patient. The black patient can be better understood, and the psychiatrist can communicate and treat all patients more empathically.

Lifelong Learning and Maintenance of Certification

There are many factors to account for why misinterpretations and miscommunications between physicians and their patients continue to arise, including racism and racial ignorance. The need for cross-cultural knowledge is noted in the professionalism and psychopathology sections of the "Milestones in Psychiatry" residency training (Psychiatry Milestone Group 2015). Though it is a significant challenge for practicing psychiatrists to find the time to continue postgraduate "lifelong learning," ongoing training is a necessity and must include components of cultural influences in therapeutic interventions. The continuity of training offers a method to improve empathy and understanding, and this should improve patient care and help to decrease the cultural and racial disparities in healthcare. Postgraduate lifelong learning should include quality improvement modules that include more comprehensive consideration of culture, specifically as it relates to diagnosis and treatment challenges in diverse populations. Ongoing emphasis on racial, cultural, and understanding of social determinants of mental health is a necessary part of medical education throughout training and afterward.

Conclusion: Components of Training in Cross-Cultural Psychiatry

Teaching cross-cultural psychiatry to residents and fellows should include the following components:

1. Appreciation of the history of cross-cultural psychiatry as it serves to improve understanding, trust, and empathy in the doctor-patient relationship
2. Understanding of cultural history and how the actual translation of cultural factors into treatment may result in actual reduction in healthcare disparities
3. Recognition that culture, including socioeconomic background, influences people and the expression of mental health problems
4. Awareness of cultural humility as an empathic method that can aid in the understanding of other cultures
5. Appreciation of the necessity of a biopsychosocial, developmental, and cultural formulation for each patient in order to understand the complete patient
6. Understanding of the necessity of a standardized tool—namely, the DSM-5 CFI—in obtaining a cultural formulation
7. Recognition that clinical experiences within a diverse environment do not automatically give one empathy or provide education on cultural psychiatry

Finally, as Dr. Ranga noted earlier, we should understand that moving along the trajectory of increasing cultural sensitivity requires a multipronged approach, including series of seminars, videos, self-assessment, patient care, and reflection. A lack of cultural understanding has an impact on appropriate diagnosis and treatment in patients from different cultural backgrounds. One can learn to understand and appropriately empathize with "the other," and this will help address the disparities in healthcare. Including these components in the training of future psychiatrists will go a long way in ensuring that the mental health of black Americans and others will be improved with a better understanding of cross-cultural psychiatry.

References

American Psychiatric Association: Diagnostic and Statistical Manual of Mental Disorders, 4th Edition. Washington, DC, American Psychiatric Association, 1994

American Psychiatric Association: Diagnostic and Statistical Manual of Mental Disorders, 5th Edition. Arlington, VA, American Psychiatric Association, 2013

Berry J: Globalization and acculturation. Int J Intercult Relat 32(4):328–336, 2008

Butterfield LH (ed): Benjamin Rush, "To the Pennsylvania Abolition Society," January 14, 1795. Letters of Benjamin Rush, Vol 2. Princeton, NJ, Princeton University Press, 1951, pp 756–759

Cartwright S: A report on the diseases and peculiarities of the Negro race. New Orleans Medical and Surgical Journal May 1851

Covey S, Merrill R, Merrill R: First Things First. New York, Fireside/Simon & Schuster, 1994

Greenwald AG, McGhee DE, Schwartz JL: Measuring individual differences in implicit cognition: the Implicit Association Test. J Pers Soc Psychol 74(6):1464–1480, 1998 9654756

Hall A: Performance improvement plans, in Residency Program Files. Memphis, University of Tennessee Health Science Center Graduate Medical Education Office, 2017

Hook JN, Davis DE, Owen J, et al: Cultural humility: measuring openness to culturally diverse clients. J Couns Psychol 60(3):353–366, 2013 23647387

Jones BE, Lightfoot OB, Palmer D, et al: Problems of black psychiatric residents in white training institutes. Am J Psychiatry 127(6):798–803, 1970 5482873

Kleinman AM: Depression, somatization and the "new cross-cultural psychiatry." Soc Sci Med 11(1):3–10, 1977 887955

Kramer BM: Racism and metal health as a field of thought and action, in Racism and Mental Health. Edited by Willie CV, Kramer BM, Brown BS. Pittsburgh, PA, University of Pittsburgh Press, 1973, pp 3–23

Lueke A, Gibson B: Mindfulness meditation reduces implicit age and race bias: the role of reduced automaticity of responding. Soc Psychol Personal Sci 6(3):284–291, 2015

McDermott F, Andrade N: People and Cultures of Hawaii: The Evolution of Culture and Ethnicity. Honolulu, University of Hawaii Press, 2011

Psychiatry Milestone Group: The Psychiatry Milestone Project. Chicago, IL, Accreditation Council for Graduate Medical Education, 2015. Available at: https://www.acgme.org/Portals/0/PDFs/Milestones/PsychiatryMilestones.pdf. Accessed January 14, 2018.

Regier DA, Myers JK, Kramer M, et al: The NIMH Epidemiologic Catchment Area program: historical context, major objectives, and study population characteristics. Arch Gen Psychiatry 41(10):934–941, 1984 6089692

Rush B: Observations intended to favour a supposition that the black color (as it is called) of the Negroes is derived from the leprosy. Trans Am Philos Soc 4:289–297, 1799

Saha S, Beach MC, Cooper LA: Patient centeredness, cultural competence and healthcare quality. J Natl Med Assoc 100(11):1275–1285, 2008 19024223

Sharpley RH: Treatment Issues: Foreign Medical Graduates and Black Patient Populations. Cambridge, MA, The Solomon Fuller Institute, 1977

Spurlock J: Black Americans in Cross-Cultural Psychiatry. Edited by Gaw A. Littleton, MA, John Wright, 1982, pp 163–178

Tweedy D: The case for black doctors. The New York Times (Sunday Review), May 15, 2015

Wittkower ED: Perspectives of Transcultural Psychiatry. Isr Ann Psychiatr Relat Discip 2:19–26, 1964 14270617

CHAPTER 19
A SEAT AT THE PSYCHIATRIC TABLE

Increasing the Workforce Presence of Blacks

Frank Clark, M.D., FAPA

THE BLACK COMMUNITY, like the communities of other racial and ethnic groups, desires peace, prosperity, and longevity. These pursuits become challenging in the face of limited access to high quality and affordable healthcare, resulting in shorter life expectancies. Furthermore, the lack of diversity in the physician workforce is problematic and poses a barrier to achieving health equity and improving outcomes. Unfortunately, these themes have become the status quo instead of an anomaly among a demographic that historically has been mistreated and marginalized. Unequal treatment as it relates to the healthcare system has been pervasive throughout this community, prompting a call for action.

Currently, African Americans compose 13% of the United States population, and that number is expected to double by 2060 (U.S. Census Bureau 2016). More than 16% of this population—roughly equal to 6.8 million people—experienced a diagnosable mental illness in the past year (Substance Abuse and Mental Health Services Administration 2014). Presently, African American physicians are 4% of the total physician workforce, which is less than half when comparing the overall percentage of this demographic in the United States (Rao and Flores 2007). Therefore, it is imperative that we reconcile the mental health disparity gap in the black community. A "seat at the table" is a key that gives our brothers and sisters hope for a better today and a brighter tomorrow.

Current State of Mental Health in Black America

Mental illness can be quite debilitating and stigmatizing for individuals regardless of demographic background. However, research has shown that blacks experience lower rates but increased severity of mental illness compared to whites (Williams et al. 2007). Furthermore, studies indicate that African Americans experience more barriers to accessing care. They are also high utilizers of inpatient services and low utilizers of outpatient services compared with whites (Williams et al. 2007). There are a multitude of factors that contribute to the more severe forms of mental illness and barriers to care experienced by this vulnerable population. These manifest themselves in the forms of homelessness, incarceration, exposure to violence, distrust of the healthcare system, and attitudes and misconceptions about mental illness, to name a few.

Homelessness remains a public health crisis that has a significant impact on individuals' mental and physical health. It is important to highlight the intersectionality of homelessness, race/ethnicity, and mental illness. It is estimated that between one-fourth and one-third of homeless individuals have a serious mental illness (Folsom and Jeste 2002). African Americans compose a large majority of the homeless population. According to a report by the Institute for Children, Poverty, and Homelessness (Da Costa et al. 2012), "Intergenerational Disparities Experienced by Homeless Black Families," in 2010, black families were seven times more likely to reside in homeless shelters compared with white families.

Another disenfranchised subgroup of African Americans comprises those who are incarcerated in jails and prisons. Historically, there have been a disproportionate number of blacks in the penal system, and the majority of this population does not receive treatment to address mental health needs. Roughly 50% of all U.S. inmates in jails and prisons are black, with one in six inmates being diagnosed with a mental illness (Noonan et al. 2016). According to a Bureau of Justice Statistics survey, in 2005 more than 1.2 million prisoners had a mental health problem, with African Americans being overrepresented (James and Glaze 2006). The lack of access to mental health services for incarcerated minority populations is unacceptable and does not allow for persons of color to achieve recovery and access rehabilitation services that are essential when they prepare to reenter society.

Violent victimization, defined as rape, aggravated assault, simple assault, and robbery, appears to be the status quo instead of an anomaly in black communities. In 2007, the Bureau of Justice Statistics presented the following findings from their report examining the risk of nonfatal violent victimization among blacks from 2001 through 2005 (Harrell 2007):

- Males had a higher propensity to violent victimization compared with females.
- Individuals experiencing violent victimization tended to be younger.
- Blacks who were single had a higher likelihood of being victims of violence compared with those who were married.
- Households with higher incomes tended to experience less violent victimization compared with households with lower incomes.
- Higher rates of violent victimization were noted among individuals residing in urban areas compared with suburban and rural areas.

The link between violent victimization and a proclivity toward developing a psychiatric illness is well established. The U.S. surgeon general's report *Mental Health: Culture, Race, and Ethnicity* is replete with evidence from two decades of research that supports this link (U.S. Department of Health and Human Services 2001). For example, Fitzpatrick and Boldizar (1993) found that greater than 25% of African American youth exposed to violence had symptoms that would a support a diagnosis of posttraumatic stress disorder. The sequelae of violent victimization include emotional and physical distress, which further impact the ability of individuals in vulnerable communities to function and thrive.

While it is imperative to raise awareness regarding the fact that African Americans are overrepresented in vulnerable populations, as noted, there are other factors that contribute to the mental health disparities that this demographic has faced. There has been a pervasive pattern of mistrust between the black community and the healthcare system. The best example to illustrate this phenomenon is the Tuskegee Syphilis Study, which was conducted between 1932 and 1972 by the U.S. Public Health Service. The purpose of this experiment was to examine the natural progression of syphilis. African American males living in Macon County, Alabama, were recruited for the study. The principal investigators for this study withheld treatment from nearly 400 men in order to look at the progression of syphilis. The study eventually lost funding, but for these men, it was a much greater loss that remains palpable for modern-day black communities. This study violated the core ethical principles that we as healthcare providers adhere to in the following ways (Heintzelman 2003):

- The nearly 400 men were under the impression that this study would last 6 months. However, in reality, it lasted 40 years.
- These men were never informed that they would not receive treatment, even after funding for the study was lost.
- The men who tested positive for syphilis were never told that they had contracted the disease.

- Treatment for syphilis was withheld from these men, even after the discovery of penicillin, which proved to be an effective treatment for this disease.

Today, the relationship between black communities and mental healthcare providers remains fractured, resulting in underutilization of services and poor health outcomes. Less than 25% of African Americans receive evidence-based treatment, including psychopharmacological or psychotherapeutic interventions for mental health disorders (Wang et al. 2000). Furthermore, African Americans are also less likely to be offered lifesaving treatments such as electroconvulsive therapy. One of the underlying themes that connect these examples of disparity and discrimination among black people is provider bias. Acknowledging our own stereotypes/biases and increasing knowledge and understanding in regard to cultural sensitivity are essential if we, as providers, desire to improve the therapeutic alliance and foster trusting relationships.

The current state of mental health in black America is also influenced by attitudes of the black community toward mental illness, which can interfere with seeking treatment. A study conducted by Ward and colleagues in 2013 provides a useful overview related to this topic. Here are a few of the findings:

- Core beliefs regarding stigma and failure to acknowledge signs and symptoms of psychological distress are not uncommon in the community.
- Individuals who have increased knowledge of and exposure to mental illness may be more likely to modify core beliefs regarding their symptoms.
- Men are especially concerned about stigma.

The information presented here must embolden communities to sow seeds of mentorship and advocacy. Black communities are in need of innovative and passionate young leaders to champion the fight for health equity. What are the ingredients needed to replace scarcity with abundance in regard to this demographic in medicine? The answer lies within the willingness from people of all backgrounds to acknowledge the need for diversity in medicine. Furthermore, this recipe for changing attitudes of the black community toward mental illness calls for a transformation of the psychiatric physician workforce. This transformation requires that physicians spend more face time with young black men and women and increase their exposure to what a physician looks like in America.

Transforming the Psychiatric Physician Workforce: The What, Why, and How

Before transformation can occur, it is important to recognize the physician workforce shortages the country is currently facing. The following are key findings from the report *The Complexities of Physician Supply and Demand: Projections From 2015 to 2030,* prepared by the Association of American Medical Colleges (2017):

- Physician shortages are estimated to be between 40,800 and 104,900 by 2030.
- The estimated shortages for physicians in primary care will range from 7,300 to 43,100 physicians by 2030.
- Non–primary care specialty (e.g., surgery, psychiatry) shortages will range from 33,500 to 61,800 by 2030.

The field of psychiatry is in desperate need of replenishing and diversifying its physician workforce. During the period of 1995 through 2013, the physician workforce increased by 45%. Meanwhile, the psychiatry workforce, including adult and child psychiatrists, rose by only 12%, from 43,640 to 49,070 (Sederer 2015). Fifty-nine percent of psychiatrists are age 55 or older and will be nearing retirement and/or reducing their workload (Association of American Medical Colleges 2012). To further complicate matters, there are about 4,000 areas nationwide where there is only one psychiatrist for every 30,000 patients (Health Resources and Services Administration Data Warehouse 2017). Underrepresented minorities, defined as African Americans, Latinos, and American Indians/Alaska Natives, are more likely to practice in medically underserved areas compared with their white counterparts. These findings further highlight and reiterate the importance of workforce diversity in the effort to improve health outcomes and eliminate health care disparities.

It would be an unrealistic expectation to think that health equity and workforce diversity in psychiatry can be achieved for blacks when only 2% of psychiatrists in the United States are African American. One could also make the case for increasing the number of blacks in the physician workforce via examining the concept of racial concordance and how it applies to the physician-patient relationship. As mentioned earlier, the mistrust between individuals in the black community and the healthcare system has created deep-seated wounds that unfortunately have yet to be healed. Racial concordance is critical to accessing equitable care for minority populations and may help close the diversity gap. Sitting across from a provider of similar racial/ethnic background can speak volumes to the patient who is longing to be understood and cared for in a manner consistent with his or her cultural values. A study by Cooper et al. (2003) demonstrated that patients in race-concordant care were more satisfied with their providers and rated their providers' performance higher compared with patients in race-discordant visits.

The data regarding physician shortages and the need for narrowing the diversity gap in the psychiatric workforce require a pragmatic, goal-oriented approach from all stakeholders at the table that is specific, attainable, measurable, realistic, and timely. The question that has echoed throughout medical institutions and healthcare systems for decades is, why is there a paucity of African American physicians?

We enter this world as infants with veils of naiveté and innocence. Unfortunately, these veils are removed by society in early childhood when our parents or guardians are unable to shield us from injustices in our schools, communities, and the world. I was born and raised in a middle-class neighborhood on the south side of Chicago in a two-parent household. My mother, now retired, worked as a teacher in the Chicago public school system for 35 years, and my father, now deceased, was a minister. I grew up in a home where ambition, resilience, and perseverance were embedded in my DNA at an early age. I knew at the age of 15 that I wanted to pursue a career in healthcare. My mother recognized my love and passion for science at an early age and was intentional in her approach to ensure that I was immersed in a culture that was both similar and distinct from mine. The majority of my summers in elementary and high school were spent in science programs that fostered discovery and innovation, in addition to doing research in laboratories at prominent universities. Despite the early exposure to medicine, I still faced challenges on my road to becoming a physician. I distinctly remember a middle-aged Caucasian woman with a background in education discouraging me from applying to medical school because my Medical College Admissions Test score was not up to par. She said, "I think you should consider another career." Statements like this can deflate one's self-confidence. There may have been an underlying racial undertone to what she was saying. If it were not for the support of my family and peers, there is a strong likelihood that I would have taken this lady's advice and pursued a different career. My story is not uncommon, as many of our black youth today may still feel discouraged from pursuing their dreams because of others' preformed biases that are not rooted in reality. The pursuit of higher education can be achieved with the aid of positive reinforcements. These include our teachers and administrators, who are of the belief that all children, regardless of demographic background, can and will be successful.

Rao and Flores (2007) sought to address the lack of African American physicians by understanding African American high school student perspectives on the barriers to pursuing a career in medicine. The participants in the study identified 27 barriers, which the authors broke down into the following 11 categories: financial challenges, time commitment, stress/difficulty, limited opportunities and exposure to medicine, lack of family support, lack of peer support, perceptions of physicians, lack of knowledge about medicine, lack of interest, negative normative cultural values and traditions, and perceived racism in the medical field and healthcare institutions.

The barriers that these students mentioned continue to reveal themselves in the current medical school, residency, and organized medicine cultures, and all seek to find innovative ways to become more diverse and inclusive. The Association of American Medical Colleges (2016) report *Facts & Figures 2016: Diversity in Medical Education* examined some of the current and longitudinal trends in medical education related to race and ethnicity. Here are some of the findings pertaining to blacks or African Americans:

- Between 1974 and 2015, the number of black or African American applicants increased by 78% (2,295 to 4,087).
- The number of black or African Americans accepted into medical school has remained stagnant from the period of 1996 (1,268) to 2015 (1,394).
- The acceptance rate for this demographic has been below 40% since 2007.
- Black or African American applicants had the lowest acceptance rate to medical school (34%) compared with white (44%), Hispanic or Latino (42%), and Asian (42%) applicants in 2015.
- The percentage of black or African American female medical school graduates increased 53% from 1986 to 2015, while the percentage of males declined by 39.4%.
- The percentage of black or African American medical school graduates in 2015 was roughly 6%, with whites and Asians representing the majority of graduates.

Once these medical students graduate and enter into specialty residency programs such as psychiatry, it is hoped that they will encounter a diverse educational and practice environment. This would include faculty and peers who resemble their racial/ethnic backgrounds to provide guidance and mentorship as they progress throughout their careers. This is essential, given that black physicians face emotional and social challenges during their postgraduate training years in the form of *microaggressions,* which is a term coined by one of the luminaries in psychiatry, the late Dr. Chester Pierce. Utilization of a support network is vital to surviving the subtle and overt forms of racism and discrimination that remain evident in the workplace. However, seeking support becomes problematic, given that only 4% of full-time faculty in academic medicine identify as an underrepresented minority (Association of American Medical Colleges 2016).

Psychiatry is becoming a more attractive and competitive field. Based on a press release in 2017 by the National Residency Matching Program, psychiatry's overall fill rate was 99.7%. The number of positions has increased by 34% from 2012 to 2017 (National Resident Matching Program 2017). While this is encouraging news for our field, the paucity of black resident psychiatrists remains depressing; only 6.6% of the nation's psychiatry residents identify as black or African American according to a survey by the American Psychiatric Association (APA). This percentage must increase if our field hopes to meet the needs of the nation's increasingly diverse population.

Throughout the years of rigorous training, a cohort of medical students and resident physicians will seize the opportunity to help shape policies that will impact the lives of the communities they serve. Their involvement in organized medicine affords them the ability to accomplish their goals at the state and national level. They have a "seat at the table." However, it can be difficult to attract and persuade African American medical students and early-career physicians to become a part of organized medicine given the history of racial bias and discrimination that our predecessors encountered when attempting to join national organizations like the American Medical Association (AMA). This type of injustice plagued the medical community for more than 100 years. In response to the callousness displayed by these predominately white organizations at the time, African American physicians refused to accept defeat. They responded by forming the National Medical Association (NMA) in 1895 so that African American physicians would have a voice to advocate for their patients. The NMA is the largest and oldest organization representing African American healthcare professionals (Baker et al. 2008).

The beginnings of the reconciliation process occurred with a collaborative effort by the AMA, NMA, and National Hispanic Medical Association (NHMA) to form the Commission to End Health Care Disparities, which had its first meeting in July 2004. This commission was inspired by the Institute of Medicine report *Unequal Treatment,* which provided recommendations to help eliminate healthcare disparities (Smedley et al. 2002). Another step in the healing process occurred in 2008 when the AMA offered a formal apology to the NMA. However, as with the Tuskegee experiment, wounds take a while to heal. While I am a proud member of the AMA and NMA, I still have a hard time convincing my black colleagues from myriad specialties of the value of joining these organizations.

The culture of healthcare delivery and access cannot be improved for black communities without a grassroots effort and classrooms ripe with encouragement, confidence, and rigorous curricula that will help prepare young men and women for any career they choose to pursue. Early exposure to STEM (science, technology, engineering, and mathematics) pipeline programs starting in elementary school is essential to increasing the workforce presence of blacks in healthcare. I am a product of pipeline programs like the Chicago Area Health and Medical Careers Program, which is still in existence. Programs like this helped pave the road for me on my journey to becoming a physician.

Physicians, medical institutions, and other organizations also have a role to play in making sure the access to the pipeline extends beyond elementary and high school. It is a collaborative effort. Florida State University College of Medicine's program SSTRIDE (Science Students Together Reaching Instructional Diversity and Excellence) is a good example of this strategy. Its program has a precollege and college track for individuals who are interested in pursuing careers in STEM.

The Student National Medical Association, founded in 1964, is the largest student-run medical organization. Its mission is to address the needs of black medical students through programs such as the Pipeline Mentoring Institute (PMI). The PMI was established to help prepare underrepresented minority students for careers in healthcare. The PMI is divided into five different programs: 1) Pre-medical Minority Enrichment and Development (PMED), 2) Minority Association of Pre-medical Students (MAPS), 3) Health Professions Recruitment Exposure Program (HPREP), 4) Youth Science Enrichment Program (YSEP), and 5) Brotherhood Alliance for Science Education (BASE).

A program near and dear to my heart is the AMA's Doctors Back to School (DBTS) Program, which was developed by the AMA's Minority Affairs Section (MAS). Throughout my 5 years of service on the MAS Governing Council as resident representative, young physician representative, vice chair, and now chair, I have been fortunate to help shape policies that impact minority patient populations in addition to participating in pipeline programs like DBTS. The purpose of this program is to motivate and mentor underrepresented minority students who have aspirations of pursuing a career in healthcare. The DBTS program exemplifies the importance of physician stewardship and sowing seeds of hope in the communities we serve. Through collaborative efforts from multiple governing council members, a National Doctors Back to School Day Program was established and takes places annually in May. This program has been well received by students and teachers at their local schools. I have many times heard students voice amazement that this is the first time they have ever met a black physician, let alone a psychiatrist. It is a fun experience for my colleagues and me to share our stories of resilience and perseverance for students, who may be the first in their family to attend college. I have no doubt that this program will continue to have an impact in the black community at large.

In regard to the field of psychiatry, the APA recognizes the importance of attracting blacks to the profession and providing incentives to help with recruitment and retention among this demographic. The APA's Division of Diversity and Health Equity strives to search for innovative ways to diversify the mental health physician workforce in the form of fellowships, grants, and networking opportunities. There are currently more than 77 fellowship programs individuals can apply for on an annual basis. The APA's Minority Fellowship Program comprises three fellowships: the Diversity Leadership Fellowship, the Substance Abuse Mental Health Services Administration (SAMHSA) Minority Fellowship, and the SAMHSA Substance Abuse Minority Fellowship. Additionally, there are travel scholarships available for underrepresented minority medical students who have an interest in pursuing a career in psychiatry to attend the Institute on Psychiatric Services' Mental Health Services Conference in October or the annual APA meeting in May. Underrepresented minority medical students interested in psychiatry and in working with under-resourced communities can also apply to the APA's Summer Mentoring Program. Finally, the APA's newest pipeline program, Black Men in Psychiatry, provides a conduit to help increase the number of black men entering the field of psychiatry. This is achieved through partnerships with historically black colleges and universities and other organizations like the NMA and 100 Black Men of America.

Conclusion

We live in a world filled with opportunities to embrace a melting pot of cultures and experiences. The physician workforce is in search of leaders in our community to fill the vacancies at a table that must increase awareness and champion efforts related to healthcare disparities. Increasing the presence of black physician leaders is essential to help meet the needs of a growing diverse population. We, as African American healthcare providers, are the change agents who can and must continue to use our voices to advocate and restore the health and longevity of our communities. Furthermore, we must stay encouraged, increase our knowledge base, and remain hopeful and steadfast with the goal of achieving health equity for current and future generations.

References

Association of American Medical Colleges: 2012 Physician Specialty Data Book. Center for Workforce Studies. Washington, DC, Association of American Medical Colleges, 2012. Available at: https://www.aamc.org/download/313228/data/2012physicianspecialtydatabook.pdf. Accessed October 2017.

Association of American Medical Colleges: AAMC Facts & Figures 2016: Diversity in Medical Education. Washington, DC, Association of American Medical Colleges, 2016. Available at: http://www.aamcdiversityfactsandfigures2016.org/. Accessed October 2017.

Association of American Medical Colleges: 2017 Update. The Complexities of Physician Supply and Demand: Projections From 2015 to 2030. Final Report. Washington, DC, Association of American Medical Colleges, 2017. Available at: https://aamc-black.global.ssl.fastly.net/production/media/filer_public/a5/c3/a5c3d565-14ec-48fb-974b-99fafaeecb00/aamc_projections_update_2017.pdf. Accessed October 2017.

Baker RB, Washington HA, Olakanmi O, et al: African American physicians and organized medicine, 1846–1968: origins of a racial divide. JAMA 300(3):306–313, 2008 18617633

Cooper LA, Roter DL, Johnson RL, et al: Patient-centered communication, ratings of care, and concordance of patient and physician race. Ann Intern Med 139(11):907–915, 2003 14644893

Da Costa N, Adams R, Simonsen-Meehan M, et al: Intergenerational disparities experienced by homeless black families. ICPH Vol 3.1, Spring 2012. Available at: http://www.icphusa.org/wp-content/uploads/2015/01/ICPH_UNCENSORED_3.1_Spring2012_TheNationalPerspective_IntergenerationalDisparitiesExperiencedbyHomelessBlackFamilies.pdf. Accessed October 2017.

Fitzpatrick KM, Boldizar JP: The prevalence and consequences of exposure to violence among African-American youth. J Am Acad Child Adolesc Psychiatry 32(2):424–430, 1993 8444774

Folsom D, Jeste DV: Schizophrenia in homeless persons: a systematic review of the literature. Acta Psychiatr Scand 105(6):404–413, 2002 12059843

Harrell E: Black victims of violent crime. Bureau of Justice Statistics Special Report NCJ 214258, August 2007. Available at: https://www.bjs.gov/content/pub/pdf/bvvc.pdf. Accessed October 2017.

Health Resources and Services Administration Data Warehouse: Health Professional Shortage Areas (HPSA) by Discipline–Total and Health Professional Shortage Areas by Geographic Area–Total, 2017. Available at: https://dataware-house.hrsa.gov/topics/shortageAreas.aspx#chart. Accessed October 2017.

Heintzelman CA: The Tuskegee syphilis experiment and its implications for the 21st century. The New Social Worker (online) 10(4), 2003. Available at: http://www.socialworker.com/feature-articles/ethics-articles/The_Tuskegee_Syphilis_Study_and_Its_Implications_for_the_21st_Century/. Accessed October 2017.

James DJ, Glaze LE: Mental health problems of prison and jail inmates. Bureau of Justice Statistics Special Report NCJ 213600, September 2006. Available at: https://www.bjs.gov/content/pub/pdf/mhppji.pdf. Accessed October 2017.

National Resident Matching Program: Press release: 2017 NRMP Main Residency Match the largest match on record. More than 43,000 applicants registered and more than 31,000 positions offered. The Match, March 17, 2017. Available at: http://www.nrmp.org/press-release-2017-nrmp-main-residency-match-the-largest-match-on-record/. Accessed October 2017.

Noonan AS, Velasco-Mandragon H, Wagner F: Improving the health of African Americans in the USA: an overdue opportunity for social justice. Public Health Rev 37(12):1–20, 2016

Rao V, Flores G: Why aren't there more African-American physicians? A qualitative study and exploratory inquiry of African-American students' perspectives on careers in medicine. J Natl Med Assoc 99(9):986–993, 2007 17913107

Sederer L: Where have all the psychiatrists gone? Doctors are struggling to meet the growing demand for psychiatric help across the U.S. U.S. News and World Report, September 15, 2015. Available at: https://www.usnews.com/opinion/blogs/policy-dose/2015/09/15/the-us-needs-more-psychiatrists-to-meet-mental-health-demands. Accessed October 2017.

Smedley B, Stith AY, Nelson AR: Unequal Treatment: Confronting Racial and Ethnic Disparities in Health Care. Washington, DC, National Academies Press, 2002

Substance Abuse and Mental Health Services Administration: Racial and Ethnic Minority Populations. Substance Abuse and Mental Health Services Administration website, 2014. Available at: http://www.samhsa.gov/specific-populations/racial-ethnic-minority. Accessed October 2017.

U.S. Census Bureau: Quick Facts. U.S. Census Bureau website, 2016. Available at: https://www.census.gov/quickfacts/fact/table/US/PST045216. Accessed October 2017.

U.S. Department of Health and Human Services: Mental Health: Culture, Race, and Ethnicity. A Supplement to Mental Health: A Report of the Surgeon General. Rockville, MD, Substance Abuse and Mental Health Services Administration, 2001

Wang PS, Berglund P, Kessler RC: Recent care of common mental disorders in the United States: prevalence and conformance with evidence-based recommendations. J Gen Intern Med 15(5):284–292, 2000 10840263

Ward EC, Wiltshire JC, Detry MA, et al: African American men and women's attitude toward mental illness, perceptions of stigma, and preferred coping behaviors. Nurs Res 62(3):185–194, 2013 23328705

Williams DR, González HM, Neighbors H, et al: Prevalence and distribution of major depressive disorder in African Americans, Caribbean blacks, and non-Hispanic whites: results from the National Survey of American Life. Arch Gen Psychiatry 64(3):305–315, 2007 17339519

CHAPTER 20
ADDRESSING THE MENTAL HEALTH NEEDS OF AFRICAN AMERICAN YOUTH IN THE NEW MILLENNIUM

Intersections and Visions for the Future

Racquel E. Reid, M.D.

Millennials and the New Millennium

African Americans make up 12.6% of the U.S. population.[1] According to 2015 Pew Research Center data, the black population is generally a young one (Fry 2018). The median age is 33 years, with most individuals being 24 years old; 25% are classified as "millennials" (classified as ages 18–35 in 2015), and a further 26% of the black population is classified as "postmillennials" (ages 0–17).

---

[1]The term *African Americans* is defined as all members of the African diaspora living within the United States. Colloquially, they are all individuals who would identify as "black" on the census, and the terms *black* and *African American* are used interchangeably throughout this chapter.

These combined generations account for approximately 51% of black individuals within the United States. Examination of millennials' and postmillennials' perceptions of their world and their mental health is imperative in order to address their mental health needs in the coming decades.

Varied studies have elucidated the state of black mental health over the past few decades. Much of this research addressed the behavior of black Generation X and the baby boomers; however, the trends in usage of mental health services by them have not changed significantly. Black adults struggle with depression and serious mental illness at rates similar to those of whites and tend to rate their depression as more severe (Molina and James 2016). They use mental health services at a much lower rate compared with those in the general population, access care later, and frequently have negative experiences after receiving treatment. Intracommunity stigma against psychiatry persists as a mechanism to preclude accessing care (Sullivan et al. 2017).

It is notable that black welfare and health cannot be separated from American social justice efforts, suffrage, resistance to Jim Crow, and the Civil Rights Movement, or battling the War on Crime. These events continually shape the way black people in the United States see the world and how people of color fit within it, and understanding these perspectives is necessary to providing culturally competent care. Several researchers have uncovered the connections between persistent racism within American society—institutional, personal-mediated, and internalized—and the resultant increases in psychopathology and overall lower quality of life for people of color (Molina and James 2016).

Much of the research on perceived discrimination has appropriately focused on depression and anxiety because of the large disease burden of major depressive disorder as well as the health implications of that burden on an already medically marginalized population. Less well examined is the state of black mental health in youth as it relates to the ever-evolving political and social landscape, especially in relation to the advent of social media. Experientially, conversations regarding black people's sociopolitical position in U.S. society frequently occur on social media sites, often with accompanying conversations relating to depression and suicide. The relative dearth of specific research within the medical community investigating how black people with mental illness approach social media offers a significant challenge. Historically, medical investigators have deferred this topic to the social sciences, but as social media becomes more ensconced in the network of American life, the interplay between social media's impact on society and vice versa cannot be reasonably ignored by physicians. The examination of black American youth in this chapter aims to evaluate social media use, bring insight to their voiced concerns via social media about the world around them, and explore mechanisms for bridging gaps and providing perceptively delivered mental healthcare.

Social Media and Youth

Social media is broadly defined as Internet-based tools or applications that allow users to generate and communicate information rapidly, including blogs, microblogs, social networking sites (SNS), and video-sharing sites. To visualize users' experience of social media, we can imagine a conference hall where many different talks are simultaneously under way. There is natural engagement between speakers and their audiences, among audience members, and intermittently between audience members and speakers in different rooms. Social media creates an online paradigm for users to engage in any number of conversations in a similar manner throughout the course of the day. Within this chapter, discussion of social media is limited to that regarding SNS, which include well-known sites such as Facebook, Reddit, Twitter, Tumblr, YouTube, Google Plus, Instagram, Snapchat, Pinterest, Vine, Kik, and LinkedIn.

Researchers studying SNS have primarily used ethnographic research methods to evaluate interactions on social media platforms. In this way they examine exchanges without the observer interference typically plaguing face-to-face methods (Naslund et al. 2014). Much of the data describing trends in use of social media are collected in this manner, which limits access to private messages and deleted posts and tends to focus on trigger words. However, collected data still provide insight into how teenagers interact online.

Usage of SNS occurs in a naturalistic manner, with individuals reporting about events as they experience them. Development of LiveJournal and Myspace spurred a community of young people using these sharing spaces to discuss common occurrences but also pressing social issues, for better or worse. Despite the rapid decline in use of these platforms in the mid-2000s, the motivations behind such engagement remain unchanged. Common Sense Media, in its 2012 survey-based report "Social Media, Social Life: How Teens View Their Digital Lives," detailed that 90% of teenagers and young adults reported use of a social media site (Common Sense Media 2012). Approximately 75% had their own account, and most accessed the site at least once daily. Users engage multiple sites to share the mundane and ridiculous nuances of daily life alongside pop culture references, politics, and shared peer interests. Additionally, many individuals use multiple social media sites daily and navigate each platform in particular ways unique to each site—certain posts that would garner thousands of notes (reactions, including "Likes" and "Reblogs") on Tumblr would not be appropriate for Facebook (Primack and Escobar-Viera 2017). Young users prefer the ease of Snapchat for private messages because they disappear shortly after being viewed.

Popular opinion portrays millennials and postmillennials as irretrievably narcissistic and apathetic, yet they find global issues similarly engaging and react to them just as deeply. They often use the online world to provoke thoughtful discourse on changing societal norms, discussing sex and sexuality, gender identity, discrimination, and marginalization with the same depth as do older generations. They are simultaneously fascinated by and overwhelmingly disappointed with our current political landscape, while yet believing in American exceptionalism. They observe and document our changing society and the dishonest application of American ideals both within the United States and abroad (American Psychological Association 2017). Despite fears of unattainable attractiveness, they use selfies as reclamation of their bodies as beautiful in a society that continues to prioritize Eurocentric standards; they spur body positivity. They see the effects of the stock market crash of 2008 and the reemergence of fascism globally, and they continue to root for their favorite artists while praying that things are better for their own children.

Teenagers and young adults utilize social media to understand the world around them and make connections online as deeply as in face-to-face interactions. They additionally feel judicious concerning their social media use and voice a desire to disconnect when necessary. Furthermore, they generally see social media interactions as a supplement to their offline life, not a replacement (Romer et al. 2013). Particularly notable is that they do all of this within the context of the normal stressors of adolescence and early adulthood.

Blackness and Social Media Use

Pew Research Center, in a 2012 report, found that Twitter use is especially high among black, non-Hispanic people, urban populations, and young adults (ages 18–29) (Smith and Brenner 2012). According to the Knowledge Networks survey, which produced the Common Sense Media (2012) report, Twitter was voted by teens to be the "most important" social network, despite Facebook dominating in SNS, with 68% of all teens reporting they use Facebook as their main networking site. African American teens disclosed using other platforms than Facebook, and 19% of black teens reported using Twitter as their primary SNS. As of 2011, 92% of college students used SNS (Lamblin et al. 2017), with Facebook being the most popular in that demographic. Sixty-six percent of Twitter users are age 25 or younger, and the biggest demographic differences in its use are ethnic (Common Sense Media 2012).

There is no doubt that the experiences of young, urban black youth are different from those of other populations, and these youth demonstrate those dissimilarities by their conversations on social media. Namely, they discuss their general distrust in the idea that those in power look out for their well-being. The Black Youth Project, established in response to the death of Trayvon Martin, produced an independent study based on Department of Labor statistics to illuminate the priorities of black millennials. The study discovered that black millennials in particular discuss feeling empowered to advocate for their own health, education, and safety. However, they are perceived as nonchalant by politicians and older generations, despite being the most politically active of all millennial racial groups (Rogowski and Cohen 2015). In 2014, after the deaths of Michael Brown and Freddie Gray, the hashtag #BlackLivesMatter appeared in various iterations all over SNS. Independent activists discussed #BlackLives-Matter online and the desperation they tend to feel regarding police harassment and violence. Increased use of the hashtag and mobilization around support of families and communities suffering from extrajudicial deaths of black young men and women persisted all throughout 2015, and the organization Black Lives Matter was established soon after.

In addition to affirming the humanity of black lives online, black millennials discussed microaggressions, coded racialized language such as the word "thug," and weaponization of typical black urban behavior against those most vulnerable to violence (Smiley and Fakunle 2016). They additionally expressed distress over the seemingly ubiquitous videos of black deaths, often at the hands of police. An American Psychological Association study released in early 2017 confirmed that 71% of black Americans studied indeed worried about police violence, and found that millennials reported higher levels of stress overall than older generations regarding not only this but also work and money (American Psychological Association 2017). The collective consciousness of black people regarding medicine as a whole was an additional part of the Black Youth Project study, and black millennials noted feeling poor overall health but desiring more coverage for Americans in spite of not always feeling valued in the medical system (Rogowski and Cohen 2015). The stigma of psychiatry remains, and many within the black community still struggle with the belief that mental illness is not real and diagnosable. In 2016, in response to online bullying by fans of Kyrie Irving, singer Kehlani attempted suicide. Many online saw her attempt as simply a cry for attention, and she was subsequently bullied again online, mainly by black youth. Yet in the midst of disbelief regarding mental illness, many black millennials find the up-to-date coverage of mass shootings and sexual assault particularly triggering. Furthermore, evidence suggests that this type of consistent coverage encourages individuals to believe in lower levels of safety. They share stories online of feeling as though they are always in danger yet continue to feel that seeing mental health practitioners is either unnecessary or dangerous.

The absolute truth persists that spaces delivering mental health care continue to pose danger to black people for dehumanization. Practitioners may inadvertently provide unsafe spaces if they do not know the lived experiences of the patients they follow. Black millennials consistently share these stories on social media, and this phenomenon corresponds to research describing increased rates of incorrect diagnoses among black individuals, less overall satisfaction, and high dropout rates (Mays et al. 2017). What is persistently evident is the necessity to discuss mental health and its impact on a global scale and how global events affect mental health.

Mental Illness and Social Networking Sites

Overall, adolescents cite their social media use (including SNS) to be a positive factor in their lives. Among the most depressed teens surveyed in the Common Sense Media (2012) report, 18% noted that social media worsens their depression, and 13% reported lessening of their depressive symptoms. They feel SNS improve their relationships and interactions with family members and friends and allow them to connect to peers with common interests. They still prefer to interact with people face-to-face and acknowledge that social media can be a barrier. Finally, most teenagers feel they are in good emotional shape: they report positive relationships with parents and peers, engage in a number of varied activities, feel as though they generally like themselves, and understand themselves as largely "normal" (Common Sense Media 2012). However, according to Centers for Disease Control and Prevention (2017) data, one in five young people younger than 25 years has symptoms that meet criteria for a diagnosable mental illness in any given year, and 80% of the individuals in that population do not receive treatment. Most mental illness, including substance use disorders, arises within adolescence, making it a delicate time for brain development and social connectedness. Given that 72% of all teens and young adults report daily social media use, no conversation regarding the mental health of young black children and adolescents can exclude patterns of social media utilization. Specifically, the Internet is widely used as a source for finding health-related information, and many youth turn to SNS because social media is increasingly seen as a credible source of information (Harris et al. 2014).

Although adolescents assert positive overall impact of social media in their lives, negative interactions frequently temper positive exchanges. Teens of all races report encounters with hate speech, including sexist (43%), homophobic (44%), and overt racist (43%) comments, with 24% noting that they see such comments "often" (Common Sense Media 2012). In her 2016 study, Rosenthal and colleagues uncovered numerous negative Facebook interactions, ranging from bullying to unwanted contact. More than 60% of the young people studied disclosed having four or more negative experiences on this platform, which some voiced as contributing to their depression (Rosenthal et al. 2016). There have also been studies suggesting that shared emotional valence can also be transmitted through social media (Kramer et al. 2014). This presents the conundrum that while depressed teens use the Internet more frequently, they may do so to their detriment, despite appreciating positive encounters.

Users with mental illness likely engage in social media use in different ways than those without. Evidence suggests that depressed teens engage in more frequent Internet usage than those without the diagnosis (Romer et al. 2013). According to a 2011 Swiss study, there is a U-shaped correlation between intensity of social media use and adolescent self-report of poor mental health, with heavy Internet users and nonusers both reporting high depressive scores (Lamblin et al. 2017). Adolescents report disclosing more personal information online than they do in person and appear to make connections online that are sometimes deeper than friendships in the "real world." Teenagers with depression do so more frequently than those without serious mental illness. There is research detailing a wide range of behaviors contributing to and resulting from usage of SNS, including isolation from friends and family as well as community building and development of a sense of accomplishment (Common Sense Media 2012). The most depressed teens in the Common Sense Media (2012) survey reported that despite the propensity for social media to make a percentage of them more depressed (18%), they felt that social media made them more confident, more popular, and less shy. In a 2017 qualitative study, depressed teens appear to use the Internet to create connection, for creative release, and often solely for distraction or entertainment, particularly when feeling more depressed (Radovic et al. 2017).

Users range in anonymity on SNS outside of Facebook, and this appears to make teens more willing to disclose information on platforms such as Twitter and Kik. Twitter users typically do not know the majority of their followers— or even of the people they follow—offline and therefore see it as less worrisome to voice what might be seen as "private" information. On Facebook, sharing mental health symptoms may be seen as a faux pas, akin to sharing personal health information at a dinner party. The "Facebook effect" promotes sharing of users' best experiences and encourages users to engage in prosocial behavior (Ziegele and Reinecke 2017). Identifiability is notably part of this phenomenon, as users are connected primarily by people they know offline. Some studies have identified that this may also contribute to depressed teens believing that others' lives are happier than theirs.

Notably, depressed individuals tend to have more emotional connections with users who are not known to them personally (Ybarra et al. 2005). In a 2016 study, Cavazos-Rehg and colleagues (2016) collected over 1.5 million tweets related to depression over the course of slightly less than 1 month. Several tweeters divulged feelings of depression, including at least one symptom meeting a criterion for major depressive disorder. Most of the users were younger than 25 years, and black users were 35% of the tweeters who reported depressive symptoms. The authors expressed concern about the high number of tweets with suicidal thoughts, especially in the context of increasing suicide numbers nationwide.

However, disclosure by users with mental illness can create connections with others based on common lived experiences and foster a space for sharing sentiments, including negative emotions, without fear of censure. Some groups of young adults with mental illness create pockets where they self-diagnose based on experienced symptoms, often voicing doing so because of limited access to care. They effectively create peer support networks on SNS by linking with individuals with similarly endorsed symptoms and building connections based on shared struggles. For those with particularly stigmatizing illnesses, such as persons with personality disorders, schizophrenia, or autism spectrum disorders, the advocacy and community found by peers using SNS are paramount for reducing negative perceptions of those illnesses (Naslund et al. 2014). SNS create niches where young people confess similar symptoms and have their experiences validated by other users. Those who have concerns about self-diagnosis point to the fact that all information shared by online celebrities or even peers is not always accurate and can contribute to stigma. However, the continued benefit of SNS is the ability to correct and delete incorrect posts, and in recovery spaces users work hard to avoid dissemination of incorrect information.

Self-deprecating humor continues to thrive, namely because some youth may post negatively in order to spur reaction from peers (Radovic et al. 2017). At any given time on Twitter, a user can observe dark humor about wanting to die in any manner of ways. The phenomenon includes individuals poking fun at themselves for the ways they cope with their mental illness even in the context of getting treatment. For example, users have described dissociating during therapy sessions, telling their physician that they feel "just fine" to avoid hospitalization, and asking tough questions about survival in the face of all they see around them. This is very different from the concerning pro-ana blogs of the late 1990s, in which anorexic patients fervently generated increasingly clever ways for others to disguise their illness while convincing their caretakers they had improved. Rather, users here poke fun at the nuances of care—cost, time, travel, and effort of maintaining good coping skills. They additionally discuss lack of equity, minimal cultural competency of providers, or the stigma that comes along with having to seek mental health care in their community and the possible fallout if their family members ever became aware of their need for support.

Areas for further research are limitless but include examination of race-specific posting behavior, especially as it pertains to illnesses other than depression and anxiety. Further investigation of preferred social networking site use could illuminate why certain ethnicities prefer a particular site and whether such a preference is gender specific. Additional exploration of trauma, and the responses of black youth to traumatic content as SNS use becomes more ubiquitous, might explain experiential reports of increasing trauma-related symptoms after exposure to triggering content.

Intersections

In 1989, Kimberlé Williams Crenshaw created a new discourse regarding the interplay of people's identities in U.S. society. She coined the word *intersectionality,* which has been expanded by many authors, including I.H. Meyer, who used the minority stress model to describe the way lesbian, gay, bisexual, transgender, and queer (LGBTQ) individuals experience compounded oppressions (Meyer 2003). Young people using social media describe their intersections (e.g., gay, transgender, disabled) and how these social categorizations intensify marginalization and systemic violence. Sexual minority youth find online social support a common and helpful space, especially if they have low social support offline (Ybarra et al. 2005). Like cisgender heterosexual youth, they use online spaces to voice microaggressions but additionally discuss injustices resulting from their unique experiences within the black community and build a family of choice. It is not surprising that the founders of Black Lives Matter are black women who identify as queer. The Black Youth Project survey identified that black millennials advocate for equity for LGBTQ individuals more than other racial groups and desire that this equal access extend to healthcare, jobs, and reduction of disease burden (Rogowski and Cohen 2015). They are more willing than the Generation X or baby boomer population to identify as LGBTQ as well. While many black non-LGBTQIA millennials still maintain prejudicial attitudes toward LGBTQIA individuals in the community, they understand that the latter's needs are important and intrinsic to black liberation, as LGBTQ+ people often lead reformative work.

Engagement of Black Youth

To assess mental health for black millennials and postmillennials, practitioners need to understand the complex views of these populations and their society. They must acknowledge that millennials are politically active, engaged in their communities more than young people of any other race, and actively seeking out avenues for activism. Furthermore, providers must acknowledge that available statistics detailing the current use of SNS are likely underestimations. Utilizers of mental health services, even youth and persons with serious mental illness, are likely to have accounts on Internet-based platforms and use them frequently. Furthermore, through social multiplier effects, the reach of posts on SNS tends to extend to other areas of social media as well as offline. Unless providers explicitly ask, it is difficult to determine if the patient receiving care has a wide following on any SNS and will specifically discuss the quality of that care, anonymously or otherwise. All in all, providers can reasonably expect that their patients and clients discuss their mental healthcare, especially if they are disappointed in the care they are receiving.

The current landscape of physician social media engagement is overwhelmingly directed toward professionalism for the practitioner and tends to overlook the perspective of younger practitioners, especially as they engage their patients. It focuses on physicians' need to tweet to improve public health while maintaining effective boundaries. While professionalism is paramount to any discussion regarding communication, especially ones involving the cloak of anonymity and risk of doctor-patient relationship blurring, it is additionally important to discuss the ways prospective patients use the Internet to talk about their care, engagement with providers, and advocacy. In a world where physicians are rated by their care, there is a lot of concern that engagement on the Internet would damage the austere perception of physicians, open up possibility of critique, and blur the lines of professionalism, but the population at large deserves physicians willing to engage the public in these realms.

Conclusion

Providers should ask about young patients' interactions online and whether they feel those interactions are overall positive or negative experiences. Screening for cyberbullying is additionally vital in depressed and anxious clients. They should be offered solutions to online bullying and abuse that include taking appropriate breaks from the Internet, with genuine understanding about the difficulty of doing so. Specifically, recommending absolute avoidance of Internet interactions would not likely be a feasible goal; suggesting breaks from certain platforms or adjustment of privacy settings may be more appropriate. Providers should endeavor to ask young black patients about the issues most pressing to them, including references to elections and recent public traumas (e.g., triggering of patients who have suffered from sexual assault resulting from seeing increasing amounts of #MeToo posts, or more depressive symptoms after the suicide of a teenager in a Netflix drama). While this may appear to take more time during appointments, engagement of black teenagers as similarly affected and knowledgeable members of society will in fact improve rapport and make teens and young adults more willing to trust their physicians. Gaining knowledge of the use of social media admittedly takes time and effort, but the rewards reaped in patient care are without measure.

References

American Psychological Association: Stress in America: Coping With Change. Stress in America Survey. Washington, DC, American Psychological Association, 2017. Available at: https://www.apa.org/news/press/releases/stress/2016/coping-with-change.pdf. Accessed June 8, 2018.

Cavazos-Rehg PA, Krauss MJ, Sowles S, et al: A content analysis of depression-related tweets. Comput Human Behav 54:351–357, 2016 26392678

Centers for Disease Control and Prevention: Children's Mental Health. Atlanta, GA, Centers for Disease Control and Prevention, 2017. Available at: https://www.cdc.gov/childrensmentalhealth/basics.html. Accessed December 5, 2017.

Common Sense Media: Social Media, Social Life: How Teens View Their Digital Lives. San Francisco, CA, Common Sense Media, 2012. Available at: https://www.commonsensemedia.org/research/social-media-social-life-how-teens-view-their-digital-lives. Accessed July 14, 2017.

Crenshaw K: Demarginalizing the intersection of race and sex: a black feminist critique of antidiscrimination doctrine, feminist theory and antiracist politics. University of Chicago Legal Forum, Vol 1989, Issue 1, Article 8, 1989. Available at: http://chicagounbound.uchicago.edu/uclf/vol1989/iss1/8.

Fry R: Millennials projected to overtake Baby Boomers as America's largest generation. Pew Research Center, March 1, 2018. Available at: http://www.pewresearch.org/fact-tank/2018/03/01/millennials-overtake-baby-boomers/. Accessed June 8, 2018.

Harris JK, Moreland-Russell S, Tabak RG, et al: Communication about childhood obesity on Twitter. Am J Public Health 104(7):e62–e69, 2014 24832138

Kramer AD, Guillory JE, Hancock JT: Experimental evidence of massive-scale emotional contagion through social networks. Proc Natl Acad Sci USA 111(24):8788–8790, 2014 24889601

Lamblin M, Murawski C, Whittle S, et al: Social connectedness, mental health and the adolescent brain. Neurosci Biobehav Rev 80:57–68, 2017 28506925

Mays VM, Jones AL, Delany-Brumsey A, et al: Perceived discrimination in health care and mental health/substance abuse treatment among blacks, Latinos, and whites. Med Care 55(2):173–181, 2017 27753743

Meyer IH: Prejudice, social stress, and mental health in lesbian, gay, and bisexual populations: conceptual issues and research evidence. Psychol Bull 129(5):674–697, 2003 12956539

Molina KM, James D: Discrimination, internalized racism, and depression: a comparative study of African American and Afro-Caribbean adults in the US. Group Process Intergroup Relat 19(4):439–461, 2016 28405176

Naslund JA, Grande SW, Aschbrenner KA, et al: Naturally occurring peer support through social media: the experiences of individuals with severe mental illness using YouTube. PLoS One 9(10):e110171, 2014 25333470

Primack BA, Escobar-Viera CG: Social media as it interfaces with psychosocial development and mental illness in transitional age youth. Child Adolesc Psychiatr Clin N Am 26(2):217–233, 2017 28314452

Radovic A, Gmelin T, Stein BD, et al: Depressed adolescents' positive and negative use of social media. J Adolesc 55:5–15, 2017 27997851

Rogowski J, Cohen C: Black Millennials in America. Chicago, IL, Black Youth Project, 2015. Available at: http://agendatobuildblackfutures.org/wp-content/uploads/2016/01/BYP-millenials-report-10-27-15-FINAL.pdf. Accessed November 4, 2017.

Romer D, Bagdasarov Z, More E: Older versus newer media and the well-being of United States youth: results from a national longitudinal panel. J Adolesc Health 52(5):613–619, 2013 23375827

Rosenthal SR, Buka SL, Marshall BD, et al: Negative experiences on Facebook and depressive symptoms among young adults. J Adolesc Health 59(5):510–516, 2016 27546886

Smiley C, Fakunle D: From "brute" to "thug": the demonization and criminalization of unarmed black male victims in America. J Hum Behav Soc Environ 26(3–4):350–366, 2016 27594778

Smith A, Brenner J: Twitter use 2012. Pew Research Center, May 31, 2012. Available at: http://www.pewinternet.org/2012/05/31/twitter-use-2012/. Accessed July 14, 2017.

Sullivan G, Cheney A, Olson M, et al: Rural African Americans' perspectives on mental health: comparing focus groups and deliberative democracy forums. J Health Care Poor Underserved 28(1):548–565, 2017 28239018

Ybarra ML, Alexander C, Mitchell KJ: Depressive symptomatology, youth internet use, and online interactions: a national survey. J Adolesc Health 36(1):9–18, 2005 15661591

Ziegele M, Reinecke L: No place for negative emotions? The effects of message valence, communication channel, and social distance on users' willingness to respond to SNS status updates. Comput Human Behav 75:704–713, 2017

CHAPTER 21
TRAINING IN THE EFFECTS OF IMPLICIT RACIAL BIAS ON BLACK HEALTH

Tiffany Cooke, M.D., M.P.H., FAPA
Nzinga A. Harrison, M.D., DFAPA

OVERT DISCRIMINATION, while still in existence, has been frowned upon. Unconscious implicit racial bias persists, however, and has far-reaching and overarching implications for blacks in the United States, from interactions with law enforcement to our healthcare system. Implicit racial bias affects various areas of the healthcare system: juvenile, adult, and elderly behavioral health; correctional health; and HIV/AIDS care. In this chapter we discuss the necessity for educating trainees and practitioners about unconscious racial bias that can impact clinical care and outcomes for blacks in the United States.

What Is Implicit Racial Bias?

Simply stated, *implicit racial bias* is a form of prejudice. It is the unconscious and unintentional negative evaluation of one racial group and its members relative to other racial groups. As psychiatrists, we recognize the importance of separating thoughts from feelings from behaviors. Implicit racial bias is the unconscious automatic thought process that leads to rapid emotional responses, including fear and mistrust or compassion and warmth, depending on whether the bias is for or against the individual encountered. The valence of the emotional response, positive or negative, then informs interpersonal behaviors—both discriminatory and supportive (Figure 21–1). Importantly, one must separate implicit racial bias—which is unconscious and quickly activated, may be in conflict with beliefs and values, and often leads to unintentional discriminatory behaviors—from *explicit racial bias*—which is conscious, is firmly rooted in beliefs and values, and requires time and motivation to manifest in discrimination. Racial bias in healthcare, both implicit and explicit, dates back to ancient times and has been a long-standing tenant of Western medicine.

History of Implicit Racial Bias in Healthcare

Bias in medicine and healthcare has recently gained substantial attention and has become an ever-growing area of research, particularly since the authors of the Institute of Medicine report *Unequal Treatment* (Smedley et al. 2002) noted that minorities receive lower quality of care than whites, even after researchers controlled for sociodemographic factors. The report authors also suggested that bias on the part of the healthcare provider may lead to disparate care among nonwhites and whites. Because prior disparities research was heavily focused on lifestyle factors, social determinants, and other factors on the part of the healthcare recipient, the report sparked new dialogue regarding the role of the provider. Many healthcare professionals pride themselves on providing equitable care; thus, acknowledging the presence and impact of implicit healthcare bias can initiate the process of actively working to reduce it and its potentially deleterious health outcomes.

Although implicit bias in healthcare is a relatively new, flourishing field of study, the presence of bias in Western medicine dates back millennia. In its earliest form this bias was overt, explicit, and typically race and/or class based. Byrd and Clayton (1992) extensively outlined the history of racial inequities in Western medicine. As they elucidated, healthcare bias against blacks and its resultant consequences have been present in every period from the Greco-Roman, when Plato and Aristotle assigned lower taxonomy rankings to blacks, to the present. In their contribution to *Unequal Treatment*, Byrd and Clayton (2002) note that the slavery of the Moors, along with the Mediterranean and Atlantic slave trades, were filled with inferior healthcare for blacks and slaves. North American English colonial slaves were often "overutilized for surgical, medical demonstration, and dissection purposes" (p. 500). During the Civil War and

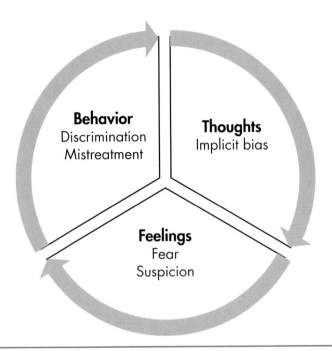

FIGURE 21–1. Relationship between implicit racial bias and discrimination.

the period following, black Union soldiers received discriminatory and sub-standard care, and care for newly freed slaves was initially virtually nonexistent. A resultant separate, substandard system of care was formed. The Civil Rights period ushered in Medicaid and Medicare, supported by the National Medical Association and initially opposed by the American Medical Association, along with the legal desegregation of hospitals. Post–Civil Rights, although advances in medical care and technology have skyrocketed, health disparities for blacks have persisted and in some cases have worsened (Byrd and Clayton 1992; Smedley et al. 2002).

While much of this historical perspective denotes explicit bias, it is important to highlight for many reasons: Even as people's explicit racial views change, their implicit racial biases remain. Explicit bias breeds stereotypes, and knowledge of stereotypes is enough to trigger implicit bias (Chapman et al. 2013). Though explicit bias is said to be socially unacceptable, implicit bias is ever persistent.

Literature has shown that most physicians hold significant pro-white bias, with the exception of African American doctors (Chapman et al. 2013). Implicit bias has a significant impact on patient health outcomes, treatment decisions, treatment adherence, and patient-provider interactions (Hall et al. 2015), which means provider implicit bias has the potential to negatively impact the health of blacks and perpetuate disparities.

Impact of Implicit Racial Bias on Health Outcomes

A significant literature on the impact of implicit racial bias on health disparities began to build in the early 2000s. In response to growing evidence and awareness about the ways in which healthcare providers' implicit racial bias could affect judgment, clinical decision making, and behavior, the Institute of Medicine published, in 2002, a comprehensive report on implicit bias, the conclusion of which was that implicit bias may contribute to health disparities but that additional research was needed (Smedley et al. 2002). Since that report, the medical literature has continued to build, and the relationship between medical provider implicit racial bias and negative health outcomes has been further elucidated, with researchers noting at least four healthcare domains that can be affected: patient-provider interactions, treatment decisions/quality of care, patient treatment adherence, and patient health outcomes (Hall et al. 2015).

In general, implicit racial bias has been shown to contribute to longer wait times for treatment for nonwhites, more time spent with white patients, and preferential requests—for example, extending visiting hours for some patients while limiting visiting hours for others. Additionally, black patients consistently react less positively to physicians with high implicit bias, even when relative to their reaction to physicians with high explicit bias (Hall et al. 2015). For example, an early study found that black patients reported less satisfaction with physicians who had low explicit racial bias but high implicit racial bias (Penner et al. 2010). This suggests that patients are able to detect implicit bias, even in the absence of explicit bias.

Physician bias has been shown to affect psychosocial outcomes for black patients, including integration, prevalence, and treatment of depression and life satisfaction. In the following subsections, we focus specifically on the impact of implicit racial bias on health outcomes among black patients in juvenile and behavioral health, adult and elderly behavioral health, correctional health, and HIV/AIDS care.

Juvenile and Behavioral Health

Most investigations of the effect of implicit racial bias on health outcomes have been conducted in adult populations. However, one study did demonstrate racial bias against black children at levels similar to those held against black adults.

Importantly, the specialty of the resident physician did not affect the level of bias, suggesting that pediatric residents are also at risk for holding implicit racial bias against black children.

While the effect of implicit racial bias against black children has not been rigorously explored in the literature, there is a small literature developing regarding the impact of racism on the health outcomes of black children. The majority of that literature reports on the association of racism with behavioral and mental health issues as opposed to physical health conditions. Exposure to racism has been associated with depressive symptoms, anxiety symptoms, conduct disorder, and low self-esteem in both preadolescents and adolescents. Interestingly, parental exposure to racial discrimination has been demonstrated to be independently associated with increased general anxiety and depression among black adolescents. In addition to generalized anxiety, depressive, and conduct disorder symptoms, there is a strong correlation between number of drinks an adolescent takes per day and perception of and anger due to racial discrimination (Pachter and Coll 2009). Finally, it is well characterized in child and adolescent psychiatry that children and adolescents may respond to stressors by internalizing or externalizing problem behaviors, leading to differing symptom patterns. Both types of problem behaviors have been associated with experiences with racism.

As discussed earlier in this chapter, racism and discrimination are behavioral manifestations of the underlying cognitive processes that include implicit and explicit bias. Just as black adults are sensitive to the presence of implicit bias in their healthcare providers, children and adolescents are likely sensitive to the effects of implicit bias on their relationships with healthcare providers as well. As psychiatrists, we understand the important relationship among thoughts, feelings, and behaviors and as such can draw the connection between implicit racial bias (thoughts) and racial discrimination against child and adolescent patients (behaviors). Given the evidence that experience with racial discrimination results in negative health outcomes for anxiety, depression, internalizing and externalizing behaviors, and alcohol use, as well as the evidence indicating that resident physicians carry implicit racial biases that may underlie the manifestation of racially discriminatory behavior, we must concentrate efforts specifically on evaluating the effects of implicit racial bias on pediatric and adolescent health, so as to inform training opportunities for undermining that bias.

Adult and Elderly Behavioral Health

There is a small but significant medical literature addressing the effects of implicit racial bias on health outcomes in black adults. There is considerably less investigation specifically regarding health outcomes of elderly black adults; however, much of the information available can be applied to the elderly black population as well.

Historically, it has been demonstrated that black patients are disproportionately diagnosed with psychotic disorders. In a recent review article, Schwartz and Blankenship (2014) reported that this phenomenon remains true, with black patients diagnosed with psychotic disorders at a rate on average three to four times higher than white patients. It is believed that implicit racial bias is playing a role in that disparity.

Regarding depression in black adults, 5%–10% of black men are believed to have experienced a depressive episode. However, treatment rates remain low in the black community. We noted earlier that patients are astute to the presence of implicit racial bias among their physicians. It has been further posited that black patients, as a result of historical experiences and ongoing experiences, have a larger mistrust of healthcare services and therefore underutilize such services (Suite et al. 2007), a pattern that perpetuates mental health disparities in black populations.

The mistrust and underutilization seen among adult black patients extend into later life as well. Although most studies suggest a higher or equivalent prevalence of depression in older black adults when compared with white adults, there are also lower rates of recognition and treatment of depression. Not surprisingly, many studies report worse depression outcomes for elderly black adults than for elderly white adults. It is quite possible that implicit racial bias among mental health providers is contributing to the reduced recognition and treatment of depression in older black adults. This is a relationship that needs further exploration.

Correctional Health

There are currently more than 2 million people incarcerated in the United States, and this excludes the millions under correctional control in the form of either probation or parole. Of these, 650,000 reenter the community each year. The incarcerated population is particularly vulnerable, yet in many cases physicians have insufficient training in clinical interaction with incarcerated or formerly incarcerated persons. Prisoners, the only individuals with a constitutional right to healthcare, often find themselves with significant unmet needs. Conditions such as HIV infection, hepatitis C, tuberculosis, diabetes, hypertension, asthma, influenza, substance use, and myriad other illnesses disproportionately affect incarcerated persons. We have already discussed the general physician pro-white bias. Thus, given the disproportionate amount of black incarcerated persons and their health risks, the impact of implicit bias can have substantial impacts on health outcomes of such a vulnerable population. These factors, along with the barriers to care that incarcerated persons face upon release, make this a susceptible population in dire need of quality healthcare but at high risk for not receiving it.

Lack of didactic curricula, pervasive social stigma, and the marginalization of this group make the potential for explicit and implicit bias great. The potential becomes even higher if there are differences in race between provider and patient. Given the punitive aspect of incarceration, explicit bias against prisoners may not be as frowned upon as racial bias. As mentioned previously, explicit bias lends itself to the formation of cultural stereotypes. Awareness and reinforcement of stereotypes lead to implicit bias (Hall et al. 2015).

As the American College of Emergency Physicians (2006) noted, "Many healthcare providers (including nurses, physicians, and technicians) view incarcerated patients as unreliable (especially with regard to providing honest personal histories), dangerous, and manipulative malingerers. Even more troublesome are beliefs by some healthcare workers that the incarcerated are essentially 'social outcasts' whose diseases are well deserved." Although there is a dearth of correctional healthcare physicians, the field is growing. Whereas stereotypes about the incarcerated, as well as about the physicians who treat them, may have precluded many from entering the field, desires for a consistent salary, benefits, and low to no overhead or malpractice have caused some to reconsider. The use of telemedicine has made it an easier transition for physicians who wish to avoid on-site work at a correctional facility. As the field and, unfortunately, the number of incarcerated persons grow, so does the need to train physicians in recognizing and lessening their implicit bias.

Correctional healthcare didactics and clinical sites would allow for medical student and resident training and also decrease the unmet health needs of the incarcerated and those for whom reentry is approaching. The literature regarding implicit healthcare bias in the United States, specifically as related to the incarcerated, is scant. Furthering studies in this area is another way to engage trainees in learning more about recognizing their biases while simultaneously expanding the body of literature in this much-needed area.

The disruption in family structure, housing, and income and the disease burden associated with such disruption have a significant impact on not only the individual but also the community. The mental and physical well-being of incarcerated persons is not a "them" issue. As previously stated, implicit bias affects health outcomes, and nowhere is this more important to consider than in the vulnerable black incarcerated/formerly incarcerated individual, who has higher risk of disease burden due to race and incarceration. Therefore, physicians have a duty to check their implicit bias and provide the best-quality care possible to this group both while incarcerated and upon reentering their communities.

HIV/AIDS Care

According to the Centers for Disease Control and Prevention (2017), in 2015, blacks composed 12% of the U.S. population but represented 45% of the population with HIV diagnoses. Even as HIV/AIDS has now come to be viewed as a chronic, manageable condition rather than a "death sentence," blacks do not appear to be reaping the benefits of advanced treatment options as compared with whites. Blacks continue to have the highest disease burden from HIV/AIDS, with myriad proposed attributing factors. One must consider the role of the healthcare provider, especially given that there is disparate care for blacks compared with whites in terms of providers prescribing antiretroviral therapy and judgments of adherence to antiretroviral therapy (Bogart et al. 2001; Cargill and Stone 2005; Fleishman et al. 2012). Because antiretroviral therapy can decrease morbidity and mortality associated with HIV, it is crucial that we work to eliminate prescribing discrepancies and inaccurate perceptions about treatment adherence. We must also inform trainees and current practitioners about the necessity of focusing on individual patient characteristics when making treatment considerations. Although there is a need to further elucidate the role of such factors as insurance status, provider trust, and satisfaction, these findings are still concerning.

Implicit HIV prejudice has the potential to negatively impact both physical and mental health (Miller et al. 2016). Coupled with the racial prejudice blacks may experience, along with general implicit healthcare bias, black persons living with HIV/AIDS face a unique set of stressors. The substance use, psychiatric disorders, and physical comorbidities that can occur with HIV/AIDS can have far-reaching implications to the individuals, their families, and the community, particularly in blacks given the disease burden. Thus, prevention is key.

Pre-exposure prophylaxis is now being recognized as a pharmacological method of reducing the chances of contracting HIV in negative individuals at high risk for acquiring it. Calabrese et al. (2014) reported that medical students exhibited decreased willingness to prescribe pre-exposure prophylaxis to a black versus a white male patient. This was due to the perception that the black patient would be more likely to engage in unprotected sex while on the treatment, despite a lack of empirical evidence showing this to be true, and in the absence of other barriers such as access to care and insurance.

Such misconceptions speak poignantly and specifically to the need to engage trainees in implicit bias training as part of the medical school curriculum. Because medical training may emphasize population, racial, or group characteristics that might inadvertently perpetuate implicit bias, it is imperative to encourage medical students to make individualized assessments of a person. Current providers must be allowed and must advocate for adequate physician-patient time to avoid the unconscious bias that is more likely to occur under time constraints. This is especially key in a time when insurance and clinical mandates limit contact between patients and providers. Time constraints coupled with implicit bias can lead to poor patient-provider communication, subsequent dissatisfaction with care, and lower likelihood of engaging.

Research highlights the effects of implicit bias on both treatment and prevention of HIV infection, contributing to the black-white disparity. While insurance, barriers to care and social determinants play a substantial role in disparities, physicians who are charged with providing equitable care must examine and seek to eliminate implicit bias as a source of adverse health outcomes.

Undermining Implicit Bias in Healthcare

In this chapter, we have defined implicit racial bias as the development of unconscious, automatic thoughts that individuals develop in response to members of a particular racial group. We have reviewed the specific effects of implicit racial bias among healthcare providers on juvenile, adult, and elderly mental health, correctional, and HIV/AIDS populations. The question remains, can implicit racial bias be undermined? A growing literature suggests yes.

Cultural competency has long been a requirement of undergraduate medical education; however, implicit racial bias training has not been a component of that training. There are evidence-based interventions for reducing implicit racial bias and the discriminatory behavior that flows therefrom. Such interventions are grounded in psychodynamic and cognitive-behavioral strategies well known to psychiatrists.

Psychodynamic interventions focus on bringing to light the impact of past experiences and relationships on current interpersonal functioning. The same principle can be applied to implicit racial bias, which is an unconscious cognitive process rooted in past exposures (personal and media), experiences, and relationships with individuals in the identified racial group. When awareness of one's implicit bias is raised, and the motivation to respond without prejudice is enhanced, the risk of acting out on one's implicit biases can be reduced.

The gold-standard test for identifying implicit bias is the Implicit Association Test (IAT; Greenwald et al. 2003). The IAT presents users with photos and words and requires the user to make a series of rapid associations between the two. It is thought to measure implicit attitudes by comparing the number of negative valence and positive valence words associated with faces of different races. After an individual has identified his or her implicit racial bias, internal and external motivators to undermine that bias must be bolstered. Internal motivation to undermine implicit racial bias is primarily driven by personal values and the belief that prejudice is wrong. External motivation, on the other hand, is driven by a desire to escape the social consequences that can arise from being identified as a person who is prejudiced or racist. While our colleagues and trainees come to us with their own set of internal motivators, it is imperative that as physicians, we create a culture in our workplaces and training programs that explicitly addresses and denounces prejudicial behavior and racism, to empower the ability of external motivators to undermine implicit racial bias.

Specific strategies for undermining implicit bias that are rooted in psychodynamic principles include perspective taking and increasing opportunities for contact with individuals of the racial group against which bias is held. During perspective-taking exercises, individuals are encouraged to take the perspective, in first person, of a member of the stereotyped group. The experience of speaking the perspective using the pronoun "I" is thought to increase psychological closeness to the stigmatized group and thereby undermine negative, automatic, group-based thoughts that may arise as a result of previous experiences or exposures to members of the stigmatized group. Similarly, increasing opportunities for positive contact with members of the stigmatized group alters the negative cognitive representations one may hold as a result of previous experiences or exposures by replacing them with positive cognitive representations of the stigmatized group. One strategy workplaces and training programs use to increase opportunities for positive contact is to focus on racial diversity of medical staff and resident trainees.

Cognitive-behavioral interventions focus on 1) reducing risk factors that increase the risk of acting out on implicit biases and 2) challenging stereotypes. Identified risk factors that increase the risk of acting out on implicit biases are completely congruous with the work state that traditional training programs create for trainees. Namely, being busy, being distracted, and being stressed reduce the functioning of the prefrontal cortex and leave physicians at the mercy of unconscious, automatic thought processes, including implicit racial bias.

Because we know that physician work and training environments cannot be completely rid of business, distraction, and stress, it is important to evaluate other strategies for undermining implicit racial bias as well—for example, challenging stereotypes. Cognitive strategies that focus on reducing stereotypes, including stereotype replacement, individuation, and perspective taking, have been applied to efforts to undermine implicit racial bias. Stereotype replacement involves raising one's awareness that a reaction one is having to an individual is based on a stereotype. The physician then intentionally labels his or her own response as stereotypical, reflects on why that response occurred, considers how the biased response could be avoided in the future, and intentionally replaces the biased response with an unbiased response. A psychiatrist will recognize this intervention as the application of cognitive strategies—thought stopping and thought replacement.

Given there are evidence-based strategies for undermining implicit racial bias, the question becomes, how do we apply those interventions to undergraduate, graduate, and continuing medical education? A six-point framework has been proposed. The key features of the framework are creating a safe and nonthreatening learning context, increasing knowledge about the science of implicit

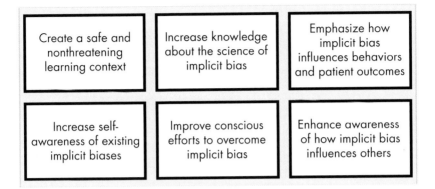

FIGURE 21–2. A framework for integrating implicit bias recognition into health professions education.

bias, emphasizing how implicit bias influences behaviors and patient outcomes, increasing self-awareness of existing implicit biases, improving conscious efforts to overcome implicit bias, and enhancing awareness of how implicit bias influences others (Sukhera and Watling 2018) (Figure 21–2). As more medical schools, residency training programs, and professional organizations begin requiring implicit racial bias training as part of undergraduate, graduate, and continuing medical education, we may see a reduction of the portion of mental health disparities in blacks that can be attributed to implicit racial bias among physicians.

Conclusion

Although explicit racial bias continues to decline, rates of implicit racial bias among healthcare providers have not shown such a decline, and the effects of implicit racial bias on the health outcomes of black populations are beginning to be well documented. We have an opportunity to incorporate implicit racial bias training into undergraduate, graduate, and continuing medical education in order to undermine the effects of implicit racial bias on healthcare decisions.

References

American College of Emergency Physicians: Recognizing the Needs of Incarcerated Patients in the Emergency Department. American College of Emergency Physicians website, 2006. Available at: https://www.acep.org/administration/resources/recognizing-the-needs-of-incarcerated-patients-in-the-emergency-department/. Accessed December 1, 2017.

Bogart LM, Catz SL, Kelly JA, et al: Factors influencing physicians' judgments of adherence and treatment decisions for patients with HIV disease. Med Decis Making 21(1):28–36, 2001 11206944

Byrd WM, Clayton LA: An American health dilemma: a history of blacks in the health system. J Natl Med Assoc 84(2):189–200, 1992 1602519

Byrd WM, Clayton LA: Racial and ethnic disparities in healthcare: a background and history, in Unequal Treatment: Confronting Racial and Ethnic Disparities in Health Care. Edited by Smedley BD, Stith AY, Nelson AR. Washington, DC, National Academies Press, 2002, pp 455–527

Calabrese SK, Earnshaw VA, Underhill K, et al: The impact of patient race on clinical decisions related to prescribing HIV pre-exposure prophylaxis (PrEP): assumptions about sexual risk compensation and implications for access. AIDS Behav 18(2):226–240, 2014 24366572

Cargill VA, Stone VE: HIV/AIDS: a minority health issue. Med Clin North Am 89(4):895–912, 2005 15925655

Centers for Disease Control and Prevention: HIV Among African Americans. Centers for Disease Control and Prevention website, October 26, 2017. Available at: https://www.cdc.gov/hiv/group/racialethnic/africanamericans/index.html. Accessed December 14, 2017.

Chapman EN, Kaatz A, Carnes M: Physicians and implicit bias: how doctors may unwittingly perpetuate health care disparities. J Gen Intern Med 28(11):1504–1510, 2013 23576243

Fleishman JA, Yehia BR, Moore RD, et al; HIV Research Network: Disparities in receipt of antiretroviral therapy among HIV-infected adults (2002–2008). Med Care 50(5):419–427, 2012 22410406

Greenwald AG, Nosek BA, Banaji MR: Understanding and using the Implicit Association Test, I: an improved scoring algorithm. J Pers Soc Psychol 85(2):197–216, 2003 12916565

Hall WJ, Chapman MV, Lee KM, et al: Implicit racial/ethnic bias among health care professionals and its influence on health care outcomes: a systematic review. Am J Public Health 105(12):e60–e76, 2015 26469668

Miller CT, Varni SE, Solomon SE, et al: Macro-level implicit HIV prejudice and the health of community residents with HIV. Health Psychol 35(8):807–815, 2016 27505199

Pachter LM, Coll CG: Racism and child health: a review of the literature and future directions. J Dev Behav Pediatr 30(3):255–263, 2009

Penner LA, Dovidio JF, West TW, et al: Aversive racism and medical interactions with Black patients: a field study. J Exp Soc Psychol 46:436–440, 2010 20228874

Schwartz RC, Blankenship DM: Racial disparities in psychotic disorder diagnosis: a review of empirical literature. World J Psychiatry 4(4):133–140, 2014 25540728

Smedley BD, Stith AY, Nelson AR (eds): Unequal Treatment: Confronting Racial and Ethnic Disparities in Health Care. Washington, DC, National Academies Press, 2002

Suite DH, La Bril R, Primm A, et al: Beyond misdiagnosis, misunderstanding and mistrust: relevance of the historical perspective in the medical and mental health treatment of people of color. J Natl Med Assoc 99(8):879–885, 2007 17722664

Sukhera J, Watling C: A framework for integrating implicit bias recognition into health professions education. Acad Med 93(1):35–40, 2018 28658015

CHAPTER 22
HISTORICALLY BLACK COLLEGES AND UNIVERSITIES AND AFRICAN AMERICAN PSYCHIATRY

Past, Present, and Future

Curley L. Bonds, M.D., DFAPA

FROM THE MOMENT they were established and continuing through their many decades of existence, the role of historically black college and university (HBCU) departments of psychiatry has grown and transformed alongside the communities that they serve. The four institutions in this country that make up this group are Howard University College of Medicine in Washington, D.C.; Meharry Medical College in Nashville, Tennessee; Charles R. Drew University (CDU) of Medicine and Science in Los Angeles, California; and Morehouse School of Medicine in Atlanta, Georgia. While CDU's medical school was founded in 1966 prior to the establishment of Morehouse's in 1975, it does not technically qualify as an HBCU. This is because the Higher Education Act of 1965 required HBCUs to have been chartered before 1964. Since Morehouse's parent institution (Morehouse College) was founded in 1867, it meets the HBCU criteria established by the 1965 legislation. CDU has been recognized as a historically black graduate institution by the U.S. Department of

Education and has always been considered informally to belong to this group. While each of these institutions is unique, they share similar missions and values that have shaped their evolution over time.

Historically Black College and University Missions

It is notable that all four of the institutions, in their formal mission statements, make strong references to serving underserved populations and/or reducing healthcare disparities:

Howard University Mission Statement

To lead in the advancement of healthcare and health equality locally and globally.

Meharry Mission Statement

MMC is an academic health sciences center that exists to improve the health and health care of minority and underserved communities by offering excellent education and training programs in the health sciences. True to its heritage, Meharry places special emphasis on providing opportunities for people of color, individuals from disadvantaged backgrounds, and others regardless of race or ethnicity; delivering high quality health services; and conducting research that fosters the elimination of health disparities.

Charles R. Drew Mission Statement

Charles R. Drew University of Medicine and Science is a private, non-profit, student-centered University that is committed to cultivating diverse health professional leaders who are dedicated to social justice and health equity for underserved populations through outstanding education, research, clinical service, and community engagement.

Morehouse Mission Statement

We exist to: Improve the health and well-being of individuals and communities; increase the diversity of the health professional and scientific workforce; address primary health care through programs in education, research, and service, with emphasis on people of color and the underserved urban and rural populations in Georgia, the nation, and the world.

In addition, Howard and CDU's missions both reference health equality. It is also notable that several of these schools proudly embrace concern with not only their local communities but also the health of the entire country and the world. Underserved people, regardless of their location, have always been a priority for these institutions. The HBCUs had the highest social mission scores among all private and public U.S. medical schools in a 2010 study published in the *Annals of Internal Medicine* (Mullan et al. 2010). The authors took into account three different dimensions to calculate a school's social mission score: the percentage of graduates who practice primary care, the percentage of graduates who work in health professional shortage areas, and the percentage of graduates who are underrepresented minority group members. These social missions extend to the departments of psychiatry within the respective institutions as well and have influenced the contributions that these departments have made to American psychiatry. The missions of the HBCUs are further reflected in the diversity of their faculty and trainees and by the locations of the hospitals and clinics with which they are affiliated.

All of the HBCUs were initially established to provide training opportunities for African American physicians seeking to practice medicine who found it difficult (if not impossible) to matriculate at established majority institutions. As a result of this goal, HBCUs have amassed an impressive collection of distinguished faculty leaders with clinical and research careers dedicated to addressing the problem of limited access to psychiatric services for minorities and the multitude of health disparities disproportionately affecting this population. Psychiatry departments within these institutions emerged with congruent goals and were instrumental in training more psychiatrists of color than majority institutions. However, it is important to note that these schools not only opened their doors to African American trainees but also welcomed a larger percentage of women, non-black minority physicians, and graduates of foreign medical schools compared with their peer institutions. This tradition of diversity contributes to HBCU departments of psychiatry having alumni that are more likely to reflect the global community than are majority institutions. This chapter highlights some of the HBCUs' contributions and sheds light on how these institutions have evolved over time as well as speculating on their future prospects.

Innovative Institutions

Howard University College of Medicine

Howard University College of Medicine was established in 1868, making it the oldest HBCU medical school. Howard celebrated its sesquicentennial year in 2017. The university's department of psychiatry encompasses a broad range of clinical programs serving the metropolitan Washington, D.C., area and is ranked as one of the top 50 most-funded psychiatric research facilities in the entire country. Howard possesses an impressive legacy as an important training ground for black psychiatrists who were pioneers in the field (Spurlock 1999). Among them was Ernest Y. Williams, M.D., a medical student at Howard University from 1926 to 1930, who ultimately became the founder of Howard's department of neurology and psychiatry in 1940. Another pioneer was Charles

Prudhomme, M.D., who graduated from Howard University's School of Medicine in 1935. Dr. Prudhomme is credited as a major force behind desegregating the Tuskegee Veterans Administration Hospital. In addition, he is also recognized as the first black African American psychoanalyst, having completed psychoanalytic training at the Washington Psychoanalytic Institute in 1956. Another major contribution of Dr. Prudhomme was his significant involvement in the landmark school desegregation case *Brown v. Board of Education of Topeka, Kansas* (347 U.S. 483 [1954]).

Howard's department of psychiatry has a long and storied tradition of playing a central role in developing innovations in the field. Maxie Maultsby Jr., M.D., founded an innovative method of psychotherapy focused specifically on African Americans called *rational behavior therapy*. Dr. Maultsby, a prolific and well-respected author of several books, wrote extensively on the subject of self-help techniques. He also served as chair of the department of psychiatry and was a professor who taught residents at St. Elizabeth's Hospital (Spurlock 1999). Other notable Howard faculty include Alyce Gullattee, M.D., who established one of the first substance abuse programs for a medical school in the District of Columbia area; and Evaristus Nwulia, M.D., who developed and patented a novel medication delivery system as well as a unique and groundbreaking diagnostic system for depression. Perhaps one of the most distinguished faculty members to head Howard's psychiatry department was William Lawson, M.D., Ph.D. Dr. Lawson is credited with well over 200 published works and helping to secure more than $10 million in research funding in addition to bringing several large and prestigious awards to the university, including three highly coveted R01 grants. He has had a long career as a prolific researcher credited with many significant findings, including helping uncover the underlying genetics of schizophrenia and bipolar disorder. Dr. Lawson continues to break ground in creating and testing evidence-based practices, including medication-assisted therapies for addictions and novel treatments for cocaine addiction. During his period of leadership at Howard, Dr. Lawson was highly respected by his peers, having been elected as president of the Washington Psychiatric Society and president of the DC chapter of Mental Health America.

Meharry Medical College

Meharry was the second HBCU medical school to be established and was initially founded in 1876, 11 years after the end of the Civil War, to train slaves in the healing arts. Meharry's department of psychiatry would become established nearly 90 years later and was founded by Dr. Lloyd Elam in 1963. Dr. Elam was first appointed as an assistant professor in internal medicine, but he became the first chair of the department of psychiatry and advanced to the rank of full professor of psychiatry in 1963. He served in this capacity before ascending the ranks to become first dean and later president of the college in 1968. During Dr. Elam's time as chair, the inpatient psychiatry and psychiatry residency programs were established, and Meharry pioneered one of the first psychiatric day treatment programs in the country. During his tenure, the school experienced enormous growth in the form of a successful $88 million capital campaign, allowing the college to erect a significant number of much-needed new buildings, as well as established graduate studies programs in public health, biochemistry, and several other health-related fields. In 1981, Dr. Elam was appointed as chancellor for the college. Meharry's eponymous Lloyd C. Elam Mental Health Center is a fitting tribute to his unparalleled legacy and continues to provide exceptional psychiatric services and substance abuse treatment (The HistoryMakers 2007).

Another notable Meharrian is Jeanne Spurlock, M.D. (U.S. National Library of Medicine 2015). Dr. Spurlock became chair of the department of psychiatry at Meharry in 1968 after leaving a position at Michael Reese Hospital in Chicago. She went on to become a highly respected author and outspoken political activist with numerous books and articles to her name. After her time at Meharry, she ascended the ranks in organized American psychiatry and was named deputy medical director of the American Psychiatric Association (APA), a position that she held for 17 years. During her long and impressive career, Dr. Spurlock contributed greatly to our understanding of sexism, racism, and cultural competence within the mental health field. She was a passionate and fierce advocate for all children and adolescents and coauthored the landmark work *Culturally Diverse Children and Adolescents: Assessment, Diagnosis, and Treatment* with Ian Canino in 1994 (Canino and Spurlock 1994). In 1999, Dr. Spurlock also published the seminal *Black Psychiatrists and American Psychiatry*, which as of this writing continues to be the best-known and most often quoted compendium on African American psychiatrists. In 1992, she was awarded a Presidential Commendation Award from the APA, along with other well-deserved acknowledgments of her career accomplishments, including the Solomon Carter Fuller Award and APA Distinguished Service Award. In addition to her work at Meharry, Dr. Spurlock also taught as a clinical professor at George Washington University and Howard University.

Another distinguished faculty member and chair of the Meharry department of psychiatry was Rahn Bailey, M.D., a graduate of Morehouse College. Dr. Bailey's many accomplishments include serving as the 113th president of the National Medical Association and receiving recognition by the same organization for his exemplary efforts to coordinate much-needed medical care for the victims of Hurricane Katrina.

Charles R. Drew University of Medicine and Science

Charles R. Drew Post Graduate Medical School was founded in Los Angeles in 1966 as the only minority-focused health sciences university located west of the Mississippi River. It was formed in the aftermath of the 1965 Watts riots to address the egregious lack of medical facilities in the impoverished and crime-ridden South Los Angeles region. Martin Luther King Jr. Hospital was established by the same legislation that created the medical school and was located adjacent to the school. The vision was for the two institutions to cooperatively train physicians to work in the underserved Watts-Willowbrook area, the poverty-stricken communities in which the institutions are located. Together, the institutions were commonly referred to by the moniker "King/Drew Medical Center." In 1987 the school became a university and officially changed its name to the Charles R. Drew University of Medicine and Science (CDU) to reflect its expanded identity and role in the community as a resource for training a wide variety of health professionals. CDU is named for the brilliant and visionary African American physician Charles R. Drew, who is still widely revered to this day for his pioneering work in blood preservation.

Psychiatric services at King/Drew Medical Center would have not existed in their present form if not for the efforts of George L. Mallory, M.D. Having completed his medical education at Howard University in 1953, Dr. Mallory later relocated to Los Angeles, where he completed his psychiatry residency training and then went on to hold prestigious faculty positions at the University of Southern California and the University of California, Los Angeles (UCLA). Dr. Mallory was recruited to become one of the initial members of the CDU faculty and the founding chair of the department of psychiatry and human behavior. He was the key author of the concept paper that established the Augustus F. Hawkins Mental Health Building on the Martin Luther King Jr. Hospital campus. Dr. Mallory's name became synonymous with psychiatric education at CDU during his tenure of more than 30 years of continuous service from 1959 to 1989. Dr. Mallory started as a staff psychiatrist, and his leadership qualities were soon recognized. He went on to serve as the chief of adult psychiatry at MLK hospital as well as the director of residency training for the Drew adult psychiatry residency. Dr. Mallory's association with Drew did not end after his retirement, as he generously agreed to serve as interim chair on multiple occasions after 1989. His guidance and wisdom were much sought after by local, regional, and national leaders throughout his extraordinary career, and he was the well-deserved recipient of the Lifetime Achievement Award by Black Psychiatrists of America in 2014.

Morehouse School of Medicine

Founded in 1975, Morehouse School of Medicine is the newest HBCU. Initially it was known as the Medical Education Program at Morehouse College, but in 1981 it became an independently chartered institution. Dewitt C. Alfred Jr., M.D., joined the faculty at Morehouse in 1984 and was appointed head of the psychiatry department in 1978 (Legacy.com Obituaries 2006). Prior to joining the Morehouse faculty, Dr. Alfred was the first African American professor of psychiatry at Emory University School of Medicine and the first African American president of the Georgia Psychiatric Association (Spurlock 1999). During his time at Morehouse, Dr. Alfred secured millions of dollars in grants that provided funds that helped the institution flourish by establishing clinical services and residency programs. As a testament to his enduring legacy, a scholarship and annual research symposium at Morehouse bear Dr. Alfred's name today.

Collaborations and Challenges

An important part of the history of HBCUs is their relationships with departments at majority schools. At times these relationships have been forged from the outset as strong intentional collaborations. Such is the case with CDU and UCLA. In fact, the CDU charter dictates that 50% of the medical school's faculty hold concurrent appointments at UCLA. The funding for CDU's medical school came jointly from Los Angeles County and the University of California and supported both infrastructure and medical student education. Today, CDU medical students are also considered UCLA students, and many of the CDU faculty participate in a variety of research projects that bridge the two institutions. The residency program at CDU began as a combined program but eventually became independent. In many instances, the two universities share clinical facilities, grants, and other resources, to the benefit of both patients and the institutions.

However, the HBCU medical schools have not always enjoyed harmonious relationships with neighboring majority institutions. Although Meharry and Vanderbilt have both existed since the mid-1870s, the schools were completely separate until the advent of the Meharry Vanderbilt Alliance in 1999. Prior to this, a very public and contentious battle was fought by Mcharry to gain access for its trainees to the federally owned Veterans Hospital of Nashville and the General Hospital of Nashville (Stuart 1982). At the time, Vanderbilt (a predominately white institution) had a much smaller student enrollment than Meharry but had eight to nine times the number of patients available to its students than did Meharry. President Ronald Reagan was asked to intervene on Meharry's behalf to help save the school, which was in the midst of struggling to preserve its accreditation. Fortunately, this unprecedented intervention resulted in a $55.6 million financial aid package that salvaged Meharry from closure in 1982. Now, through the Alliance, the two institutions have partnered together to support undergraduate medical education, residency training, and community-based research and training programs. This collaborative partnership has helped to identify some of the barriers to minority participation in clinical research and many other important findings (https://www.vumc.org/meharry-vanderbilt/).

Atlanta's 125-year-old Grady Memorial Hospital is the largest public hospital in Georgia and the only Level-1 trauma center within 100 miles of the Atlanta metropolitan area, home to 5.7 million people. Both Morehouse and Emory schools of medicine provide doctors for the hospital that serves the most disadvantaged residents of the area (Lawley and Higginbotham 2007). In 2007 the hospital's survival was threatened by critical budget shortfalls that resulted in a failure to pay vendors on time. In an editorial to the *Atlanta Journal-Constitution,* the deans of both schools concluded that the situation at Grady was grave and called for a change of governance (Epps et al. 1994). At the time, the hospital system owed a total of $54 million jointly to both institutions and faced a $120 million cash shortfall overall. In 2008 the situation was reversed when the hospital was made into a nonprofit corporation and several foundations pledged millions of dollars to rescue it (Blau 2013).

Grady Memorial is not the only public hospital supporting HBCU training to have suffered adversity. King/Drew Medical Center, mentioned previously, was forced to close its doors in 2007 after a series of unfortunate and highly publicized lapses in care. The hospital was beleaguered by government bureaucracy and years of mismanagement that led to its acquiring the sullied reputation as a dangerous place for patients and the infamous nickname "Killer King." The death knell occurred after federal regulators withdrew funding when the hospital lost accreditation from the Centers for Medicare & Medicaid Services, forcing its closure. CDU's psychiatry program voluntarily closed, along with 15 other postgraduate medical training programs on the campus. These dire circumstances exacerbated the already serious shortage of community psychiatrists in Los Angeles's inner city. Fortunately, the CDU College of Medicine survived and went on to develop new partnerships with other community institutions that allowed medical students to continue training. Kedren Community Mental Health Center and Hospital, founded in the 1960s in response to social injustice affecting residents of South Los Angeles, now serves as a teaching hospital for the school. The Affordable Care Act and the Mental Health Services Act of California (MHSA) have provided new revenue streams and an expanded base of newly insured patients that will support a new residency training program slated to open in the summer of 2018. The MHSA, also known as the "Millionaire's Tax" or Proposition 63, imposes a 1% income tax on personal incomes in excess of $1 million. Since its inception in 2005, the MHSA has generated over $14.6 billion in revenue and has allowed for the creation of more than 1,000 innovative programs that range from prevention and early intervention to infrastructure, technology, and workforce development, including residency training. The South Los Angeles community has warmly embraced the new program focused on addressing the social determinants of health led by

Curley Bonds, M.D. (department chair) and Cee Freeman, M.D., M.P.H. (residency training director).

Past, Present and Future Roles of Historically Black Colleges and Universities

In addition to their historical role in training African American physicians to serve the community, HBCUs have played a critical role in increasing access to training for other underrepresented minority groups, including women and international graduates. Over the past three decades a large percentage of residents training at the HBCUs came from foreign medical schools in Asia, Africa, and the Middle East, among other regions around the world. This trend reflected the fact that training positions in psychiatry were often left unfilled by U.S. graduates. This meant that applicants who had difficulty entering more competitive specialties chose psychiatry, a specialty that openly welcomed and appreciated cultural diversity (Majeed et al. 2017). HBCU departments evaluated foreign graduates based on their individual achievements and credentials, with an eye toward building a workforce equipped to address the growing underserved immigrant populations in urban centers. International medical graduates (IMGs) are more likely to practice in underserved communities and rural areas where low-income, immigrant, and minority patients receive care (see Chapter 8 in this book). However, the barriers caused by limited language proficiency, poor understanding of American culture, and the complexity of the American healthcare system have at times led to tensions between IMGs and African American patients. This has resulted in a recent effort to recruit and attract U.S. graduates or at least those with U.S. clinical experience, preferably those who share similar culture and values to the communities in which they will serve.

The futures of the HBCU departments of psychiatry have been secured in recent years by an increasing appreciation for the vitally important role that behavioral interventions play in reducing overall healthcare costs. These institutions' role in training medical students and psychiatric residents is critically important to ensure a workforce that is capable of addressing our society's multitude of health disparities. This function is closely linked to their role in nurturing academicians who dedicate their careers to social and health justice, advocacy, and a greater understanding of the unique needs of underserved populations in the United States as well as around the globe.

Healthcare legislation such as the Affordable Care Act and MHSA in California has created generous new revenue streams that have resulted in countless programs that benefit HBCUs and the communities that they treat. Hospitals and clinics have seen an astonishing increase in demand for psychiatric services with the advent of parity laws that require behavioral health and substance abuse treatments to be offered alongside general medical and surgical interventions. As a result, HBCUs have expanded their staff and facilities. In California alone, the Affordable Care Act allowed more than 5 million people to obtain health insurance coverage for the first time. Similar gains across the country could be reversed by elected leaders with political agendas that do not place a high priority on universal access to healthcare. California's Welfare and Institution Code requires counties to spend down MHSA funds within 3 years, but doing so can be a challenge given the complex bureaucracy governing how the monies are spent. As a result, some counties have found themselves with unspent reserves that are at risk of being returned to the state to be allocated for other uses through a process known as "reversion." Academicians and leaders at HBCU institutions will undoubtedly be at the forefront of helping to maintain the hard-fought gains of the Affordable Care Act through focused research demonstrating the benefits of increased access to behavioral health care for all Americans, and their leaders will once again play the role of strident advocates and serve as a united voice for minority communities whose services are at risk.

The history and legacy of the HBCU departments of psychiatry are rich with tales of triumph over adversity. These institutions were built by an impressive group of gifted academicians who tirelessly worked to ensure equal access to care for all patients, including those of African descent. HBCUs have always been and will continue to be leaders in developing and implementing specialized, culturally relevant psychiatric interventions. Their continued survival will ensure that psychiatry examines, understands, and addresses the needs of the most vulnerable people in our nation.

References

Blau M: How Grady Memorial Hospital skirted death. Creative Loafing, February 28, 2013. Available at: http://www.creativeloafing.com/news/article/13072642/how-grady-memorial-hospital-skirted-death. Accessed January 3, 2018.

Canino IA, Spurlock J: Culturally Diverse Children and Adolescents: Assessment, Diagnosis, and Treatment. New York, Guilford, 1994

Epps C, Johnson D, Vaughan A: African American Medical Pioneers. Rockville, MD, Betz, 1994

The HistoryMakers: Education Makers: Dr. Lloyd C. Elam. The HistoryMakers (website), March 14, 2007. Available at: http://www.thehistorymakers.org/biography/dr-lloyd-c-elam-41. Accessed January 3, 2018.

Lawley TJ, Higginbotham EJ: Medical schools are overlooked keys to Grady puzzle. Emory Report, September 10, 2007. Available at: http://www.emory.edu/EMORY_REPORT/erarchive/2007/September/Sept10/FirstPerson.htm. Accessed January 3, 2018.

Legacy.com Obituaries: Dewitt C. Alfred Jr. The Atlanta Journal-Constitution, March 15–17, 2006. Available at: http://www.legacy.com/obituaries/atlanta/obituary.aspx?pid=17088757. Accessed January 3, 2018.

Majeed MH, Ali AA, Sudak DM: International medical graduates and American psychiatry: the past, present, and future. Acad Psychiatry 41(6):849–851, 2017 28707232

Mullan F, Chen C, Petterson S, et al: The social mission of medical education: ranking the schools. Ann Intern Med 152(12):804–811, 2010 20547907

Spurlock J (ed): Black Psychiatrists and American Psychiatry. Washington, DC, American Psychiatric Press, 1999

Stuart R: Meharry Medical College of Nashville fights Vanderbilt for hospital rights. The New York Times, April 26, 1982. Available at: http://www.nytimes.com/1982/04/26/us/meharry-medical-college-of-nashville-fights-vanderbilt-for-hosptial-rifgts.html. Accessed January 3, 2018.

U.S. National Library of Medicine: Biography: Dr. Jeanne Spurlock, in Changing the Face of Medicine (online exhibition). Bethesda, MD, U.S. National Library of Medicine, 2015. Available at: https://cfmedicine.nlm.nih.gov/physicians/biography_306.html. Accessed January 3, 2018.

PART IV

Psychiatric Research and Blacks

CHAPTER 23
THE IMPORTANCE OF "BENT NAIL" RESEARCH FOR AFRICAN AMERICAN POPULATIONS

Carl C. Bell, M.D., DLFAPA, FACPsych

THERE ARE THREE basic ways of knowing: we can know things rationally by thinking about them; we can know empirically, which is knowledge based on our perceptions; and we can know metaphorically, in which we grasp things intuitively. It is in the metaphor that one finds wisdom (Kopp 1971). The purpose of this chapter is to describe a process the author is convinced can improve the quality and quantity of knowledge on African American mental health and wellness. For lack of a better label, the process is metaphorically known as "bent nail" research.

In his youth the author was given a book filled with challenges and adventures—for example, how to make a snow brick maker for building an igloo, how to build a portable reading desk, and how to make a telephone from scratch. Like most African American youth, being curious, industrious, and having a strong drive toward active mastery, he would try to build various items in the book, but there was one major challenge—he was too poor to afford the proper tools or building materials. For example, one year he tried to construct a bookcase to display his plastic models. By rummaging through various alleys in Chicago, he was able to obtain the wood necessary for the shelves and vertical supports, and by using used bent nails and hammering them straight to be re-used, he was able to construct the bookcase. Of course, it was a bit off center, because it leaned a bit to the right; but more importantly, it was functional and able to display the models. It was a "bent nail" bookcase. During the author's psychiatric career, like many black psychiatrists, he found himself in similar cir-cumstances—that is, he would be curious about a common clinical observation and would want to research it. However, like most clinical, black psychiatrists, the author did not have the sophisticated infrastructure or funding to do pris-tine, formal academic research. Drawing on the metaphor of the "bent nail" book-case, the author's various research teams have done research projects on African Americans using the resources they could scrounge up from their day-to-day clinical settings. For example, in a compilation of the author's early published research work (Bell 2004), there is an early 1980 point-prevalence study in the psychiatric outpatient clinic at Jackson Park Hospital exploring the number of African Americans who had bipolar disorder but were misdiagnosed as being schizophrenic. Fortunately, around the same time, Dr. Billy E. Jones was also interested in the misdiagnosis of African Americans with bipolar disorder. He asked similar questions: "How many of our clinic's African American patients who had bipolar disorders [had] been misdiagnosed with a schizophrenic diag-nosis?" (Jones et al. 1981). Dr. Jones's research also found that the misdiagnosis of black patients who had bipolar disorder was a problem. The author's and Dr. Jones's work was not competitive but cooperative, because their goal was serv-ing African Americans, not building formal academic research careers. Perhaps having both trained at Meharry Medical College, both authors were "profession-ally socialized" somewhat differently from many in standard medical schools (Griffith and Delgado 1979). Neither of them was clawing for the limited grants required to do pristine, formal academic research. Their studies were designed to determine the prevalence of a specific psychiatric disorder in an African Amer-ican clinical population and to understand why so many were misdiagnosed so that they would be in a better position to help their patients.

In addition to highlighting how to get research funding for academic research, using the "bent nail" metaphor, this chapter illustrates how rudimentary, basic clin-ical research—that is, "bent nail" research—can have a meaningful impact on the dearth of knowledge regarding African American psychiatric issues. The author recommends this approach to black psychiatrists, most of whom are in clinical set-tings taking care of black psychiatric patients (as noted by a "bent nail" research project done by Jones and Gray [1985]). Clearly, it is neither the amount of funding behind a research project nor the sophistication of the biostatistics that makes research useful. Rather, it is the insight and creativity contained in the research question and the poignancy of the basic sciences and clinical obser-vations driving the questions. There are many unanswered questions when it comes to African American mental health and wellness, and if African American psychiatrists, from their unique perspectives, do not explore these questions, no one will do it from the unfettered, honest view that black psychiatrists have about African Americans. There is a danger that black psychiatrists may glamorize, minimize, or misinterpret African American mental health and wellness issues. However, the author would rather take chances with black psychiatry leading research on African Americans than trust the skewed and deficit approach most European Americans take. The ideal would be if everyone could be trusted to be evenhanded, but sadly this is not a present-day reality.

Early Beginnings of "Bent Nail" Research

When the author started medical school at Meharry Medical College in 1967, he was struck with the health disparities between African Americans and whites. (Back then, the only two "cultural, racial, and ethnic" groups being considered were blacks and whites.) In Meharry's *Textbook of Pediatrics* (Nelson 1966, p. 1233), it was stated that "familial retardation" or "subcultural retardation" was the largest group of mental retardation (25%–40% of institutionalized "retardates" and 60%–75% of the mentally retarded living in the community). Nelson's (1966) chapter noted "limited intellectual stimulation and the relatively inferior environment such a situation [i.e., being in the lowest economic and cultural strata] usually affords play important parts in determining the social inadequacy such children exhibit" (p. 1233). It was taught at Meharry that mild mental retardation was two to three times more prevalent in African American youth compared with white youth. However, from an African American perspective this did not make sense, because in lower economic and cultural strata, a great deal of intellectual capacity is required to flourish. Nearly 50 years later, mild *intellectual disability,* a neurodevelopmental disorder formerly known as *mental retardation*, continues to be diagnosed in African American, non-Hispanic children at least two times the rate, and in Hispanic children 1.5 times the rate, that it is in white, non-Hispanic children (Boat et al. 2015). It was also taught that the prematurity rates among African Americans were twice the rates among whites. The explanations for these differences continue to be framed in a psychosocial, and not a biological, manner, when the reality is that there are cultural, social, psychological, and biological determinants of such differences. For far too long African American physicians have backed away from the biological determinants of health for fear that focusing on this will call up an old enemy, eugenics. There seems to be a lack of recognition that social determinants of health can result in "acquired biology"—that is, biology that is acquired during pregnancy and after which is not genetic in nature but comes from toxic environments.

The question was always, "Why?" There were some social and psychological hypotheses for these observations, but they were not backed by scientific study. Rather, the explanations were supported by poorly developed opinions by clinicians and scientists that were for the most part unsubstantiated and untested. Furthermore, these explanations just did not make sense. For example, "subcultural retardation" was proposed to be due to the lack of books in African American homes, but thoughtful African Americans knew there was a well-read Bible in most African American homes.

Before the era of sophisticated research, significance was determined by Student's t-test, Chi Square tests of independence, and tests of correlation (r), and usually there were only two variables being considered, so research was not very sophisticated. In addition, the requirements for Institutional Review Board (IRB) approval were not as stringent. Now regression analysis is available, so multiple variables can be considered in an experiment (after all, behavior is multidetermined), and IRBs are a requirement. Another limitation of earlier research is that it was monochromatic—the research was predominantly on white, middle-class, male issues; there was little in the literature about African American issues with the exception of supposed African American deficits. This problem continued until the sixteenth Surgeon General's report on culture, race, and ethnicity was published in 2001 exposing this disparity (U.S. Department of Health and Human Services 2001). The documentation of this cultural, racial, and ethnic research disparity stimulated some further research on African American issues, but not to any significant scale. Sadly, research questions continue to stem from monocultural ethnocentrism, and deficit questions instead of strength-based questions continue to abound in U.S. mental health and wellness research. For example, the reasons why African American females have the lowest suicide rate in the United States is still poorly explored (U.S. Department of Health and Human Services 2012). Furthermore, it has only been recently that the important major public health questions surrounding the reasons African Americans are reported to have twice the rates of mild intellectual disability and of Alzheimer's disease are gradually being brought to light.

Of course, one of the earliest "bent nail" African American psychiatrist researchers was Dr. Ernest Y. Williams, M.D., chairman of the department of psychiatry at Howard University in the 1940s and 1970s (Williams 1967). Dr. Williams's work is well represented in PubMed and goes from 1939 to 1971, with many of his papers published in the *Journal of the National Medical Association*. It was almost as though he had taken Booker T. Washington's adage of "cast down your bucket where you are" to heart. Much of the research Dr. Williams did was very useful rudimentary, basic clinical research, or "bent nail." For example, he was not in a position to use randomly selected, representative samples, but because the kinds of issues in the African American patients he was seeing were representative of black Americans in general, his observations filled a void. Similarly, in addition to highlighting the misdiagnosis of African Americans, Billy E. Jones, M.D.'s research team was very instrumental in highlighting that black psychiatrists were treating black patients in psychotherapy and white psychiatrists had very little experience with these patients. Four other "bent nail" African American researchers whose clinical observations were telling were James H. Carter, M.D.; Dr. James L. Collins, M.D.; Orlando B. Lightfoot, M.D.; and Jeanne Spurlock, M.D. Of course, before these six "bent nail" researchers, America's first black psychiatrist, Solomon Carter Fuller, was busy developing staining techniques in Alzheimer's lab that helped delineate the neurobiology of Alzheimer's disease. Because he was a Negro, Dr. Fuller was relegated to doing the dirtiest work in pathology—that is, dealing with brain pathology—but he took advantage of his relegation to these duties as an adventure in uncharted territory.

There were several reasons for the lack of sophisticated research on African Americans in addition to the lack of research resources. One such reason touted the most is that African Americans do not trust research because of the infamous Tuskegee experiments. In her book *Medical Apartheid,* Washington (2006) does an excellent job of highlighting United States' repeated medical ethics violations on African Americans before the Tuskegee experiments were revealed in 1972. She documented that African American distrust of research has long-standing and deep roots that predate the Tuskegee experiments. She also documented the U.S. government's violation of medical ethics by not informing syphilitic black men in Tuskegee, Alabama, that there was lifesaving treatment for their condition (Washington 2006). However, consistently since medical school, the author's experience with African American research subjects is that they are more than willing to participate in research if it is made clear that African American researchers, who have a solid African American identity and integrity, are leading the research. In addition, the author's experience is that by actively involving African Americans at all levels of research, African Americans are more than willing to participate.

The author's involvement in "bent nail" research on African Americans began in medical school in 1968 when the author studied nutrition in 50 African American youth in North Nashville, Tennessee (Bell 2004). Informed consent was a major component of the study, because the author was studying children as young as 6 months. There were very few refusals. One of the main findings of the study was that 8% of the sample had been born prematurely (Bell 2004), a finding that did not make sense until recently (Bell and Chimata 2015), when it became clear the prematurity rates were likely due to fetal alcohol exposure— a major disregarded cause of prematurity in people. Reflecting on this research, it was being done by a black medical student from a black medical school that had a tradition of serving the black community in North Nashville. Meharry's motto was "Serving God by Serving Man." There was little thought about exploiting African Americans, and the institution placed high value on pragmatic public health. Meharry intuitively knew the only real way to address health disparities was through prevention, a lesson learned from the polio epidemic. The aims of the research were to learn the quality of African American youths' nutrition so there could be an understanding and policies could be put in place to correct and prevent medical and psychiatric problems in African Americans.

The author and colleagues continue to use this formula, and it has served them well in their studies beginning in 1980 on the prevention of violence in African Americans (Bell 2017b), starting in 1982 on African American children exposed to violence (Bell 2004), beginning in 1984 on isolated sleep paralysis in African Americans (Bell 2004), and during our 1984 studies on head injury in African Americans (Bell 2004), to name a few. These studies could all be described as "bent nail" research, which spurred the development of multiple formal academic research projects to confirm the original "bent nail" research observations.

Matriculation Into Formal Academic Research

Formal academic research is more than a notion, and although the emphasis in this chapter is on doing "bent nail" research, formal academic research is essential to confirm the results of "bent nail" research. To fit the definition of evidence based, the findings of a research project have to be verified by at least three independent research groups—after all, we are scientists. The research in the twenty-first century is far more sophisticated than the "bent nail" research of Drs. Fuller, Williams, Carter, Collins, Lightfoot, and Spurlock.

Although the author was a "bent nail" researcher whose "bent nail" research had significant public policy impact during most of his early career, when he mistakenly thought "bent nail' research was passé, he consulted with a successful formal academic researcher to learn how to get funding required to do research that would be more respected in the twenty-first century. The author learned that most often psychiatrists who are in the formal academic research club also have a doctoral degree (Ph.D.). Having this degree illustrates to funding bodies, public or private, that the applicant has had training in all the skills necessary to do quality research worth funding. Accordingly, because blacks with "M.D., Ph.D.s" are "as scarce as hens' teeth," many African American researchers are psychologists and not psychiatrists. For example, one of the most successful teams of African American researchers in psychology is led by Dr. James Jackson (an outstanding African American social psychologist) at the University of Michigan. The University of Michigan houses the Program for Research on Black Americans (PRBA), which conducts excellent psychosocial research on African Americans. This is a necessary perspective on African American health and mental health issues, as many of these issues are driven by social context and social determinants of health. However, there are biological considerations as well, and although PRBA has had some psychiatric input, biology/medicine is not a major thrust of its program. The nation needs black psychiatrists who are biologists interested in research if progress is to be made.

It is possible for African American psychiatrists without Ph.D.s to break into the formal academic research world. There are several ways to do this. Several psychiatric training programs offer formal research training for psychiatrists, but such positions are extremely competitive. To become a formal academic researcher there is a long and tortuous research pathway that often involves finding a mentor who knows and can teach the budding African American psychiatric researcher the techniques necessary to get funding. Just to name a few, these skills consist of 1) developing a "burning research question"; 2) doing pilot studies; 3) presenting clear, concise, doable aims; 4) carrying out sampling and subject recruitment; 5) using or developing valid and reliable measures; 6) developing an appropriate research design; 7) managing the data and doing statistical analysis; 8) developing the grant proposal; 9) ensuring that the research is ethical; 10) managing the grant funds; 11) writing the paper; and 12) preparing the next grant to stay involved in formal academic research. In the twenty-first century, formal academic research requires diverse teams.

These skills are often taught in formal research training programs. Another path to becoming a National Institute of Mental Health R01–funded researcher (one taken by the author) is by starting out with "bent nail" research and discovering something important—for example, the large numbers of children exposed to violence (Bell 2004) or strategies to prevent violence in African Americans (Bell 2004)—and then getting invited to participate in formal academic research as a coinvestigator (see Flay et al. 2004). This path, although not formal research training, affords the budding African American psychiatric researcher an opportunity to learn necessary research skills and develop a record of accomplishment that a review committee looks for before awarding a grant to a research proposal.

Naturalistic Large-Scale Public Health Research

Another aspect of research that is important and in which black psychiatrists should involve themselves is "naturalistic large-scale public health research" (O'Connell et al. 2009, p. 333). The reality is that although pristine, formal academic research designs have internal validity, making them important for the furtherance of science, they do not always have good external validity. For example, because of the risks involved, actively suicidal patients are often excluded from randomized, double-blind, control trials, and while this makes sense, it prevents any formal academic research on patients who are actively suicidal. In addition, the findings from pristine, formal academic research are rarely applied and used in real-life circumstances. However, the work of James P. Comer, M.D., Felton (Tony) J. Earls, M.D., Mindy T. Fullilove, M.D., and Carl C. Bell, M.D., has exemplified work in the area of population-based prevention in mental health.

Science can often benefit from the experience of everyday clinical observations. For example, in 1982 when clinical observations in a predominately African American community mental health setting found an extraordinary number of children exposed to violence, a plethora of formal academic scientific research projects confirmed this observation. Following the confirmation of these findings, it was discovered that "risk factors were not predictive factors due to protective factors," culminating in several large-scale strategies to prevent these children from developing mental health sequelae (Primm and Lawson 2010, p. 27). This is another example of how "bent nail" research can be "directionally correct." In addition, communities are more likely to implement formal academic psychosocial programs if, on the ground floor, these programs involve significant community input in the design and implementation of the research (Bell 2004). Research designed to test empirically programs being implemented in naturalistic environments can also identify approaches that are readily implementable by other communities.

Randomized, controlled prevention trials can also inform public health practice. For example, a violence prevention trial, Aban Aya (Flay et al. 2004), informed a Chicago public school violence prevention initiative (Bell 2017b), "which demonstrated significant reductions in pregnant teenage dropout rates" (O'Connell et al. 2009, p. 334). Accomplishing such tasks often involves having a black psychiatrist, like Drs. James P. Comer at Yale or Carl C. Bell formerly at the Community Mental Health Council Inc. in Chicago, who has done formal academic research and also has cachet with public systems and community and is in a position to influence public policy.

Prominent African American Formal Academic Researchers

At the risk of leaving someone out, the prominent African American formal academic psychiatric researchers are Chester M. Pierce, M.D. (recently deceased), formerly at Harvard, who did a lot of his earlier work in the Navy, where enuresis and somnambulism were issues, so he studied them; Charles Pinderhughes, M.D., who did psychoanalytic research; Charles B. Wilkinson,

M.D. (deceased), at the Greater Kansas City Mental Health Foundation, who studied the collapse of two skywalks in the lobby of the Hyatt Regency Hotel in Kansas City, Missouri; James Lincoln Collins, M.D. (deceased), at Walter Reed Army Medical Center and Howard University; Victor R. Adebimpe, M.D. (deceased) at University of Pittsburgh Western Psychiatric Institute and Clinic; Fran Baker, M.D., at the University of Maryland; Pamela Y. Collins, M.D., M.P.H., formerly at the National Institute of Mental Health and currently at the University of Washington, Seattle; James P. Comer, M.D., at Yale; Felton J. Earls, M.D., at Harvard; Mindy T. Fullilove, M.D., at New School/ Parsons; Ezra E.H. Griffith, M.D., at Yale; Helena B. Hansen, M.D., Ph.D., at New York University; David C. Henderson, M.D., at Boston University; William B. Lawson, M.D., Ph.D., at Dell Medical School; and Donald H. Williams, M.D. (retired), at Michigan State University. Although the author had an R01 grant to study HIV infection prevention in Durban, South Africa, he would not include himself in this august list. Taking a play from Booker T. Washington's and Solomon Carter Fuller's (America's first African American psychiatrist) playbook, the author has essentially designed and developed "naturalistic, large-scale health research" in whatever clinical practices he has been involved in delivering. In the author's opinion, others such as Drs. Fran M. Baker, Ezra E.H. Griffith, Billy E. Jones, and Donald H. Williams have done the same. This path involves doing "bent nail" research on the clinical population that the African American clinical psychiatrist is serving. This list would not be complete without mentioning of James Ralph, M.D. (deceased), at the National Institute of Mental Health, who did a great deal to support research on African Americans when he was head of the Center for Minority Group Mental Health Programs.

The Value of Research on Black Americans to America

Unfortunately, because so little research on African American issues is done, it is difficult to recognize the value of black research to America. If psychiatrists were better able to solve research questions on African Americans, the entire nation would benefit. For example, if the nation had taken a public health approach to the opioid epidemic in African Americans that presaged the opioid epidemic in European Americans, the nation would already have some answers as to what to do about the European American problem. African American health and mental health issues represent a "canary in the coal mine" opportunity to see a problem before it hits. If we understood how African American women are better able to resist suicide, we would be in a better position to help our veterans.

A Both/And Approach to Doing Research on African Americans

The author's experience suggests that both "bent nail" and pristine, formal academic research are necessary to make progress in solving African American public health challenges. Therefore, instead of an either/or approach, a both/and approach is recommended. While it is true that some pristine, formal academic research is not specifically focused on African American issues, some studies may be useful to solve African American issues. However, the reality is that many African Americans find themselves in unique social contexts, and these contexts may influence acquired biological realities that shape psychiatric illness and wellness. Unfortunately, these acquired biological realities are not usually considered in current pristine, formal research agendas. It is the author's opinion, based on his own experience, that this reality heightens the need for "bent nail" research. There is a plethora of untested African American research ideas that need exploration—for example, the reason for the high rates of Alzheimer's disease in African American elders, the impact of higher rates of head injury in African Americans, and the solution to the high rates of mild intellectual disability and prematurity in African Americans.

Sometimes "bent nail" and formal academic research can support each other to clarify reality. For example, Dr. Robert Freedman's research at the University of Denver, Colorado, suggests, based on findings on the gene *CHRNA7*, that prenatal choline might prevent schizophrenia, autism, and attention-deficit/hyperactivity disorder (Freedman and Ross 2015). The "bent nail" research by Dr. Bell's team suggests that choline deficiency brought on by fetal alcohol exposure effect results in patients with neurobehavioral disorder associated with prenatal alcohol exposure (ND-PAE, also known as *fetal alcohol spectrum disorders*) being misdiagnosed as having schizophrenia, bipolar disorder, and depression (Bell and Chimata 2015). The social determinant of health of living in poor, ghetto neighborhoods with an overabundance of liquor stores resulting in excess ND-PAE may be a major variable that is responsible for the high rates of prematurity and mild intellectual disability seen in some African American communities (Bell 2017a). Thus, the "bent nail" and pristine, formal academic research observations are aligned, as both point to choline when given as a prenatal supplement as being a protective factor (Bell and Ajula 2016), a conclusion arrived at from two entirely different vantage points.

Unless there are some radical changes in the way research is done, black psychiatrists are going to have to figure out how to work together to create synergy regarding needed research on African American issues. To date, the investment of European American researchers in African American issues has been minimal. Accordingly, it is up to black psychiatric researchers to figure out the greater risk and protective factors of African Americans' mental health and wellness issues, and good old-fashioned "bent nail" research can lead the way for the more sophisticated research to follow.

Another issue is the replication of research findings on African Americans. For example, replication of the potentially illuminating finding of high rates of fetal alcohol exposure in African Americans, heretofore only thought to occur in Native Americans, has not been pursued by any of the predominantly black medical schools, despite entreaties to do so.

Conclusion

This chapter proposes a different approach to research on African Americans. While recognizing the importance of pristine, formal academic research, the author advocates for "bent nail" research, or rudimentary, basic clinical research, as a solution to the paucity of knowledge about African American mental health. Furthermore, there is a need for large-scale public health research on African American issues. It is not enough to find answers to public health problems of African Americans; black psychiatrists must thrust evidence-based strategies that benefit African American public health into the public eye to create the political will to enact the solutions into public policy. Having seen firsthand an evidence-based intervention that reduced the number of African American children going into foster care from 40/1,000 down to 11/1,000 in McLean County, Illinois (Redd et al. 2005), only to see the harvesting of black children continue despite the success of the naturalistic, large-scale public intervention, illustrates the need for political will.

References

Bell CC: The Sanity of Survival: Reflections on Community Mental Health and Wellness. Chicago, IL, Third World Press, 2004

Bell CC: Fetal alcohol spectrum disorders in African American communities: continuing the quest for prevention, in Perspectives on Health Equity and Social Determinants of Health. Edited by Bogard K, Murry VM, Alexander C. Washington, DC, National Academy of Medicine, 2017a, pp 181–198

Bell CC: Lessons learned from 50 years of violence prevention activities in the African American community. J Natl Med Assoc 109(4):224–237, 2017b 29173929

Bell CC, Ajula J: Prenatal vitamins deficient in recommended choline intake for pregnant women. J Fam Med Dis Prev 2(6):2–48, 2016

Bell CC, Chimata R: Prevalence of neurodevelopmental disorders among low-income African Americans at a clinic on Chicago's south side. Psychiatr Serv 66(5):539–542, 2015 25726976

Boat T, Wu J; Committee to Evaluate the Supplemental Security Income Disability Program for Children With Mental Disorders: Mental Disorders and Disabilities Among Low Income Children. Washington, DC, National Academies Press, 2015

Flay BR, Graumlich S, Segawa E, et al: Effects of 2 prevention programs on high-risk behaviors among African American youth: a randomized trial. Arch Pediatr Adolesc Med 158(4):377–384, 2004 15066879

Freedman R, Ross RG: Prenatal choline and the development of schizophrenia. Shanghai Arch Psychiatry 27(2):90–102, 2015 26120259

Griffith EE, Delgado A: On the professional socialization of black residents in psychiatry. J Med Educ 54(6):471–476, 1979 448697

Jones BE, Gray BA: Black and white psychiatrists: therapy with blacks. J Natl Med Assoc 77(1):19–25, 1985 3968711

Jones BE, Gray BA, Parson EB: Manic-depressive illness among poor urban blacks. Am J Psychiatry 138(5):654–657, 1981 7235063

Kopp SB: Guru: Metaphors From a Psychotherapist. Palo Alto, CA, Science and Behavior Books, 1971

Nelson WE (ed): Mental retardation, in Textbook of Pediatrics, 8th Edition. Philadelphia, PA, WB Saunders, 1966, pp 1232–1243

O'Connell ME, Boat T, Warner KE (eds): Preventing Mental, Emotional, and Behavioral Disorders Among Young People: Progress and Possibilities. Washington, DC, National Academies Press, 2009

Primm AB, Lawson WB: Disparities among ethnic groups—African Americans, in Disparities in Psychiatric Care. Edited by Ruiz P, Primm AB. Baltimore, MD, Wolters Kluwer/Lippincott Williams & Wilkins, 2010, pp 19–29

Redd J, Suggs H, Gibbons R, et al: A plan to strengthen systems and reduce the number of African-American children in child welfare. Illinois Child Welfare 2(1–2):34–46, 2005

U.S. Department of Health and Human Services: Mental Health: Culture, Race, and Ethnicity. A Supplement to Mental Health: A Report of the Surgeon General. Rockville, MD, Substance Abuse and Mental Health Services Administration, 2001

U.S. Department of Health and Human Services: National Strategy for Suicide Prevention: Goals and Objectives for Action. A Report of the U.S. Surgeon General and of the National Action Alliance for Suicide Prevention. Washington, U.S. Department of Health and Human Services, 2012

Washington H: Medical Apartheid. New York, Harlem Moon, 2006

Williams EY: The Howard department of neurology and psychiatry. J Natl Med Assoc 59(6):447–454, 1967 4867387

CHAPTER 24
RACISM AND MENTAL HEALTH

Pathways, Evidence, and Needed Research

David R. Williams, Ph.D., M.P.H.
Ayesha McAdams-Mahmoud, M.P.H.

RACISM IS AN organized system premised on the categorization and ranking of social groups into races. The actors in this system devalue, disempower, and differentially allocate desirable societal opportunities and resources to racial groups they regard as inferior (Williams and Mohammed 2013). The crystallization of this ideology of inferiority into multiple aspects of society leads racism to be foundational to the structures and processes of society and its institutions and not primarily centered in individual beliefs and behaviors. However, racism also leads to the development of negative attitudes and beliefs toward racial out-groups, which manifest themselves as prejudice and stereotypes that can be measured at both the societal and the individual level. In turn, this deeply embedded cultural racism triggers *discrimination*, the differential treatment of racial out-groups by both individuals and social institutions (Williams and Mohammed 2013). Accordingly, through multiple mechanisms, the racist ideology that is deeply embedded in the floorboards of a nation creates racial inequality that becomes evident in a type of societal equivalent to sick building syndrome that has implications for the health of everyone in the house (Malat et al. 2018). In fact, research reveals that in race-conscious societies, such as Australia, Brazil, South Africa, the United Kingdom, and the United States, nondominant racial groups tend to have worse health than their more advantaged peers and elevated exposure to risk factors for poor mental and physical health.

In this chapter we provide an overview of empirical research that delineates the multiple mechanisms by which racism, by unfairly advantaging some groups and disadvantaging others, can adversely affect community and individual mental health. First, institutional racism can lead to societal policies that reduce access of the socially stigmatized to desirable opportunities and resources in society. Second, a large and growing body of evidence indicates that experiences of racial discrimination are an important type of stressful life experience that can adversely affect mental and physical health. Third, cultural racism can initiate and sustain negative racial stereotypes that can lessen support for egalitarian policies, trigger health-damaging psychological responses such as internalized racism and stereotype threat, and facilitate explicit and implicit biases that restrict access to desirable resources, including medical care. We end the chapter with a consideration of some research priorities and evidence of promising interventions.

Institutional Racial Discrimination and Mental Health

Racism is deeply imbedded in the institutions of society, which enables discrimination to persist in institutional structures and policies, even if there are marked declines in individual-level racial prejudice and explicit discrimination (Williams and Mohammed 2013). The persistence of racial inequalities in society must be understood in the context of persistent racialized social structures that can affect mental health status and access to opportunities that promote mental health. One of the most powerful institutional (or structural) mechanisms of racism is residential segregation (Williams and Collins 2001). The term *residential segregation* refers to the occupancy of different neighborhood and community environments by race that was developed in the United States to ensure that whites were protected from living in the same residential environments as blacks (or African Americans). The forced removal and relocation of American Indians to reservations is another example of institutionalized isolation of a stigmatized racial population. The physical separation of races by enforced residence is an institutional mechanism shaped by multiple social forces—political, legal, economic, religious, cultural, and historical events (Williams and Collins 2001).

This enforced residence in separate areas developed in both northern and southern urban areas in the late nineteenth and early twentieth centuries and has remained strikingly stable since then, but with small declines in recent years (Massey and Denton 1993). Although segregation has been illegal since the Fair Housing Act of 1968, it is perpetuated today through an interlocking set of individual actions, institutional practices, and governmental policies. In the 2010 U.S. Census, residential segregation was at its lowest level in 100 years, and declines in segregation were evident in all of the nation's largest metropolitan areas (Glaeser and Vigdor 2001). However, recent declines in segregation have been driven by a few blacks' moving to formerly all-white census tracts, and have had little impact on the very high percentage black census tracts, the residential isolation of most African Americans, and the concentration of urban poverty (Glaeser and Vigdor 2001). Although most immigrant groups have experienced some residential segregation in the United States, no immigrant group has ever lived under the high levels of segregation that currently exist for the black population, making the experience of being black in American spaces unique and distinctive (Williams and Collins 2001).

Segregation affects mental health in multiple ways (Williams and Collins 2001). Segregation is a critical determinant of socioeconomic status (SES), as measured by income, education, occupational status, and wealth. SES, in turn, is a strong predictor of variation in a broad range of psychiatric disorders. For example, national studies in the United States have documented that the prevalence of DSM disorders, both for persons in treatment and for those not in treatment, is inversely related to income and education.

Research reveals that segregation is a key determinant of economic well-being in adulthood by reducing access to high-quality elementary and high school education, preparation for higher education, and employment opportunities. For example, research finds that segregated schools have lower levels of teacher quality, educational resources, and per-student spending and higher levels of neighborhood violence, crime, and poverty. Segregation has also reduced access to employment opportunities by triggering the exodus of low-skill, high-pay jobs from areas of minority concentration and by facilitating discrimination based on place of residence.

Accordingly, because of segregation, there are large racial differences in SES as measured by income, education, occupational status, and wealth. According to a Census Bureau report (Proctor et al. 2016), for every dollar of income that white households received in 2015, Hispanics (or Latinos) earned 72 cents and blacks earned 59 cents. Stunningly, this black-white income gap is identical to the one in 1978—the peak year of the gains from the Civil Rights Movement and the antipoverty policies of the 1960s and 1970s. However, racial differences in income understate the magnitude of racial differences in economic resources. Income captures the flow of resources into the household, but wealth or assets reflect the economic reserves that families have to cushion shortfalls of income. Another Census Bureau report indicated that for every dollar of wealth that white households have, Hispanics have seven pennies, and blacks have six pennies (U.S. Census Bureau 2014). Not surprisingly, one national study, using rigorous statistical analyses, found that the elimination of segregation would erase black-white differences in income, education, and unemployment and reduce racial differences in single motherhood by two-thirds (Cutler and Glaeser 1997). These data illustrate that racial differences in SES are not randomly occurring social patterns but are the direct result of the successful implementation of discriminatory social policies.

Segregation can also adversely affect mental health, because the concentration of poverty and poor-quality housing and neighborhood environments that characterize segregated spaces leads to elevated exposure to chronic and acute stressors and reduced access to a broad range of resources that enhance mental health. A recent qualitative study of Baltimore residents illustrated how segregation can lead to multiple stressors that can have negative mental health consequences (Turney et al. 2013). The study found that residents had high levels of exposure to stressors linked to the social environment, including pervasive violence and criminal activity, shootings, drug activity, the need to resort to violence to defend oneself, high levels of break-ins and theft, incessant shouting and cursing, poor role models for children, unsafe places to raise children, and the resultant constant worry about the safety of children. In addition, stressors linked to the physical environment included broken elevators, roach and rodent infestation, trash buildup, dampness in the walls, extremely hot (or cold) interior temperatures, the absence of green open spaces, crumbling sidewalks, graffiti, litter, and inadequate lighting. A study of a representative sample of adults in Chicago found that compared with whites, blacks and U.S.-born Latinos had more exposure to a broad range of acute and chronic psychosocial stressors and greater clustering of multiple stressors. Moreover, this elevated stress exposure accounted for some of the racial differences that persisted in symptoms of depression and anxiety after income and education were taken into account.

Research reveals that segregation directly and indirectly contributes to lower access to care and poorer quality of healthcare, including mental healthcare (White et al. 2012). Segregation has historically played a major role in configuring the location of healthcare facilities and services. Accordingly, healthcare access varies across neighborhoods, with low neighborhood SES impeding one's ability to access high-quality healthcare services. Research has found that the utilization of different hospitals by blacks and whites contributes substantially to observed racial disparities in healthcare. Although the distribution of patients within the facilities may reflect the underlying segregation pattern of the neighborhood, some evidence also suggests that the degree of segregation within healthcare institutions also contributes to racial healthcare disparities, independent of neighborhood-level segregation. Research has also found that pharmacies located in segregated neighborhoods are less likely to stock sufficient medication to meet community needs compared to those located in less segregated areas. Other research indicates that retail clinics, which hold the potential for better access to care for underserved populations, are disproportionately located in more socioeconomically advantaged neighborhoods. These differences in quality and resource availability are likely to play a strong role in differential healthcare outcomes.

Characteristics of healthcare providers are another pathway linking residential segregation to healthcare outcomes. The magnitude of segregation of a neighborhood has been associated with the availability, affordability, and quality of healthcare providers. Recruitment and retention of both primary care and specialty physicians in underserved areas are often a challenge. Studies have found that segregated areas have reduced access to both primary care and specialty physicians, and the referral patterns of physicians vary by degree of segregation (White et al. 2012). Physicians serving neighborhood areas with a high concentration of blacks or Hispanics are less likely to be board certified and more likely to report that they are unable to refer their patients to needed specialty services within those neighborhoods. Moreover, providers in predominantly black neighborhoods are more likely to be confronted with clinical, logistical, and administrative challenges. Thus, the poor mental health of minorities can be further exacerbated by racial differences in access and quality of care linked to place of residence. Instructively, research finds that even when blacks have equivalent or lower rates of mental disorders compared with whites, once diagnosed with a disorder, blacks tend to have higher rates of persistence or chronicity, more severe symptoms, higher levels of impairment, and lower rates of treatment.

Interpersonal Discrimination and Mental Health

High-quality scientific evidence documents that racial discrimination is persistent and pervasive in contemporary society (Pager and Shepherd 2008). In audit studies, researchers select, match, and train individuals to be equally qualified in every respect but to differ only in race. Audit studies in employment document that a white job applicant with a criminal record is more likely to be offered a job than a black applicant with an identical resume whose record is clean. Similarly, job applicants with distinctively black names (e.g., Latisha and Darnell) are less likely to get callbacks for job interviews than applicants with identical resumes who have distinctively white names (e.g., Alison and Brad). Other audit studies reveal the existence of racial discrimination in purchasing homes and cars, renting apartments, obtaining mortgages and medical care, applying for insurance, and hailing taxis.

Individuals are aware of at least some of the experiences of discrimination that they encounter, and research reveals that these subjective experiences of being treated badly or unfairly are a type of stressful life experience that can adversely affect a broad range of health outcomes and health risk behaviors (Lewis et al. 2015; Williams and Mohammed 2009). Early studies of discrimination and mental health were largely U.S. based and cross-sectional and focused on symptoms of anxiety, depression, and other self-reported health indicators in adults, with special attention to black people. However, a large body of research and empirical evidence from population-based studies has now emerged documenting that discrimination is associated with poorer health status, and the association is strongest in the case of mental health. These findings are consistent across a broad range of outcomes—including psychological distress, well-being, schizophrenia, burnout, daily moods, cognitive impairment, rates of psychiatric disorders, and conduct problems—and across socially disadvantaged groups on every continent.

Many of the methodological limitations of the early studies have been addressed (Williams and Mohammed 2009). For example, a growing number of prospective studies have reported a positive association between perceived discrimination and changes in mental health symptoms. There was also concern about the extent to which subjective reports of discrimination are independent of other psychological characteristics. More recent studies have found that the association between discrimination and self-reported health remained robust after adjustment for psychological characteristics such as social desirability bias, cynical hostility, positive and negative affect, and trait anxiety.

There have also been several recent studies that have examined the association between discrimination and psychiatric disorders defined by DSM criteria (Lewis et al. 2015). Although most of these studies have been cross-sectional, they have documented a consistent association between self-reported discrimination and a broad range of psychiatric disorders, including depression, anxiety disorders, eating disorders, substance abuse, and psychotic disorders. Several of these studies analyzed these associations in populations outside the United States. For example, a national study in South Africa found that both acute and chronic discrimination were associated with an elevated risk of 12-month and lifetime rates of psychiatric disorders, even after adjustment for other stressors and potentially confounding psychological factors (Lewis et al. 2015). An early national study of African Americans found prospective associations between discrimination and major depression and documented that major depression and depressive symptoms at baseline were not associated with subsequent reports of discrimination (Brown et al. 2000). A recent United Kingdom national longitudinal study using four waves of data found a dose-response relationship between repeated experiences of racial discrimination and reductions in the mental health (measured by nonspecific psychological distress) of ethnic minority people over time (Wallace et al. 2016).

Research is also documenting that discrimination, like other stressors, can affect health and mental health through both actual exposure and the vigilance, worry, rumination, and anticipatory stress that can be triggered by the threat of exposure (Lewis et al. 2015). Recent research reveals that anticipating being a target of discrimination can lead to heightened vigilance and a failure to ever completely relax because of the perceived threat. This hypervigilance, in turn, can lead to dysregulation of both emotional and physiological functioning that can adversely affect mental and physical health. For example, a study of Baltimore adults found that black people had higher scores than whites on vigilance, and vigilance was associated with an elevated risk of depressive symptoms and contributed to the black-white disparity in depression (LaVeist et al. 2014).

Cultural Racism and Mental Health

Undergirding the institutional and interpersonal discrimination in society are the racist beliefs, stereotypes, and assumptions that are deeply embedded in American culture (Williams and Mohammed 2013). Research has shown that greater exposure to television programs that portray blacks negatively is predictive of higher levels of racial prejudice toward African Americans. Some evidence suggests that even negative nonverbal behavior (facial expressions and body language) directed toward black characters on TV leads to increases in racial prejudice among viewers. Not surprisingly, research reveals that there are high levels of negative stereotypes of racial minorities in the United States, with blacks being viewed the most negatively. A team of researchers created a database of American culture—the books, newspapers, and other materials that the average college-educated American would read in his or her lifetime (Verhaeghen et al. 2011). Analysis of these data reveals that the word *black* is most frequently paired in American culture with, in order, *poor, violent, religious, lazy, cheerful,* and *dangerous.* In contrast, *white* is most frequently paired with *wealthy, progressive, conventional, stubborn, successful,* and *educated.* Some evidence suggests that the prevalence and persistence of negative racial stereotypes contribute to the low levels of empathy for racial inequities in health and the lack of political will to address them.

This cultural racism can also affect mental health in multiple ways. First, some members of stigmatized racial populations respond to the pervasive negative racial stereotypes in the culture by accepting them to be true. This endorsement of the dominant society's beliefs about their innate and/or cultural inferiority is called *internalized racism* or *self-stereotyping.* Research indicates that internalized racism is associated with lower self-esteem and psychological well-being and higher levels of alcohol consumption, depressive symptoms, and obesity (Williams and Mohammed 2009). A recent national study found that internalized racism was positively associated with depressive symptoms and serious psychological distress among African Americans and Caribbean blacks (Mouzon and McLean 2017). In this study, higher levels of mastery or perceptions of control reduced the negative effects of internalized racism on mental health.

Second, cultural racism can lead to stereotype threat, which has significant consequences for the stigmatized group. The term *stereotype threat* refers to the expectations and anxieties that can be activated in members of a stigmatized group when negative stereotypes about their group are made salient. These anxieties can adversely affect academic performance and psychological functioning (Steele and Aronson 1995). There has been limited research on the health consequences of stereotype threat. However, some evidence suggests that stereotype threat can lead to increased anxiety that can reduce self-regulation and impair decision-making processes in ways that can increase aggressive behavior and overeating. In addition, stereotype threat can impair patients' communication abilities in the clinical encounter, and this can lead patients to discount information from the provider and have lower levels of adherence to medical advice.

Third, cultural racism can also lead to unconscious bias in the clinical encounter that can lead to minorities' receiving poorer-quality care. Research indicates that when an individual holds negative stereotypes about a social group and meets someone who fits the stereotype, she or he will discriminate against that target individual. This stereotype-linked discrimination is normal and typically activated automatically, unconsciously, and without intent, irrespective of the extent to which the individual sincerely endorses egalitarian beliefs. Clinical environments are spaces where societal racial bias can influence both the quality and intensity of care that racial minority patients receive and the quality of patient-provider interactions. Research has linked clinician implicit bias to biased treatment recommendations, poorer quality of patient-physician communication, and lower patient ratings of the quality of the medical encounter (Williams and Wyatt 2015; see also Chapter 21 in this book). Implicit bias can lead clinicians to spend less time evaluating black patients, overmedicate black patients, and provide inadequate pain medication. Other chapters in this text provide a glimpse of black patient experiences in psychotherapy (Chapter 15, by Anderson Franklin) and psychopharmacology (Chapter 16, by William Lawson) and illustrate some of the responses to racism and discrimination in the clinical context. Franklin, Newton (Chapter 14), and Lawson in their chapters provide considerable evidence of racial disparities in mental healthcare, and Fullilove (Chapter 25) proposes an undoing of inequality as a logical mental health intervention.

Future Research

A priority for future research is to understand better the mental health consequences of racial hostility that is embedded in the larger societal environment.

A recent commentary has summarized several lines of evidence that suggest events linked to the recent presidential campaign and election may have negative mental health consequences for many Americans, especially racial minorities, immigrants, and Muslims (Williams and Medlock 2017). Prior research suggests that these events may give rise to feelings of fear and anxiety that adversely affect individuals who have been direct targets of experiences that they perceive to be hostile or discriminatory. This holds as well for individuals, groups, and communities who feel vulnerable because they hold membership in a group that has been stigmatized or marginalized or has been a target of increased levels of hostile rhetoric or actions.

Several lines of evidence support this hypothesis (Williams and Medlock 2017). The election of Barack Obama led to an increase in racial resentment, animosity, division, and political polarization in the United States. Then the presidential candidacy of Donald Trump brought to the surface preexisting hostile attitudes toward racial and ethnic minorities, immigrants, and Muslims. His election led to an increase in incidents of harassment and hateful intimidation. Disturbingly, the most commonly reported location where harassment has occurred is in K–12 schools. Instructively, there is a growing body of scientific research which indicates that experiences of racial discrimination experienced by teenagers produced striking levels of biological dysregulation that are evident by their early 20s. Other recent studies have revealed that residing in communities with high levels of racial prejudice is associated with elevated risks of disease and death, especially for stigmatized racial and sexual minorities. Another line of research showed that anti-immigrant policies and initiatives can trigger hostility toward immigrants that can lead to perceptions of vulnerability, threat, and psychological distress among immigrants who were directly targeted as well as among other group members who were not direct targets. Other evidence indicated that a large proportion of American adults were stressed by the current political environment. A national survey conducted early in 2017 found that a disturbingly high proportion of American adults reported that the recent presidential election was a significant source of stress (Williams and Medlock 2017). Democrats were more likely than Republicans (72% vs. 26%), and minorities (69% of blacks, 57% of Asians, 56% of Hispanics) were more likely than whites (42%), to report that the 2016 presidential election was stressful. However, the ways in which all of these trends are directly impinging on the short- and long-term mental health status of the U.S. population and targeted subgroups and its implications for the need for mental health services are not clearly understood at this time.

Another research priority is to understand better the ways in which the racism can affect the mental health of whites. A recent review suggests that whiteness can have both positive and negative effects on the health of whites (Malat et al. 2018). On the one hand, whites' greater access to material and social resources can have positive effects on physical and mental health. Consistent with this expectation, whites have better health than blacks on most measures of physical health but have rates of suicide, depression, and other common mental disorders that are higher than blacks'. This pattern is particularly pronounced, especially in recent years of economic stagnation, for low-SES whites. Moreover, whites in the United States compare poorly on international health comparisons. Evidence is presented that suggests that some social policies supported by the ideologies and narratives of whiteness may have positive effects on the health of whites, whereas other policies may adversely affect whites' health or place ceilings on the attainable level of health for whites. Future research is needed to clarify under what conditions the system of racism can have positive and negative effects on subgroups of whites. The flip side of this research agenda is the need for redoubled efforts to understand the resilience resources and protective factors that buffer the mental health of blacks and other minorities from at least some of the negative effects of racism.

Promising Interventions

In this chapter we describe the house that racism built and the toll the multiple processes of racism has had on population and individual mental health. Unearthing effective avenues for reducing racial inequalities and discriminatory acts requires a clear recognition that racism is a system composing a set of dynamically related components and subsystems (Reskin 2012). Discrimination and disparities are products of racism's reciprocal and causal processes, which occur across multiple interdependent subsystems (Reskin 2012). Therefore, interventions that would successfully disrupt these systems and their processes must involve an exogenous force that acts on every subsystem or on key levers (such as residential segregation) that would trigger ripple effects across multiple subsystems.

Multilevel policies and interventions in homes, schools, neighborhoods, and workplaces are needed to dismantle the negative effects of institutional aspects of racism. For example, Purpose Built Communities (PBC) has developed a comprehensive model of attacking simultaneously all the underlying social problems that poor segregated communities face (Franklin and Edwards 2012). Importantly, PBC seeks to confront residential segregation and its pervasive negative consequences. The first site implementing the PBC model was East Lake, Atlanta. PBC transformed a dilapidated public housing project with high crime, welfare use, and unemployment and low-performing students into an oasis with cradle-to-college high-quality educational opportunities, mixed-income housing, early child development programs, full employment, and recreational and wellness opportunities. PBC is partnering with local organizations in multiple communities across the country to break the cycle of poverty and address institutional racism head-on. This type of comprehensive environmental intervention requires meaningful collaboration of local community members, local organizational leaders, and enlightened philanthropy. Healthcare organizations and professionals need to collaborate with other sectors of society to increase awareness about the critical role that social policies and interventions in domains far removed from traditional medical and public health policy can have in improving health and reducing disparities.

Research on the negative effects of interpersonal discrimination on health has identified several factors that can buffer at least some of its adverse consequences (Lewis et al. 2015). One line of research finds that high levels of supportive social relationships from family, friends, or others can reduce the negative effects of the chronic wear and tear of discrimination on the body. Some other studies find that high levels of religious involvement and/or church-based social support can also cushion the negative effects of discrimination on depressive symptoms. Some limited evidence also finds protective effects of psychological resources such as optimism. Future research is needed to characterize fully the range of resilience resources that can enable individuals and communities to cope with racism and the conditions under which they are more or less likely to be effective.

Recent scientific evidence also indicates that at the individual level, it is possible to reduce implicit and explicit racial prejudice. Professor Devine and her team at the University of Wisconsin (Devine et al. 2012) have developed a multifaceted approach combining, in a single program, multiple strategies that have been shown to reduce implicit bias. These strategies include stereotype replacement, counterstereotype imaging, individuation, perspective taking, and increasing opportunities for interracial contact. These researchers have shown that community resident nonblack adults can be motivated to increase their awareness of bias against blacks, increase their concerns about the effects of bias, and implement the necessary strategies. This program has been effective in producing substantial reductions in bias that remained evident 3 months later. Healthcare delivery and educational institutions need to embrace and implement such programs to reduce discrimination in the clinical context.

Conclusion

Large social inequities in mental health are unacceptable in a nation founded on the principles of liberty, equality, and justice for all. There is inadequate recognition that dismantling racial bias in all its forms is likely to be a potent health intervention. We need more research and interventions that attend to the ways we can address racism and each of the specific mechanisms through which it can negatively affect mental health.

References

Brown TN, Williams DR, Jackson JS, et al: Being black and feeling blue: the mental health consequences of racial discrimination. Race & Society 2:117–131, 2000

Cutler DM, Glaeser EL: Are ghettos good or bad? Q J Econ 112(3):827–872, 1997

Devine PG, Forscher PS, Austin AJ, et al: Long-term reduction in implicit race bias: a prejudice habit-breaking intervention. J Exp Soc Psychol 48(6):1267–1278, 2012 23524616

Franklin S, Edwards D: It takes a neighborhood: Purpose Built Communities and neighborhood transformation, in Investing in What Works for America's Communities. Edited by Andrews NO, Erickson DJ. San Francisco, CA, Federal Reserve Bank of San Francisco, 2012, pp 170–183

Glaeser EL, Vigdor JL: Racial Segregation in the Census 2000: Promising News. Washington, DC, Brookings Institute Center on Urban and Metropolitan Policy, 2001

LaVeist TA, Thorpe RJ Jr, Pierre G, et al: The relationships among vigilant coping style, race, and depression. Journal of Social Issues 70(2):241–255, 2014

Lewis TT, Cogburn CD, Williams DR: Self-reported experiences of discrimination and health: scientific advances, ongoing controversies, and emerging issues. Annu Rev Clin Psychol 11:407–440, 2015 25581238

Malat J, Mayorga-Gallo S, Williams DR: The effects of whiteness on the health of whites in the USA. Soc Sci Med 199:148–156, 2018

Massey DS, Denton NA: American Apartheid: Segregation and the Making of the Underclass. Cambridge, MA, Harvard University Press, 1993

Mouzon DM, McLean JS: Internalized racism and mental health among African-Americans, US-born Caribbean blacks, and foreign-born Caribbean blacks. Ethn Health 22(1):36–48, 2017 27354264

Pager D, Shepherd H: The sociology of discrimination: racial discrimination in employment, housing, credit, and consumer markets. Annu Rev Sociol 34:181–209, 2008 20689680

Proctor BD, Semega JL, Kollar MA: Income and poverty in the United States: 2015. Current Population Reports, P60-256 (RV). Washington, DC, US Census Bureau, Washington, DC, September 2016. Available at: https://www.census.gov/content/dam/Census/library/publications/2016/demo/p60-256.pdf. Accessed June 27, 2018.

Reskin B: The race discrimination system. Annu Rev Sociol 38:17–35, 2012

Steele CM, Aronson J: Stereotype threat and the intellectual test performance of African Americans. J Pers Soc Psychol 69(5):797–811, 1995 7473032

Turney K, Kissane R, Eden K: After moving to opportunity: how moving to a low-poverty neighborhood improves mental health among African American women. Soc Ment Health 3(1):1–21, 2013

U.S. Census Bureau: Wealth, asset ownership, & debt of households detailed tables: 2011. Available at: https://www.census.gov/data/tables/2011/demo/wealth/wealth-asset-ownership.html. Accessed June 27, 2018.

Verhaeghen P, Aikman SN, Van Gulick AE: Prime and prejudice: co-occurrence in the culture as a source of automatic stereotype priming. Br J Soc Psychol 50(3):501–518, 2011 21884547

Wallace S, Nazroo J, Bécares L: Cumulative effect of racial discrimination on the mental health of ethnic minorities in the United Kingdom. Am J Public Health 106(7):1294–1300, 2016 27077347

White K, Haas JS, Williams DR: Elucidating the role of place in health care disparities: the example of racial/ethnic residential segregation. Health Serv Res 47(3 Pt 2): 1278–1299, 2012 22515933

Williams DR, Collins C: Racial residential segregation: a fundamental cause of racial disparities in health. Public Health Rep 116(5):404–416, 2001 12042604

Williams DR, Medlock MM: Health effects of dramatic societal events—ramifications of the recent presidential election. N Engl J Med 376(23):2295–2299, 2017 28591522

Williams DR, Mohammed SA: Discrimination and racial disparities in health: evidence and needed research. J Behav Med 32(1):20–47, 2009 19030981

Williams DR, Mohammed SA: Racism and health, I: pathways and scientific evidence. Am Behav Sci 57(8):1152–1173, 2013 24347666

Williams DR, Wyatt R: Racial bias in health care and health: challenges and opportunities. JAMA 314(6):555–556, 2015 26262792

CHAPTER 25
TOWARD A LIBERATION PSYCHIATRY

Contributions From the Psychology of Place

Mindy Thompson Fullilove, M.D., Hon AIA

it was other people
those who, to me, broke the thread
therefore
the place, to me, became this way
that is the reason
why the place, to me, is no longer a place
because, to me, the thread is broken
because the thread no longer sings through the light
therefore
the place, to me, no longer feels like my place
therefore
it feels as if the place stands open before me
stands open and is empty
since, for me, the thread is broken
the place, for me, feels strange

therefore[1]

Dia!Kwain "The Broken Thread"

---

[1]Dia!Kwain, a member of the Khoikhoi nation (one of the first nations of Southern Africa), lived in the Western Cape in the mid- to late 1800s. He spoke the now extinct /Xam language. This is an unpublished translation by Robert Sember of Antjie Krog's Afrikaans version of the poem published in Krog 2002. Reproduced here by permission of Kwela Books.

DIA!KWAIN, a member of the Khoikhoi nation, one of the first nations of Southern Africa, wrote the poem in the epigraph about his experience of the arrival of other peoples who usurped the land that had once been that of his tribe. He puts forward the idea that "other people" broke the thread that no longer "sings through the light" and that therefore the place is "no longer a place." He emphasizes "to me." This remarkable poem, presented here in a translation by Robert Sember, captures the essence of the psychology of place, that we are connected to place by threads that sing through the light. When these are ruptured, we lose the connection to place, without which it no longer makes sense to us. Dia!Kwain takes us into the heart of the emotional experience of oppression, illuminating it by his focus on place. In this chapter, I hope to explore some of the key contributions the psychology of place can make to liberation psychiatry.

Frantz Fanon, Chester Pierce, Jeanne Spurlock, and other great black psychiatrists have understood that the oppression of black people not only has posed a threat to the physical and mental health of the oppressed but also has threatened the health of the oppressor. It is this Manichaean model—the oppressed and oppressor divided and therefore locked together in dysfunction—that they have worked so hard to explain.

Not only are oppressed and oppressor socially divided, they also are physically divided. In the United States, the highly elaborated system of segregation is known as Jim Crow (Zinn 1980). It was designed to separate people by race. Segregation was applied within places, like hospitals, trains, and cities, designating parts for whites and parts for blacks and other people of color. The parts for people of color were systematically denied resources, leading the U.S. Supreme Court to declare, in the 1954 *Brown v. Board of Education* ruling, "Separate is inherently unequal" (*Brown v. Board of Education of Topeka, Kansas*, 347 U.S. 483 [1954]). Despite advances on many fronts, segregation continues to plague the United States. Therefore, it is essential to understand that oppression has an inherent geography. It is this geography that makes it essential to incorporate place into our understanding of mental health.

Because of this geography of Jim Crow, I propose that the development of liberation psychiatry requires an exploration of "place," the locations in which people live, work, and love (Fullilove 1996). According to physics, matter has many definitions, but the most common is that it is any substance that has mass and occupies space. All physical objects are composed of matter, in the form of atoms, which are in turn composed of protons, neutrons, and electrons. People have physical being, are composed of atoms, and occupy space. *Space* is generally defined as open and unbounded areas. People are—and must be—located in space. Over eons people have organized space, and they have developed cultural patterns for bounding and naming it. These bounded areas are what we call "place." People live in places and experience the boundaries of place—especially the near places, like neighborhoods—as a secondary homeostatic system. Thus, the psychology of place becomes a fundamental, albeit often overlooked, part of human psychology.

In a segregated society, the boundaries of place are also markers of stratification that delineate the flows of both risks and benefits. Those in the favored strata derive extra benefit, while those in the lower strata are relatively deprived. The relative privilege of being on top obscures the fact that the constraint on flows of ideas and goods distorts the functioning of the whole society, enmeshing everyone in its caricatures of relatedness (Memmi 2013).

Using the biopsychosocial model of George Engel (1980) as a theoretical guide, my team has carried out several decades of research on the structure and process of American Jim Crow, with emphasis on the series of forced displacements that occurred in the second half of the twentieth century (Fullilove and Wallace 2011). This has led us to a dynamic model of the injuries of oppression, which occur across systems and at multiple levels of scale. Liberation psychiatry, by incorporating the psychology of place, will be positioned to implement what Wallace and Wallace (2013) have called "magic strategies," complex ecological interventions that are sensitive to time, place, and culture.

The Biopsychosocial Model Is Essential

George Engel, a psychiatrist who helped surgeons and internists understand their patients' needs, developed a concept he called the "biopsychosocial model" (Engel 1980). In contrast to the "biomedical model," which focused on what was going on inside the human body in a circumscribed biomedical sphere, the biopsychosocial model encompassed more: the biology, psychology, and sociology of illness.

Engel demonstrated this idea by describing the story of Mr. Glover, a man who had had a heart attack. The biomedical way the story would be told is something like this:

> This 55-year-old well-nourished, well-developed white man with a previous history of myocardial infarction began experiencing chest pain at 10 A.M. and was brought to the emergency department by ambulance at 11 A.M. He was hospitalized in the intensive care unit, where he experienced cardiac arrest due to ventricular fibrillation. He was successfully converted to normal rhythm. The rest of his hospital stay was unremarkable, and he was discharged to follow-up with his internist.

Engel had a completely different approach to the story (Figure 25–1). He started at the same place, acknowledging that Mr. Glover had a coronary artery occlusion, a heart attack. The coronary artery occlusion affected the cell and tissue levels of the systems hierarchy, producing the symptom of pain that Mr. Glover experienced.

But then Engel turned his attention to the time between the onset of pain and Mr. Glover's arrival at the hospital. A lot was happening in that hour that helps us understand the patient and his situation. We begin to see the myriad other systems that are going to be shaping the outcome of the problem.

While the first event is the "coronary artery occlusion," the second event is the "intervention of the employer." At first, Mr. Glover, who had had a previous heart attack, hoped that the feelings of unease and pressure inside his chest were signs of indigestion. He avoided talking to anyone in the office. As the pain increased, he realized that if he was having a heart attack, he should get his affairs in order. He started working to accomplish this. Meanwhile, the dangers of the heart attack were increasing. Finally, his employer intervened, and he agreed to go to the hospital (Figure 25–2).

In interviewing Mr. Glover, Engel learned that Glover's employer—who seemed to understand his need to preserve his dignity and sense of self—complimented him on his sense of responsibility, assured him that she and his coworkers would be able to manage because he had done such a great job, and emphasized that his most urgent responsibility was to get well so that he could continue to be the fine family man and coworker she knew him to be. This was clearly comforting to Mr. Glover. Engel showed how the processes inside Mr. Glover's body were continuing but systems outside his body were being mobilized.

Once he arrived at the hospital, Mr. Glover was admitted to the intensive care unit on a protocol for those with heart conditions. He relaxed, accepting that he had had a second heart attack and must begin to heal. At that point, the cardiac team wanted to put a catheter in Mr. Glover's artery. The residents in charge of this task were not able to perform it. After several tries, they went away to get help.

It was at that point that Mr. Glover had the near-fatal arrhythmia. Dr. Engel, in the diagram for this event, which he called "unsuccessful attempt at arterial puncture," noted that at the person level, Mr. Glover experienced a wide range of emotions, including frustration, pain, anger, self-blame, and giving up, which mobilized responses of the nervous system, including the fight-flight reaction (Figure 25–3). The nervous system, once activated, released a massive load of chemicals into the blood. This, Engel postulated, was what triggered the arrhythmia and cardiac arrest.

Happily, Mr. Glover was successfully resuscitated. The rest of his recovery was "uneventful," and he was discharged home. Yet even the return to health had implications for the patient, the family, and the community. In taking us carefully through this assessment of Mr. Glover's experience, Engel made the point that the biomedical model, which only considered the factors that are interior to the person, missed crucial events at higher levels of scale, including the patient's experience of the event and the influence of other actors on the unfolding drama. When we have the full hierarchy of systems in front of us, we have a more accurate view of what is happening.

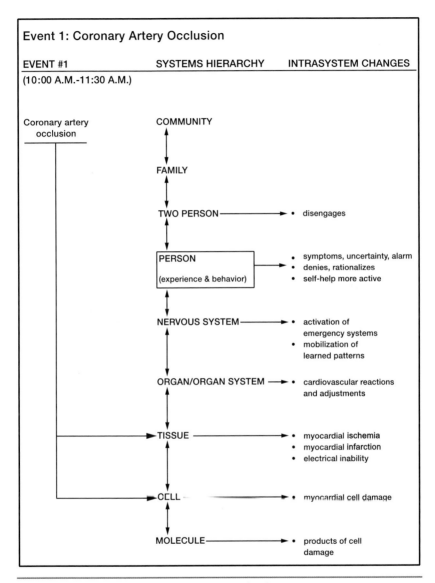

FIGURE 25–1. **Coronary artery occlusion.**

This figure is important because it shows the numerous levels of the biopsychosocial model and indicates what was happening at a number of levels at the opening of the episode of coronary artery occlusion.

Source. Reprinted from Engel GL: "The Clinical Application of the Biopsychosocial Model." *American Journal of Psychiatry* 137(5):535–544, 1980. Copyright 1980, American Psychiatric Association. Used with permission.

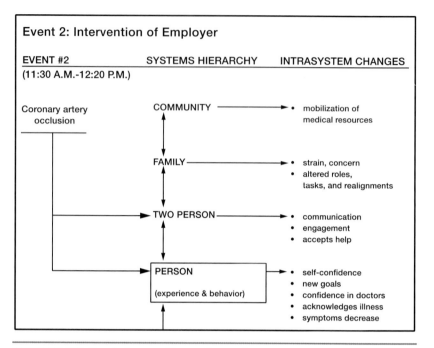

FIGURE 25–2. Intervention of employer.

This is a portion of Figure 25–1, showing the ways in which the personal problem is affecting larger social systems, specifically the two-person, family, and community systems.

Source. Reprinted from Engel GL: "The Clinical Application of the Biopsychosocial Model." *American Journal of Psychiatry* 137(5):535–544, 1980. Copyright 1980, American Psychiatric Association. Used with permission.

It is this model that can help us bring the person into relationship with the surrounding world. Engel's model used "community" to imply a set of people among whom the patient is embedded. *Community* is a useful and also a useless word. When we say "community," we think we know something. It is true that Mr. Glover was embedded in a community. Yet having said that, what do we know about his community? Of whom was it composed? Where did they live? This brings us to the problem of race in America and the study of the psychology of place.

We Live Divided

The United States—despite arguing that its revolutionary fight was for "freedom"—established itself as a slave nation, preserving and protecting the rights of slave owners, and counting slaves as only three-fifths of a person. African

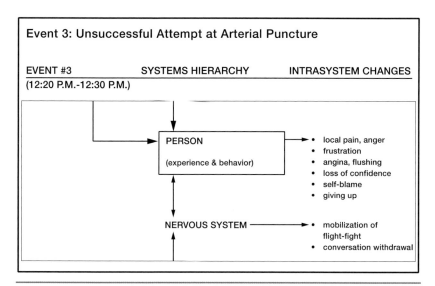

FIGURE 25–3.   Unsuccessful attempt at arterial puncture.

This diagram shows the ways in which the actions of the medical residents affected the physiology of the patient. Specifically, the failure to introduce the arterial line causes the patient to experience many emotions and mobilizes the fight-flight response, triggering ventricular fibrillation.

Source.   Reprinted from Engel GL: "The Clinical Application of the Biopsychosocial Model." *American Journal of Psychiatry* 137(5):535–544, 1980. Copyright 1980, American Psychiatric Association. Used with permission.

Americans and their white allies carried out a sustained struggle to abolish slavery and establish freedom and equality. Gains in the Reconstruction era were largely lost as inclusive democratic institutions were replaced by the Jim Crow system, which was later copied by admirers in Nazi Germany to create fascism and in South Africa to create apartheid. The long Civil Rights struggle, which we can date from W. E. B. Du Bois's and William Trotter's founding of the Niagara Movement in 1905, culminated in marked victories in the mid-1960s, with the signing of the Civil Rights Act, the Voting Act, and the establishment of Medicaid, which desegregated hospitals.

A paradox of the post–Civil Rights era has been the "urban crisis," a polite way of saying "inner-city black poverty." The impression that the Civil Rights Movement "fixed" the problem of segregation conflicted with the reality of enduring—and worsening—distress. The idea that this was a failure of "personal responsibility" took hold and was widely promoted by right-wing politicians (Harvey 2007).

The perspective of the psychology of place helps us track and interpret a different story, often overlooked in the history of the twentieth century, of a series of forced displacements that had devastating effects on inner-city communities. The psychology of place posits that there are essential connections between individuals and their place of residence as well as among residents of a given place and between and among residents of different places. These are connections of attachment, such as those described by Bowlby and others (Fullilove 1996), as well as the strong and weak social bonds that Granovetter (1973) has described.

Through the lens of psychology of place, we can appreciate the strength of segregated communities that managed to temper the ravages of racism through the Jim Crow era and build political power and many kinds of wealth. It was the power of these communities that was expressed in the Civil Rights Movement. The example of the Montgomery Bus Boycott can illuminate this point (King 2010). Rosa Parks's legendary act of civil disobedience took place on Thursday, December 1, 1955. By Monday morning, December 5, 1955, at 6 A.M., 50,000 black people were boycotting the buses. For more than a year, they endured threats and attacks, faced layoffs, organized carpools, fed many, conducted weekly rallies, and held firm until they won. Only a very well integrated, powerful community—with deep spiritual principles—could have accomplished such a feat.

It is the power of the Civil Rights Movement that raises the question: Why wasn't everything fixed by the late 1960s? Why were there terrible riots across the United States in the summers of 1967 and 1968? This is where the story of serial forced displacement, which starts with urban renewal, as carried out under the Housing Act of 1949, comes in (Fullilove 2004). Known among black people as "Negro removal," the Housing Act authorized cities to clear "blighted land," using the power of eminent domain, and sell the land at reduced cost to developers for "higher uses" such as cultural centers, universities, and public housing. During the 14 years of the urban renewal program, 993 cities participated, carrying out more than 2,500 projects. Of those residents displaced, 63% were African Americans; the areas destroyed included substantial portions of such important black cultural centers as the Hill District in Pittsburgh and the Fillmore in San Francisco.

The Kerner Commission's (1968) study of civil disorder in 1967 included urban renewal in the list of factors that triggered the rebellions. The process of urban renewal tore communities apart, destroying their accumulated social, cultural, political, and economic capital as well as undermining their competitive position vis-à-vis neighborhoods that were not disturbed (Fullilove 2004). This profoundly weakened affected neighborhoods; those harms were repeated in subsequent displacements due to planned shrinkage, mass incarceration, HOPE VI (which was directed at federal housing projects), the foreclosure crisis, and gentrification (Fullilove and Wallace 2011).

The series of displacements from neighborhoods occurred contemporaneously with deindustrialization, which undermined the economic foundations of older American cities, leaving unskilled workers at a severe disadvantage (Bluestone and Harrison 1982). This created the massive deindustrialization diaspora to the Sun Belt, destabilizing both sending and receiving cities. In the upheaval caused by these policies, the epidemics of heroin and crack cocaine took off, violence soared, and AIDS became a serious threat to health. Asthma and obesity flourished. Trauma, as a result of these accumulating disasters, became a major source of psychiatric illness.

The economic and social dismemberment of African American communities stole their wealth, their power, and their capacity to engage in problem solving. Returning to the biopsychosocial model, we can begin to name the processes that are happening at each level of scale. The experience of trauma, grief, anger, and the stress of losing one's embedding community have significant effects on the person. These can lead to psychiatric illness, the use of drugs, eating and autoimmune disorders, and infectious diseases. The vulnerability of the individual—stripped of the protection of a known and loved place—is greatly increased. When social processes of constant upheaval set in, as they did because of the serial nature of forced displacement, the individuals were not able to reestablish the beloved community. Then, new kinds of social organization developed, and new kinds of communication were employed. It is in this context, the aftermath of serial forced displacement and deindustrialization, that we find widespread social fracture, violence, addiction, and refusal of participation in larger social systems through voting and other nonviolent forms of action.

There Are No "Magic Bullets"

Human ecologists Rodrick and Deborah Wallace open their important monograph commenting that "the most effective medical or public health strategies must be analogously patterned across scale and level of organization: 'magic strategies' will almost always be synergistically, and often emergently, more effective than 'magic bullets'" (Wallace and Wallace 2013, p. v).

The Wallaces contrast "magic strategy" with "magic bullet," a term invented by Paul Ehrlich in 1900. Ehrlich hypothesized an agent that would kill specific microbes without harming the human body and named it *Zauberkugel* ("magic bullet"). As antibiotics became widely available, it was assumed that the eradication of the targeted germs could not be far behind. It turned out this was impossible. Alan Brandt (1987) detailed the unsuccessful efforts at using antibiotics for wiping out venereal disease. Rather than wiping out disease, the widespread use of antibiotics has led to resistance in the microbes, which have evolved to survive. In 2016, the World Health Organization released the following statement:

> New guidelines for the treatment of 3 common sexually transmitted infections (STIs) have been issued by WHO in response to the growing threat of antibiotic resistance.

Chlamydia, gonorrhoea and syphilis are all caused by bacteria and are generally curable with antibiotics. However, these STIs often go undiagnosed and are becoming more difficult to treat, with some antibiotics now failing as a result of misuse and overuse. It is estimated that, each year, 131 million people are infected with chlamydia, 78 million with gonorrhea, and 5.6 million with syphilis.

Resistance of these STIs to the effect of antibiotics has increased rapidly in recent years and has reduced treatment options. Of the 3 STIs, gonorrhea has developed the strongest resistance to antibiotics. Strains of multidrug-resistant gonorrhea that do not respond to any available antibiotics have already been detected. Antibiotic resistance in chlamydia and syphilis, though less common, also exists, making prevention and prompt treatment critical. (World Health Organization 2016)

It is the need for *prevention*—which is a different process from *treatment*—that implicates a magic strategy instead of simply a magic bullet. The point of the Wallaces' paper is to suggest a mechanism explaining why magic bullets alone cannot ensure public health (Wallace and Wallace 2013). Their argument hinges on some basic facts about humans: We are biological beings, systems of systems that use complex cognitive strategies to regulate our interior workings: getting food digested, air moving, blood flowing, and hormones regulated. We are also social beings, deeply interconnected with other people with whom we develop shared cultures. The interior system of systems and the exterior cultures are tightly interconnected and interpenetrating. Therefore, if we want to manage disease and promote health, the Wallaces argue, it makes sense to work at the scale of the body *and* at the scale of the society.

This analysis provides helpful clarity. Starting from the premise of curing the individual, it seems as if the public health problem is simply to cure all the individuals. This turns out to be impossible. By introducing culture into our consideration, we start to realize there are neglected issues that must be addressed. How would you get all the individuals diagnosed? How would you get them treated? What if the individuals do not want to be diagnosed or treated? What if some individuals are treated differently in society? How is that to be managed? The existence of a medicine that cures an illness is not the same as a method of managing disease at the level of society, especially a highly stratified society, like that during Jim Crow.

The Wallaces' work provides a plausible connection between the layer of person and the layers of society by linking the body's biological ability to read what's going on in society, comparing it to an internal picture of the world, and choosing an appropriate action based on that knowledge. They noted examples from numerous parts of the human body, and we cite one here:

Upon recognition of a new perturbation in the surrounding environment, emotional and/or conscious cognition evaluate and choose from several possible responses: no action necessary, flight, fight, helplessness (flight or fight is needed, but not possible). Upon appropriate conditioning, the HPA axis is able to accelerate the decision process, much as the immune system has a more efficient response to second pathogenic challenge once the initial infection has become encoded in immune memory. Certainly, hyperreactivity as a sequela of posttraumatic stress disorder (PTSD) is well known. (Wallace and Wallace 2013, p. 16)

That the human body can read—as the Wallaces note, consciously or unconsciously—the surrounding environment is the foundation for the necessity of the magic strategy. They also stress that

[f]or humans culture is absolutely fundamental.... Successful human populations have a core of tool usage, sophisticated language, oral tradition, mythology, music, and decision-making skills focused on relatively small family/extended family social network groupings. More complex social structures are built on the periphery of this basic object. The human species' very identity may rest on its unique evolved capacities for social mediation and cultural transmission. These are particularly expressed through the cognitive decision-making of small groups facing changing patterns of threat and opportunity, processes in which we are all embedded and all participate. (Wallace and Wallace 2013, p. 19)

Magic Strategies Enact Liberation Psychiatry

People can be heard to say, "It was better when we had segregation." Obviously, we still have segregation, so that is not really what has changed. What has changed is the nature of community. The Montgomery, Alabama, of 1955 had remarkable strength, as did many other black communities. Those strengths were systematically destroyed by serial forced displacement and deindustrialization. The social fracture that followed the implementation of those policies fed the downward spiral of social dissolution, hatred, and racism. The anomie was often more terrifying than the threats of illness and violence.

Yet people continued to rebuild, even in the face of constant disruption. Over decades of fieldwork, I have observed communities in their struggle to manage violence, AIDS, addiction, and homelessness. Their struggles had much in common. From my observations of the tools they used, I developed a framework of "elements of urban restoration" to repair the damage to the urban ecosystem created by Jim Crow, serial forced displacement, and deindustrialization (Fullilove 2013).

What is striking about watching people at work in community building is that people feel better long before the problems are solved. As we counter anomie, the fears of isolation and abandonment are eased. In northern Manhattan, my research team led a project called City Life Is Moving Bodies (CLIMB), which built a hiking trail from Central Park to the Cloisters. The trail passed through parks that had suffered from disinvestment, including one, Highbridge Park, that had been largely abandoned. Our project organized an annual pot-luck hiking event that culminated in a party in Highbridge Park. From the beginning, it was an occasion to see people laugh and play, relax with one another, and leave with renewed confidence that they could make their neighborhood better. We have described this as "collective recovery" (Fullilove et al. 2004). Organizations can be crucial supporters of collective recovery by incorporating an awareness of people's needs into their ongoing activities.

The other observation is the constancy of struggle: every gain for equality and democracy is immediately contested by those who wish to preserve wealth and power for the few. In fact, the setbacks from serial forced displacement and deindustrialization have been devastating for communities of people of color and working people. These processes have not been stopped. Indeed, the tax bill enacted in the 2017 Tax Cuts and Jobs Act by a Republican-controlled Congress, which sought to widen the already massive gap between the super-rich and everyone else, is doomed to cause more harm. Also, as I have noted, in this Manichaean system, the widening gap between those on top and those on the bottom served to strengthen the linking of their fates, which Wallace and Wallace (1999) have called the "paradox of Apartheid."

Conclusion

Liberation psychiatry presupposes that the world around us is influencing our mental health. Here I have argued that the psychology of place elaborates the outer systems of the biopsychosocial model and can help us understand the ways in which social, economic, and political processes actually become embodied in our hearts and minds. At the same time, empirical observation has established that people can understand their problems and will rally for change. As psychiatrists, we can make an important contribution to people's awareness that mental well-being requires a just world.

I opened this chapter with an astounding poem from a man who was one of the First People of South Africa. He observed that "other people" had broken the thread and that therefore the place was "no longer a place." This is the kind of damage that has followed serial forced displacement and deindustrialization, causing people much pain and suffering. Liberation psychiatry stands with the injured, on behalf of all of us, to repair the thread, so that it can sing once again.

References

Bluestone B, Harrison B: The Deindustrialization of America: Plant Closings, Community Abandonment, and the Dismantling of Basic Industry. New York, Basic Books, 1982

Brandt AM: No Magic Bullet: A Social History of Venereal Disease in the United States Since 1880. Oxford, UK, Oxford Paperbacks, 1987

Engel GL: The clinical application of the biopsychosocial model. Am J Psychiatry 137(5):535–544, 1980 7369396

Fullilove MT: Psychiatric implications of displacement: contributions from the psychology of place. Am J Psychiatry 153(12):1516–1523, 1996 8942445

Fullilove MT: Root Shock: How Tearing Up City Neighborhoods Hurts America and What We Can Do About It. New York, One World, 2004

Fullilove MT: Urban Alchemy: Restoring Joy in America's Sorted-Out Cities. New York, New Village Press, 2013

Fullilove MT, Wallace R: Serial forced displacement in American cities, 1916–2010. J Urban Health 88(3):381–389, 2011 21607786

Fullilove MT, Hernandez-Cordero L, Madoff JS, et al: Promoting collective recovery through organizational mobilization: the post-9/11 disaster relief work of NYC RECOVERS. J Biosoc Sci 36(4):479–489, 2004 15293388

Granovetter MS: The strength of weak ties. Am J Sociol 78(6):1360–1380, 1973

Harvey D: A brief history of neoliberalism. New York, Oxford University Press, 2007

Kerner Commission: National Advisory Commission on Civil Disorder. Washington, DC, US Government Printing Office, 1968

King ML Jr: Stride Toward Freedom: The Montgomery Story, Vol 1. Boston, MA, Beacon Press, 2010

Krog A: Met Woorde Soos Met Kerse. Cape Town, South Africa, Kwela Books, 2002

Memmi A: The Colonizer and the Colonized. New York, Routledge, 2013

Wallace R, Wallace D: Emerging infections and nested martingales: the entrainment of affluent populations into the disease ecology of marginalization. Environment and Planning A 31(10):1787–1803, 1999

Wallace R, Wallace D: Magic Strategies: The Basic Biology of Multilevel, Multiscale, Health Promotion. PeerJ PrePrints, May 21, 2013

World Health Organization: Growing antibiotic resistance forces updates to recommended treatment for sexually transmitted infections. WHO releases new treatment guidelines for chlamydia, gonorrhoea and syphilis. Media Centre, August 30, 2016. Available at: http://www.who.int/mediacentre/news/releases/2016/antibiotics-sexual-infections/en/. Accessed January 3, 2018.

Zinn H: A People's History of the United States. New York, Perennial Classic, 1980

CHAPTER 26
THE "NEW" EPIDEMIC

Trauma Among Urban Adolescents Living in Poverty

Nadia L. Ward, Ph.D.
Aaron D. Haddock, Ph.D.
Patricia Simon, Ph.D.
Michael J. Strambler, Ph.D.

ROUGHLY 16 MILLION children between the ages of 5 and 17 live in poverty in the United States. A staggering 45.8% of these children are black (National Center for Health Statistics 2016). Data from the National Center for Health Statistics (2016) further indicate that 45% of all poor children reside in female-headed households, and when the data are disaggregated by race and ethnicity, we find that 52% of poor black children, 50% of poor Hispanic children, and 36% of poor white children are being raised by single mothers. Living in poverty presents a multiplicity of challenges in communities plagued by social, economic, and environmental disadvantage. Urban minority youth are placed at high risk for engagement in risky behaviors that have implications for their healthy adjustment along cognitive, social, emotional, and behavioral domains of functioning. Youths' prolonged exposure to stressful life conditions (violence, drugs, food insufficiency, housing insecurity) severely compromises the functioning and development of emergent brain and body systems that help regulate the body's response to stress (Felitti et al. 1998).

It is not surprising that the topic of trauma among school-age children and adolescents has received increased national attention in recent years. Trauma, the "new" epidemic, is anything but new. For those working with urban children and adolescents living in poverty, trauma is a rite of passage that is inextricably connected to their early lived experiences. What is new is the acknowledgment that there is now scientific evidence that has demonstrated a link between adverse childhood experiences and long-term health consequences in adulthood. Early studies claimed that the physiological damage done to the body due to prolonged exposure to stress was intractable (Kaufman et al. 2000). However, we now know that preventive interventions coupled with the presence of a strong, caring, adult role model can, in fact, buffer and "undo" the harmful effects of toxic stress on the body (Kaufman and Charney 2001). Moreover, there are promising new approaches and clinical interventions that support youth affected by trauma in addressing their trauma histories.

In this chapter, we discuss how trauma affects the lived experience of urban adolescents in schools and the impact prolonged exposure to toxic stress has on their health and well-being. We describe the spectrum of trauma, and its associated signs and symptoms, and review targeted clinical interventions that have shown promise in buffering the negative impact of trauma on the healthy adjustment of adolescents. Although targeted interventions have demonstrated positive effects for alleviating students' symptoms of trauma, there are often challenges in implementing these types of programs in school settings. Urban public schools are woefully under-resourced and therefore lack the ability to meet the demand of providing high-quality behavioral health services to students, particularly those affected by trauma. In a climate of ever-shrinking educational funding, school districts are often forced to cut mental health services to students in desperate need of support. This translates into fewer mental health practitioners in schools, who struggle to manage large caseloads and long wait-lists while students' behavioral health needs are neglected.

This scenario creates the unique opportunity to forge partnerships between universities and school districts to address the issue of trauma in the urban community. We present details about such a collaboration—one that leveraged university and community resources to aid a district in its mission to prepare students for postsecondary education. With funding from the U.S. Department of Education, our research team implemented a multiyear district-wide educational initiative aimed at increasing high school graduation rates and college enrollment rates. What we failed to recognize were the large percentage of students in our cohort who had experienced adverse life experiences and the impact prolonged exposure to toxic stress had had on their cognitive, social, and emotional development.

We collected data about our students that helped to characterize our cohort along dimensions of stressful life events and the impact these events had on students' grades, educational engagement, and participation in enrichment and support activities. What we learned changed our conceptualization of the work and the manner in which we engage students and their families. It also informed how we recruit, train, and supervise direct service staff in their work with students exposed to trauma. Our work on this topic received considerable attention from school staff, thereby facilitating the expansion of our role in the district. It enabled our team to provide training and consultation to the district's mental health practitioners and teachers on understanding trauma and embracing a student-centered, trauma-informed approach in their work with urban youth. Finally, it provided an opportunity to dialogue with district leadership and building administrators on how to create culturally responsive and trauma-sensitive school environments conducive to student learning.

Our goal in this chapter is to describe what trauma looks like in urban communities and the role toxic stress has on students' early neurological development, learning, and behavior in school. Also outlined are student-centered approaches that help buffer students from the long-term negative effects of trauma. as well as school-wide strategies schools can implement to create learning environments sensitive to the needs of students affected by trauma. We present a case study that highlights how we used data to inform how services are designed and implemented to respond to the needs of a more vulnerable segment of our cohort.

Risky Behaviors and Urban Youth

When constantly confronted with the stressors of living in poverty, urban youth engage in risky behaviors that in the short term may alleviate stress but ultimately contribute to increased rates of morbidity and mortality (Evans et al. 2007). The Centers for Disease Control and Prevention (CDC)'s Youth Risk Behavior Surveillance Report (Kann et al. 2016) found that compared with white and Hispanic students, black students had higher prevalence rates for risky and health-undermining behaviors such as fighting, sexual promiscuity, marijuana use, overeating (that leads to obesity), and physical inactivity. The cause of these conditions and resulting inequities in health have been shown to be socially determined and a result of the complex interplay among factors such as genetics, economic disadvantage, environment, racism, and substandard education (Braveman et al. 2011). These traumas, when experienced in childhood or adolescence, increase youths' likelihood of disease and chronic health problems protracted later in life (Tough 2011).

Linking Adverse Childhood Experiences to Health Outcomes

A seminal epidemiological study conducted by the CDC and Kaiser Permanente (Felitti et al. 1998) examined the association between traumatic childhood experiences, household dysfunction, and multiple health behaviors that impact the long-term physical and mental health condition of their patients in adulthood. The Adverse Childhood Experiences (ACE) study interviewed 17,000 white, college-educated, employed adults who were screened for 10 traumatic experiences in childhood as part of a routine health screening. There were seven categories of traumatic experiences in childhood assessed as part of a routine health screening. Traumas assessed fell into two categories: Abuse (psychological, physical, sexual) and Household Dysfunction (substance abuse, mental illness, mother treated violently, criminal behavior).

Findings indicated that 70% of participants experienced at least one type of trauma during childhood. Participants who experienced four or more traumas during childhood had 4 times the risk of chronic bronchitis, over 4 times the likelihood of depression, and 12 times the risk of suicide. Furthermore, the authors found that ACE scores were directly related to early initiation of smoking and sexual activity, alcoholism, adolescent pregnancy, depression, and risk for intimate partner violence experienced later in life. The ACE study was the first to link adverse childhood experiences to health risk behaviors and disease later in life. It is likely that for urban adolescents who are living in disenfranchised communities, prolonged exposure to toxic stress places them at high risk for the health risk behaviors found in the ACE study (Felitti et al. 1998; Kann et al. 2016).

Toxic Stress

Toxic stress is described as the prolonged activation of the body's stress response systems in the absence of protective relationships (Cohen 2017). Our stress response system is our body's natural alarm that warns us of an impending threat and activates a physiological response that mobilizes us to "fight," take "flight," or "freeze" in the face of a threat. When urban youth are continuously bombarded by external threats, the brain/body's stress response system is put in a chronic state of fear or hypervigilance that activates what is referred to as the "survival brain." The survival brain actively works to distinguish between real or imagined external environmental threats. Thus, in the context of the school setting, trauma-exposed youth may be easily "triggered," thereby causing them to react as though the previous traumatic event is presently happening, even when there is no threat. Common trauma triggers that youth experience include unpredictability; sensory overload; feeling vulnerable, overwhelmed, or frustrated; and confrontation (St. Andrews 2013).

It is the body's prolonged overactivation of the stress response system that alters the biochemistry of DNA in the brain through a process called *methylation* (Kaufman et al. 2000). This process of methylation prevents the brain from properly regulating its response to stress. As a result, the normal development of neurological functioning is interrupted and affects the development of the frontal lobe, where executive functioning takes place (plan, organize, make decisions); the hippocampus, which is responsible for learning and memory; and the amygdala, which attaches emotion to memory. Other systems affected are the cardiovascular, metabolic, and immune systems, and changes in these systems increase the likelihood of long-term medical conditions such as diabetes, hypertension, obesity, cancer, depression, and substance use, which are common among racial and ethnic minorities.

The Spectrum of Trauma

Trauma is defined as an acute or chronic life event that threatens one's physical and/or emotional well-being (St. Andrews 2013). Trauma is also understood as existing on a spectrum that ranges from acute to complex. *Acute trauma* is a single time-limited event, whereas *chronic trauma* is defined as multiple traumatic exposures and/or events over extended periods of time. *Complex traumas* are multiple trauma exposures that are experienced over time. Here, the trauma often occurs within the youth's caregiving system. *Vicarious or secondary trauma* is characterized by the exposure to the trauma of those in close contact with the traumatized individual. For urban youth living in toxic environments, their experience of trauma has a profound impact on their schooling experience.

Impact of Trauma on School Functioning

Research has shown that exposure to toxic stress and traumatic experiences can have a profound impact on learning and academic outcomes for urban youth. In a comprehensive review of the literature on trauma-informed schools, Overstreet and Chafouleas (2016) found that students with extensive trauma histories demonstrated poor academic performance, increased school absences, increased expulsions and suspensions, decreased high school graduation rates, and increased delinquent behavior. Regarding social-emotional and behavioral functioning, trauma exposure has been found to be associated with increased incidence of disruptive behavior, hyperactivity, impulsivity, sexual promiscuity, and substance abuse.

A Trauma-Informed Approach to Working With Youth

A trauma-informed approach uses the recognition that certain behaviors are related to traumatic experience to drive a new set of practices at school with young people who exhibit these behaviors. When we adopt a trauma lens, we shift from a deficit model that asks "What is wrong with you?" to one that asks

"What happened to you?" With this paradigm shift, a new opportunity is offered to engage in a dialogue that shifts the school environment and classroom practices to respond more effectively to students' needs.

It is important that schools foster a sense of community and belonging that facilitates students' positive adjustment and sense of trust. Caring and trusting relationships are a precondition to effectiveness and form the foundation for cooperative, prosocial behavior and academic achievement. Without strong, positive relationships with school staff, trauma-impacted students are more likely to disengage from school. The research is clear that students who are more connected to teachers and peers demonstrate greater school engagement and more positive trajectories of development in both social and academic domains (Durlak et al. 2011). Cultivating authentic trusting relationships with students impacted by trauma helps to reverse negative working models that students have of themselves and the expectation of critical, punitive relationships from adults.

When students impacted by trauma exhibit maladaptive behaviors, it is important to take a teaching stance that enhances, rather than harms, the helping relationship. This means shifting the focus from imposing our will on the student, which often exacerbates an issue, to collaboratively engaging in problem solving and teaching adaptive skills. Greene's Collaborative Problem Solving model (Greene 2014) offers a simple and helpful multistep approach to engaging in problem solving with students that includes expressing empathy, defining the problem, and collaborative problem solving.

Evidence-Based Interventions

In a comprehensive review of psychosocial interventions that alleviate the impact of trauma, Dorsey et al. (2017) found that the strongest evidence exists for cognitive-behavioral interventions. Moreover, efficacious interventions typically include psychoeducation about trauma, training in emotion regulation, exposure (in vivo and imaginal), cognitive processing, and/or problem solving. Regarding setting, there is evidence that the disseminating trauma-focused interventions in schools can increase their reach. One study showed that youth were more likely to participate in a trauma-focused intervention if it was based at school rather than in a clinic (Jaycox et al. 2010). Later we provide an overview of well-established interventions that can be implemented in schools.

Trauma-Focused Cognitive-Behavioral Therapy

Trauma-focused cognitive-behavioral therapy (CBT) teaches youth how to manage reactions to traumatic memories. The program is implemented with parents and youth (ages 3–18 years old). Guided by the acronym PRACTICE, participants receive psychoeducation and parenting skills education, learn relaxation techniques, engage in trauma narrative development, participate in in vivo gradual exposure, complete conjoint parent/child sessions, and develop a plan for their future, with emphasis on enhancing their safety. The participant and a nonoffending caregiver typically participate in 8–20 sessions. The evidence for trauma-focused CBT is well established, with randomized controlled trials showing that it is efficacious for reducing trauma-related symptoms among youth who have survived sexual violence (Cohen et al. 2016). These findings are also supported by data from a systematic review showing that results persist 12 months posttreatment (Cary and McMillen 2012).

Cognitive Behavioral Intervention for Trauma in Schools Program

The Cognitive Behavioral Intervention for Trauma in Schools (CBITS) program is a 10-session, school-based (fifth through twelfth grade) group intervention that aims to reduce youths' trauma-related symptoms, teach them how to manage trauma-related stressors, and build their social support network. The program achieves these aims by providing psychoeducation on trauma, providing relaxation training, engaging youth in cognitive restructuring, guiding them through graduated in vivo exposure exercises, and teaching social problem solving. In addition to the standard 10 group sessions, youth may participate in up to 3 individual sessions, parents participate in 2 group sessions, and teachers participate in 1 educational session. Randomized controlled trials have shown that CBITS reduces posttraumatic stress disorder (PTSD) and trauma-related symptoms (Jaycox et al. 2010; Kataoka et al. 2003).

Multimodality Trauma Treatment

Multimodality Trauma Treatment (MMTT), also known as Trauma-Focused Coping in Schools, is a 14-session group intervention for youth ages 9–18 years. The program emphasizes cognitive-behavioral skills training and peer mediations. It is designed for youth who have been exposed to one traumatic event. Youth participants receive psychoeducation, anxiety management training, cognitive training, anger and grief management, an individual session to develop a trauma narrative, and guidance in developing a stimulus hierarchy. They also participate in group narrative exposure, receive training in cognitive and active processing of worst moments, receive training in relapse prevention, and participate in graduation. Two studies have shown that participation in MMTT is associated with reductions in PTSD and other trauma-related symptoms in diverse community settings (Amaya-Jackson et al. 2003).

Overall, there is robust evidence to support implementing trauma-focused interventions in schools, with the strongest evidence for those guided by CBT. There is a gap in research regarding implementation of these interventions among black American youth living in poverty. In the following discussion we describe our experiences implementing comprehensive services in a predominantly black, low-income community.

Yale GEAR UP Partnership Project

Our interest in the topic of trauma among urban youth was born of our experience working in an urban public school in New England. Our team received funding from the U.S. Department of Education to implement a school reform effort that sought to increase students' academic performance and access to post-secondary education. The intervention targeted a cohort of 1,600 seventh-grade students and followed them from seventh grade through their entry into college.

Our interest in trauma came from formative evaluations and feedback received from direct service staff. Data indicated a disproportionate number of students in our cohort were failing in ninth grade. Furthermore, direct service staff shared during weekly supervision that students had made meaningful connections, and as a result, had described the pain of their experiences. Personal narratives were shared by students who described incidents of sexual assault and molestation, the murder of a sibling and a peer, the death of an entire family due to arson (where the sole survivor was our student), the arrest and incarceration of a parent, and a home invasion and theft. Students also recounted stories of homelessness, food insecurity, housing instability, and gang involvement. Other stories highlighted their experience raising younger siblings, working while in school, or living with a parent struggling with substance abuse dependency and/or a co-occurring mental disorder.

After we examined service utilization data and anecdotal reports, it became evident that our students' pervasive low level of academic performance could be attributed to their trauma experiences. This explained their difficulty managing their emotions, controlling their behavior, and communicating their needs. We also learned that student planning and management teams (SPMT) (composed of mental health professionals) were so overwhelmed that it took weeks for a student to be seen by a mental health practitioner. Our direct service team required more training in trauma and counseling techniques they could use in their work with students before their triage into services provided by the SPMT. Given these observations, we designed a study that would allow us to identify specific stressors students were experiencing. The study had two aims: to characterize a cohort along dimensions of risk and protective factors and to determine how risk factors were associated with school performance and engagement in academic enrichment and support services provided by the program.

A mental health survey was administered to a sample of the tenth-grade students at the end of the 2014–2015 school year. Student exposure to stressful life events was assessed among 360 students using 47 items from the Life Events Questionnaire (LEQ; Masten et al. 1994). The LEQ assesses the number of events that a person has experienced across three dimensions: perceived consequences (negative, positive, or ambiguous), duration (discrete/acute or chronic/persistent), and independence from students' actions (independent and nonindependent). Given our interest in stress, only scales addressing negative consequences were considered; consequently, the following four scales were used: 1) Chronic, Onset Negative, Independent Scale (e.g., "There were many arguments between adults living in the house"); 2) Chronic, Onset Negative, Nonindependent Scale (e.g., "I had many arguments with my parent[s] during this past year"); 3) Discrete, Onset Negative, Independent Scale (e.g., "A parent was arrested or went to jail during this past year"); and 4) Discrete, Onset Negative, Nonindependent Scale (e.g., "I went to jail"). The number of items was added to create a total score for each scale.

The Strengths and Difficulties Questionnaire (SDQ; Goodman 2001) ($n=$ 426) is a 25-item scale that assesses five domains of functioning—conduct problems (e.g., "I fight a lot"), hyperactivity (e.g., "I am restless"), emotion symptoms (e.g., "I worry a lot"), peer problems (e.g., "other children or young people pick on me"), and prosocial traits (e.g., "I often volunteer to help others"). Each item assesses whether a given behavior is "not true," "somewhat true," or "certainly true." This was scored on a 0 to 2 scale to produce sum scores for each subscale.

In terms of associations between academic performance and life events, we found a negative association between negative discrete events that directly involve students' actions (LEQ Discrete, Onset Negative, Nonindependent Scale) and core Grade Point Average for the first semester. Grades had the strongest association with positive and negative discrete events (e.g., "I got in trouble with the law"), with lower grades being associated with negative events and higher grades being associated with higher grades. Specifically, we found that grades had a correlation of −0.19 with negative events and 0.16 with positive events. Observing this relationship in tertiles for core GPA, we found that students in the second GPA tertile differed from those in the third, with students in the second tertile reporting 1.68 negative events and those in the third indicating 1.00 event, for a difference of 0.68 events (95% confidence interval [CI] 0.21, 1.15). Those in the first GPA tertile also had more positive discrete events ($m=1.12$), such as receiving "a special award or recognition," than those in the third tertile ($m=1.74$), with a difference of 0.62 events (95% CI 0.04, 1.21).

When we examined the associations between students' grades and the SDQ, we found a positive association ($r=0.26$) between grades and prosocial behavior in that students with higher grades endorsed more prosocial behavior. Students in the first GPA tertile had a mean score of 5.21 (standard deviation [SD]=

2.70) out of a possible 10 on the Prosocial scale, and those in the third tertile had a mean score of 6.61 (SD = 2.12), for a difference of 1.40 (95% CI 0.51, 2.29).

It is notable that of the life events and strengths difficulty bivariate correlations noted, the association between grades and prosocial behavior was the strongest. Although these findings are not causal, they hold promise for supporting students' academics through developing their prosocial and other social and emotional skills. However, higher-risk students may be challenging to reach with academic support and social and emotional programming. For example, in our programming efforts, we have found that, in general, lower-performing students tend to access fewer services than higher-performing students. For example, students in the first GPA tertile received an average of 2 hours of exposure to a social development program, whereas those in the third tertile received more than 5 hours. Similarly, those in the first tertile were exposed to four fewer hours of college tours.

With these findings came the realization that a new strategy for engaging low-performing students was necessary. These students represent one-third of the cohort and require targeted behavioral health interventions aimed at preventing school dropout. Additionally, data also provided support for enhanced training and professional development for our direct service team members. The severity of stressful life events experienced by our students changed the manner in which we recruited, trained, and supervised our direct service team. Our students required a more clinically skilled team with diverse talents to support students affected by trauma. We employed individuals enrolled in master's-level graduate training programs in counseling-related disciplines. Our training strategy was theoretically driven and incorporated didactic training sessions on family systems, working with culturally diverse populations, motivational interviewing, positive youth development, and reflection. These additions, we believed, would further enhance the training team members received from their graduate training programs and provide sorely needed counseling supports to students in schools.

Finally, this new information also allowed our team to think differently about how we monitor the ongoing progress of a cohort, particularly in behavioral health domains. Thus, in addition to the process evaluation strategy, we incorporated a predictive modeling framework to identify students who are at risk of not meeting key academic and social and behavioral outcomes. By using available indicators such as school attendance, behavior, exam scores, grades, and social behavioral indicators that are collected and analyzed at regular time intervals, these approaches can help predict the likelihood of students' school failure and trigger the provision of services that would also be valuable in supporting students' academic and social-emotional needs.

Conclusion

Research has now established that prolonged exposure to toxic stress is linked to long-term health conditions in adulthood. For low-income urban adolescents living in the United States, the concomitant effect of social, economic, and environmental disadvantage places them at high risk for a range of negative developmental outcomes. Prolonged exposure to adverse childhood experiences interferes with optimal functioning of the developing brain, which in turn negatively affects students' school functioning. Fortunately, research has demonstrated that stable and responsive relationships with caring adults can protect youth from the damage done by toxic stress and promote resiliency (Cohen 2017). Adopting a trauma-informed approach and implementing evidence-based clinical interventions provide behavioral health support to students affected by trauma. Schools working in collaboration with university partners can provide critical resources to promote adolescents' academic, social-emotional, and behavioral development.

References

Amaya-Jackson L, Reynolds V, Murray MC, et al: Cognitive-behavioral treatment for pediatric posttraumatic stress disorder: protocol and application in school and community settings. Cogn Behav Pract 10(3):204–213, 2003

Braveman P, Egerter S, Williams DR: The social determinants of health: coming of age. Annu Rev Public Health 32:381–398, 2011 21091195

Cary CE, McMillen JC: The data behind the dissemination: a systematic review of trauma-focused cognitive behavioral therapy for use with children and youth. Child Youth Serv Rev 34(4):748–757, 2012

Cohen JA, Mannarino AP, Deblinger E: Treating Trauma and Traumatic Grief in Children and Adolescents. New York, Guilford, 2016

Cohen SD: Three Principles to Improve Outcomes for Children and Families. Cambridge, MA, Center on the Developing Child at Harvard University, 2017. Available at: https://developingchild.harvard.edu/resources/three-early-childhood development-principles-improve-child-family-outcomes/. Accessed December 11, 2017.

Dorsey S, McLaughlin KA, Kerns SEU, et al: Evidence based update for psychosocial treatments for children and adolescents exposed to traumatic events. J Clin Child Adolesc Psychol 46(3):303–330, 2017 27759442

Durlak JA, Weissberg RP, Dymnicki AB, et al: The impact of enhancing students' social and emotional learning: a meta-analysis of school-based universal interventions. Child Dev 82(1):405–432, 2011 21291449

Evans GW, Kim P, Ting AH, et al: Cumulative risk, maternal responsiveness, and allostatic load among young adolescents. Dev Psychol 43(2):341–351, 2007 17352543

Felitti VJ, Anda RF, Nordenberg D, et al: Relationship of childhood abuse and household dysfunction to many of the leading causes of death in adults. The Adverse Childhood Experiences (ACE) study. Am J Prev Med 14(4):245–258, 1998 9635069

Goodman R: Psychometric properties of the Strengths and Difficulties Questionnaire. J Am Acad Child Adolesc Psychiatry 40(11):1337–1345, 2001

Greene RW: The Explosive Child: A New Approach for Understanding and Parenting Easily Frustrated, "Chronically Inflexible" Children, Revised 5th Edition. New York, HarperCollins, 2014

Jaycox LH, Cohen JA, Mannarino AP, et al: Children's mental health care following Hurricane Katrina: a field trial of trauma-focused psychotherapies. J Trauma Stress 23(2):223–231, 2010 20419730

Kann L, McManus T, Harris WA, et al: Youth Risk Behavior Surveillance—United States, 2015. MMWR Surveill Summ 65(6 No SS-6):1–174, 2016 27280474

Kataoka SH, Stein BD, Jaycox LH, et al: A school-based mental health program for traumatized Latino immigrant children. J Am Acad Child Adolesc Psychiatry 42(3):311–318, 2003 12595784

Kaufman J, Charney D: Effects of early stress on brain structure and function: implications for understanding the relationship between child maltreatment and depression. Dev Psychopathol 13(3):451–471, 2001 11523843

Kaufman J, Plotsky PM, Nemeroff CB, et al: Effects of early adverse experiences on brain structure and function: clinical implications. Biol Psychiatry 48(8):778–790, 2000 11063974

Masten AS, Neemann J, Andenas S: Life events and adjustment in adolescents: the significance of event independence, desirability, and chronicity. Journal of Research on Adolescence 4(1):71–97, 1994

National Center for Health Statistics: Health, United States, 2015: With Special Feature on Racial and Ethnic Health Disparities. Hyattsville, MD, National Center for Health Statistics, 2016

Overstreet S, Chafouleas SM: Trauma-informed schools: introduction to the special issue. School Ment Health 8(1):1–6, 2016

St. Andrews A: Trauma and Resilience: An Adolescent Provider Toolkit. San Francisco, CA, Adolescent Health Working Group, 2013

Tough P: The poverty clinic. The New Yorker, March 21, 2011

CHAPTER 27
ADDICTION, DRUG POLICY, AND BLACK CLINICAL INNOVATIONS

Helena B. Hansen, M.D., Ph.D.
Jacquelyne F. Jackson, Ph.D.

By getting the public to associate the hippies with marijuana and blacks with heroin, and then criminalizing both heavily, we could disrupt those communities. . . . We could arrest their leaders, raid their homes, break up their meetings, and vilify them night after night on the evening news. Did we know we were lying about the drugs? Of course we did.

John Elulichman, Domestic Policy Chief to President Nixon (quoted in Baum 2016)

The pathologies ascribed to poor black and brown people really should be ascribed to a drug war that is pathological, that militarized police, that targets our communities.

Asha Bandele, Senior Director, Drug Policy Alliance (2018)

IN THIS CHAPTER we highlight the role of discriminatory drug policy and of addiction interventions in maintaining racial hierarchies in the United States, as well as their damaging effects on the health and community integrity of black Americans. We also point toward innovations of black mental health professionals, critical scholars, and political activists who have shifted control of interventions to black community members and redefined the causes and nature of addiction.

Race and narcotics use have been intertwined in U.S. policy and segregationist practices for more than a century. Because drug policy and the symbolism surrounding drug use are about more than just drugs—they are also a medium for American racial politics—they are at the center of movements for racial equity. For health inequalities to be rectified, mental health professionals must have a critical understanding of the implicit racial coding of addiction interventions and narcotic laws, marketing, and regulation. Drug policy, drug-related interventions, and law enforcement impede residential, educational, and economic advancement of blacks in America and maintain segregation in neighborhoods, schools, and the workplace. Examples include the disparate enforcement of narcotics surveillance, arrests, and sentencing in black neighborhoods:

- Black men are 13 times more likely to be sent to prison on drug charges than white men, despite being no more likely to use drugs than white men (Human Rights Watch 2009).
- Clinical practitioners are less likely to prescribe pain medications or other narcotics to black patients where they are medically indicated.
- Practitioners are more likely to test black than white pregnant women for narcotics use and refer black children to protective services in the setting of scarce addiction treatment options.

Black people have long been portrayed in the media and policy debates as prone to drug use. Images of black addiction and violence have fed white flight from cities to suburbs and popular support for punitive drug policies and for policies that reduce social benefits such as welfare, Social Security, and affordable housing for people with drug use histories. The result is a vicious cycle: media portrayals of blacks as prone to addiction and drug violence worsen residential segregation, disproportionate surveillance, arrests, and underinvestment in public services and infrastructure in black neighborhoods, which in turn concentrates poverty and exposure to drug trade where other sources of employment are scarce. This cycle exemplifies what social scientists term *structural violence*, which refers to institutional mechanisms that lead systemically to loss of life and suffering (Galtung 1969). Such institutional racism does not require individual acts of discrimination: it is a pernicious form of "racism without racists" (Bonilla-Silva 2017).

The institutional mechanisms underlying racial inequalities in addiction, its treatment, and outcomes are often invisible in clinical literature because the clinical unit of observation is the individual, which implies that disorders and behaviors are due to individual predispositions such as genetic inheritance or to poor choices stemming from psychological underdevelopment. For its part, drug policy almost never explicitly mentions race. Drug policy is instead crafted in terms of individual pathology that nonetheless contains hidden racial intent, in the idiom of "color-blind ideology" (Alexander 2010). Therefore, much of the research that critically examines the impact of drug policy on black communities has been generated by social scientists and historians. Scholars in these disciplines provide a systemic, contextual understanding of neighborhoods, institutions, and policies to explain the reasons individuals use drugs, population-level patterns in drug use, and the health and social consequences of such use. Given the stark racial inequalities in health, race clearly has biological correlates. However, these correlates usually signal biological effects of racism rather than biological causes of racial difference (Gravlee 2009). Therefore, to effectively address racial inequalities in addiction, practitioners must start not by identifying racially patterned biological differences to which treatments can be tailored, but by changing the social conditions that create those biological effects. This is precisely where black mental health professionals, critical scholars, and community activists have been in the forefront of shifting the target of intervention, from neuroreceptors and behavioral conditioning to communities, institutions, and public policies.

Racialized Narcotic Prohibition

Racialized narcotic prohibition has long been a driving force of inequalities in drug policy and outcomes. Its origins go back to the early twentieth century and the expediency of racial imagery to national and international politics. Narcotics, such as cocaine and opiates, had been freely available in over-the-counter "patent medications" throughout the late nineteenth century. The typical habitual user was a white Victorian housewife who initially received morphine from her private doctor for menstrual cramps or chronic conditions, and transitioned to heroin after it was marketed in the late 1800s as a "non-habit-forming" treatment for her morphine addiction, as well as an effective cough syrup for her children. Growing disillusionment among doctors regarding narcotics, scrutiny of medications after passage of the Pure Food and Drug Act of 1906, and international pressure on the United States to pass narcotic control laws following the Opium Wars in Asia coincided with increasingly racialized media portrayals. Examples of the latter were "cocaine-crazed negroes" in the South, Chinese opium dens that lured unsuspecting white women into the sex trade, and Mexican "marijuana madness" in the Southwest. Such imagery assisted the passage of narcotic prohibition, including the 1914 Harrison Narcotics Tax Act prohibiting physicians from prescribing opiates to opiate-addicted patients, the 1924 Heroin Act, the 1937 Marihuana Tax Act, and the creation of the Federal Bureau of Narcotics in 1930 (Courtwright 1982; Musto 1999).

Public officials and popular media coverage in that era amplified racial stereotypes about the identity and moral irresponsibility of narcotic users. For example, Harry Anslinger, who ran the Federal Bureau of Narcotics from 1930 to 1962, referenced "Negroes, Hispanics, Filipinos, and entertainers" as the source of narcotics and distinguished nonwhite "pushers" from the unsuspecting white youth they supposedly victimized, where white drug users were systematically pardoned in court and blacks sentenced for intention to sell (Lassiter 2015). This "reciprocal criminalization of blackness and decriminalization of whiteness" (Muhammad 2011) mirrors a longstanding distinction between legal and illegal narcotics. It provided a protected zone of legal narcotic use for the white middle class with access to private doctors, one that enabled high levels of white narcotic use in the postwar period in the form of barbiturates, stimulants, and later benzodiazepines such as Valium, colloquially known among suburban housewives as "mother's little helper." As a result, postwar narcotic overdose deaths among whites soared, exceeding the rates of the current opioid overdose crisis (Herzberg 2009).

As civil rights activism peaked in the 1960s, race riots raged in major cities where the unemployment rate among blacks was twice that of whites. Lyndon B. Johnson identified drug use as a cause of black poverty and unrest, launching drug raids in black neighborhoods with the support of the Bureau of Narcotics and Dangerous Drugs. Continuing this precedent, Richard Nixon announced the "War on Drugs" in 1971, declared drugs "public enemy number one," and, in 1973, created the Drug Enforcement Administration (DEA) to enhance drug interdiction and regulation (Alexander 2010).

Ronald Reagan reinvigorated the War on Drugs in the 1980s amid media references to the supposed violent threat that African American crack-addicted people posed to white communities. This coverage built support for the passage of the 1986 Anti-Drug Abuse Act, which mandated a minimum 5-year prison sentence for possession of 1/100th the weight of crack cocaine in comparison to powder cocaine, appropriated an additional $1.7 billion for the War on Drugs, and established 29 new mandatory minimum sentences for offenses involving drugs other than cocaine, including marijuana. After passage of the Anti-Drug Abuse Act, narcotics searches and arrests were focused on black and Latino neighborhoods and led to sharp increases in mass incarceration (Alexander 2010). This racialized neoprohibition converged with the HIV epidemic and had lethal effects in black neighborhoods that were contending with injection-related HIV. Many of the intensified law enforcement practices discouraged safe drug injection and promoted HIV transmission, such as prosecution for possession of clean injection equipment and federal bans on harm-reduction measures such as syringe exchange.

Against this backdrop, increasing opioid use among whites starting in the late 1990s—following the aggressive marketing of OxyContin as a "minimally addictive pain reliever" to primary care doctors in white suburban and rural areas—was met with a different, less punitive response. This difference was first apparent in the distinction law enforcement agencies made between manufactured opioids and heroin. Although by 2004 prescription opioids overtook heroin as the primary opiate of abuse in the United States, as of 2007 the arrest rate for illegal possession of manufactured drugs were less than one-fourth those for possession of heroin. Arrests for illegal sale of manufactured drugs was less than one-sixth that of arrest for selling heroin (Office of Justice Programs 2018). Not coincidentally, at the time, the "nonmedical use" of pain relievers was twice as high among whites as among blacks (Substance Abuse and Mental Health Services Administration 2010), while rates of heroin use among blacks, Latinos, and whites were almost identical (Office of National Drug Control Policy 2011). The subsequent shift from nonmedical use of prescription opioids to heroin use in white communities has been followed by bipartisan calls for less punitive law enforcement for heroin and an emphasis on diversion from jail or prison to treatment and supportive services—for a "kinder, gentler" drug war (Seelye 2015).

Since suburban and rural white opioid consumers were not politically supportable targets for law enforcement, the DEA and other regulators shifted their surveillance and enforcement to prescription opioid prescribers and suppliers through prescription monitoring programs. Other shifts included the following: court-sponsored diversion from sentencing to treatment, training, and engagement of police officers as first responders who administer naloxone during overdose; Good Samaritan laws protecting overdose bystanders from drug charges; support for medication-assisted treatment such as office-based buprenorphine maintenance as an alternative to stigmatized (and racialized) methadone clinics; harm-reduction measures such as pharmacy availability of naloxone without prescription; and syringe exchange programs. Racial and geographic inequalities in the implementation of these decriminalization measures, including diversion from drug sentencing and access to office-based treatment with buprenorphine, are pervasive (Vaez-Azizi et al. 2019).

Drug Policy, Black Communities, and Clinical Care

Owing to drug war–related mass incarceration, its convergence with deinstitutionalization, closure of state mental hospitals, and the fact that the majority of people with narcotic dependence have other comorbid psychiatric diagnoses, the

U.S. jail and prison systems are now the largest providers of addiction treatment and mental healthcare in the country (Swanson 2015). Thus, in the experience of many black Americans, addiction and mental health treatment have merged with the criminal justice system, fostering their mistrust of treatment providers.

A history of incarceration further marginalizes low-income black people from employment in the formal economy and increases their likelihood of involvement in the drug trade. Employers discriminate against applicants with a legal record, and a drug conviction disqualifies people from entitlements, including public housing. Welfare reform, including the Temporary Assistance for Needy Families program (established in the Personal Responsibility and Work Opportunity Reconciliation Act of 1996) limiting welfare payments to 5 years, and the 1996 discontinuation of Social Security disability benefits for people with a disabling substance dependence diagnosis have left many low-income people who have a history of drug dependence and arrest with few options other than the drug trade as a source of income (Hansen et al. 2014). The resulting cycle of concentrated drug trade, violence, joblessness, homelessness, and related chronic diseases, including HIV infection and psychiatric disorders, in low-income communities has been termed a "syndemic"—co-occurring and mutually exacerbating epidemics—and has dramatically increased disparities in life expectancy by race and neighborhood (Drucker 2013; Singer 2009).

At the same time, public policies such as urban renewal and planned shrinkage have maintained racial segregation in American cities; disintegrated urban infrastructure such as housing stock, transportation, and public space; and disrupted community support networks in black city neighborhoods through repeated dislocation of low-income residents. Widespread trauma, unstable housing, and thinning social networks are the result, and they increase the risk of narcotic dependence. Calls for "trauma-informed care" by the federal Substance Abuse and Mental Health Services Administration (SAMHSA) may not consider the capacities of public facilities that are systematically defunded and have few resources for psychosocial services.

The criminalization of mental healthcare in black neighborhoods contributes to a two-tiered system of addiction treatment in the United States. One example of this is the bifurcation of medically assisted treatment for opiate dependence, with DEA-regulated methadone clinics that require daily observed dosing concentrated in black and Latino low-income neighborhoods, and office-based buprenorphine maintenance by monthly prescription concentrated in higher-income white areas. Methadone was introduced in 1971 as Richard Nixon's first weapon in the War on Drugs, in response to white fears of rioting and violence in black city neighborhoods and their imagined connection to heroin. From its inception, methadone has been separated from mainstream medical care, stigmatized, and heavily regulated in order to prevent diversion. Buprenorphine, despite its pharmacological similarity to methadone as an opioid agonist, was legalized for private office–based prescription in the year 2000 in response to congressional concern about rising opioid use among suburban youth. The congressional testimony in support of DATA 2000 asserted that buprenorphine was uniquely appropriate for a new kind of opioid user as opposed to the system of methadone treatment, "which tends to be concentrated in urban areas, [and] is a poor fit for the suburban spread of narcotic addiction" (Alan I. Leshner, Ph.D., October 5, 1998; Congressional Record January 28, 1999, S1092). It was also asserted, in testimony related to DATA 2000, that as an alternative to methadone, buprenorphine would serve a new kind of addict, "including many citizens who would not ordinarily be associated with the term addiction" (statement of Charles O'Brien, M.D., introduced during testimony; Congressional Record, September 22, 2000, S9113)—and, implicitly, are white.

Buprenorphine, commercially known in its combination form (with naloxone) as Suboxone, was marketed to middle-class, insured patients over the Internet. Manufacturer-sponsored Web-based public service announcements featured white professionals and business owners on Suboxone (see https://naabt.org). To give additional assurance to the DEA that buprenorphine would not spill over into illicit markets, buprenorphine's manufacturer, along with SAMHSA, developed an 8-hour certification course that was required for doctors wishing to prescribe buprenorphine, a requirement that has been a significant barrier to equity in access to treatment (Jones 2018; Urada et al. 2014). As a result, the first nationally representative study of buprenorphine patients showed they were 91% white, and more than half of the patients were college educated and employed at baseline (Stanton et al. 2006). More recent studies suggest that this pattern persists (Hansen et al. 2016). This example illustrates how the racial coding of the War on Drugs and the reciprocal, decriminalized space of white drug use that it maintains also lead to racial segregation in treatment.

Drug Policy, Foster Care, and Child Welfare

Drug-war policies have harmed black communities through increased placement of black children in foster care due to alleged neglect or abuse stemming from maternal drug use. The Anti-Drug Abuse Act of 1986 was followed by dramatic increases in the imprisonment rate of women—which rose 433% from 1986 to 1991 alone—of whom 80% were sentenced under new mandatory minimum sentencing laws for low-level drug offenses and of whom 70% had children younger than 18 years (Bush-Baskette 2000).

Black women were targeted for drug testing, drug-related charges of child abuse, and child welfare system involvement (Summers 2015). Black children were placed in foster care at the highest rate of any racial group. Low-income black parents, primarily mothers, were given low priority in oversubscribed public drug treatment facilities and received low-quality services (Hser et al. 2007).

Child welfare funding structures incentivize state and local governments to maximize the number of children placed in foster care in ways that also allow those governments to retain substantial revenue in excess of the costs of providing foster care (Jackson, submitted). The basis for child removal is often the result of poverty, such as overcrowded living quarters and inadequate child supervision, rather than a consequence of abuse or willful neglect, and if the parent himself or herself was in foster care as a child, that can be counted against him or her as an indicator of risk, demonstrating that the child welfare system penalizes black mothers and their children for being poor (Roberts 2002).

Conclusion

In response to the structural forces driving the risk and outcome of addiction among blacks in America, black mental health practitioners, researchers, and activists have been at the forefront of advocating for change not only in individual patient care but also at structural levels: through community organizations; agencies providing housing, job training, and education; and organizations advocating for policy change. This approach exemplifies "structural competency": the skill and initiative to intervene on behalf of patients outside of the four walls of the clinic and to influence institutional drivers of addiction risk and addiction outcomes (Hansen and Metzl 2017).

Black mental health practitioners have innovatively integrated evidence-based medicine into recovery networks and holistic care that involves community organizations and cultural arts. For example, in 1969, black addiction medicine pioneer Dr. Beny Primm became the first physician to introduce methadone maintenance in the black neighborhoods of Harlem and Fort Greene when he founded the Addiction Resource and Treatment Corporation. Cognizant of the social determinants of addiction in those communities, Primm also introduced comprehensive care that included family therapy, job training, education, and, beginning in the 1980s, on-site HIV services as well as creative art therapies whose participants have their work featured in community art events (H. Hansen interview with B. Primm, February 12, 2011).

Building on this approach, black mental health practitioners and researchers have turned collaborations with community organizations into health interventions that take entire neighborhoods, and even cities, as their target. For example, psychiatrist Mindy Fullilove, who began her research career studying dislocation of black neighborhoods by urban renewal and planned shrinkage policies as drivers of crack cocaine use, heroin use, and HIV transmission, now works with community agencies, urban planners, and architects to redesign cities so that they are racially and socioeconomically desegregated and offer health-promoting public space such as parks and green spaces. She and colleagues make the city itself their patient: the city is the unit of analysis and of intervention (H. Hansen, interview with M. Fullilove, March 6, 2016; see also Chapter 25, this volume).

Black addictions researchers have critiqued individualist biomedical models of addiction. Neuroscientist Carl Hart, for example, called into question the "chronic brain disease" model of addiction that gained widespread purchase in clinical medicine during President George H.W. Bush's Decade of the Brain. Beginning in that period, the National Institute on Drug Abuse dedicated its resources to neurophysiological and neuroimaging research to identify the biological basis for addiction. Hart challenged the received wisdom of addiction neuroscience, arguing that its biological model had diverted attention and resources away from the social determinants that drive racial disparities in the risk of addiction and its health and social consequences (Hart 2013).

Black mental health practitioners have advocated for the decriminalization of narcotics in order to reduce drug possession–related sentencing that feeds mass incarceration. For example, in New York State, practitioners successfully lobbied to repeal mandatory minimum sentencing under punitive Rockefeller drug laws as a part of the Drop the Rock coalition, and under the auspices of the Drug Policy Alliance, black researchers have collaborated with members of the New York State Assembly Black, Puerto Rican, Hispanic, and Asian Caucus to call for racial impact assessments of new drug-related policies, based on the model of environmental impact assessments currently conducted by the federal Environmental Protection Agency. Contemporary civil rights movements, including Black Lives Matter (https://blacklivesmatter.com/), advocate decarceration: abolishing jails and prisons as a societal response to drug trade and crime. Medical students of color and their allies in turn have taken up this social justice agenda in the movement White Coats for Black Lives (http://www.whitecoats4blacklives.org/), using demonstrations and die-ins to bring attention to the impact of institutional racism on health, including through drug war policies and mass incarceration. They have compelled medical school administrators to provide training in social determinants of racial inequalities in health, and they have formed coalitions with community agencies and local health and social service administrators to document and reverse the institutional determinants of health inequalities. The best of black clinical innovation lives on in these social media platform organizers: of treating the social and political inequalities that make us sick.

References

Alexander M: The New Jim Crow: Mass Incarceration in the Age of Colorblindness. New York, The New Press, 2010

Baum D: Legalize it all: how to win the war on drugs. Harper's Magazine, April 2016, pp 24–34

Bonilla-Silva E: Racism Without Racists: Color-Blind Racism and the Persistence of Racial Inequality in America. Lanham, MD, Rowman & Littlefield, 2017

Bush-Baskette S: The war on drugs and incarceration of mothers. J Drug Issues 30(4):919–928, 2000

Congressional Record: Hearing before the Subcommittee on Health and Environment of the Committee on Commerce, House of Representatives, 106th Cong., 1999, pp 1–23

Congressional Record: Drug Addiction Treatment Act of 2000. Senate, 106th Cong., 2000, p S9111

Courtwright D: Dark Paradise: A History of Opiate Use in America. Cambridge, MA, Harvard University Press, 1982

Drucker E: A Plague of Prisons: The Epidemiology of Mass Incarceration in America. New York, The New Press, 2013

Drug Policy Alliance: When They Call You a Terrorist: A Black Lives Matter Memoir Trailer. January 4, 2018. Available at: https://www.facebook.com/drugpolicy/videos/10156381580289245/. Accessed January 15, 2018.

Galtung J: Violence, peace, and peace research. J Peace Res 6(3):167–191, 1969

Gravlee CC: How race becomes biology: embodiment of social inequality. Am J Phys Anthropol 139(1):47–57, 2009 19226645

Hansen H, Metzl JM: New medicine for the U.S. health care system: training physicians for structural interventions. Acad Med 92(3):279–281, 2017 28079725

Hansen H, Bourgois P, Drucker E: Pathologizing poverty: new forms of diagnosis, disability, and structural stigma under welfare reform. Soc Sci Med 103:76–83, 2014

Hansen H, Siegel C, Wanderling J, et al: Buprenorphine and methadone treatment for opioid dependence by income, ethnicity and race of neighborhoods in New York City. Drug Alcohol Depend 164:14–21, 2016 27179822

Hart C: High Price: A Neuroscientist's Journey of Self-Discovery That Challenges Everything You Know About Drugs and Society. New York, HarperCollins, 2013

Herzberg D: Happy Pills in America: From Miltown to Prozac. Baltimore, MD, Johns Hopkins University Press, 2009

Hser YI, Teruya C, Brown AH, et al: Impact of California's Proposition 36 on the drug treatment system: treatment capacity and displacement. Am J Public Health 97(1):104–109, 2007 17138930

Human Rights Watch: Key findings at a glance, in Punishment and Prejudice: Racial Disparities in the War on Drugs. Human Rights Watch website, 2009. Available at: https://www.hrw.org/legacy/campaigns/drugs/war/key-facts.htm. Accessed February 3, 2010.

Jackson J: America's False Rescue That Rips Black Lives to Shreds. Oakland, CA, submitted

Jones EB: Medication-Assisted Opioid Treatment Prescribers in Federally Qualified Health Centers: Capacity Lags in Rural Areas. J Rural Health 34(1):14–22, 2018 28842930

Lassiter MD: Impossible criminals: the suburban imperatives of America's war on drugs. J Am Hist 102(1):126–140, 2015

Muhammad KG: The Condemnation of Blackness. Cambridge, MA, Harvard University Press, 2011

Musto DF: The American Disease: Origins of Narcotic Control. New York, Oxford University Press, 1999

Office of Justice Programs, Bureau of Justice Statistics: Drugs and crime facts, 2018. Available at: https://www.bjs.gov/content/dcf/enforce.cfm. Accessed June 11, 2018.

Office of National Drug Control Policy: Minorities & Drugs: Facts & Figures. Office of National Drug Control Policy website, 2011. Available at: https://www.whitehousedrugpolicy.org/drugfact/minorities/minorities_ff.html. Accessed December 15, 2015.

Roberts D: Shattered Bonds: The Color of Child Welfare. New York, Basic Civitas Books, 2002

Seelye K: In heroin crisis, white families seek gentler war on drugs. The New York Times, October 30, 2015. Available at https://www.nytimes.com/2015/10/31/us/heroin-war-on-drugs-parents.html. Accessed January 3, 2018.

Singer M: Introducing Syndemics: A Critical Systems Approach to Public and Community Health. Hoboken, NJ, Wiley, 2009

Stanton A, McLeod C, Luckey B, et al: Expanding treatment of opioid dependence: initial physician and patient experiences with the adoption of buprenorphine. Rockville, MD, Substance Abuse and Mental Health Services Administration, 2006. Available at: www.buprenorphine.samhsa.gov/ASAM_06_Final_Results.pdf. Accessed March 10, 2010.

Substance Abuse and Mental Health Services Administration: Results From the 2009 National Survey on Drug Use and Health, Vol I: Summary of National Findings. Rockville, MD, Office of Applied Studies, 2010

Summers A: Disproportionality Rates for Children of Color in Foster Care (Fiscal Year 2013). Reno, NV, National Council of Juvenile and Family Court Judges, 2015

Swanson A: A shocking number of mentally ill Americans end up in prison instead of treatment. The Washington Post, April 30, 2015. Available at: https://www.washingtonpost.com/news/wonk/wp/2015/04/30/a-shocking-number-of-mentally-ill-americans-end-up-in-prisons-instead-of-psychiatric-hospitals/?utm_term=.2fc12d24ff0f. Accessed January 15, 2018.

Urada D, Teruya C, Gelberg L, et al: Integration of substance use disorder services with primary care: health center surveys and qualitative interviews. Subst Abuse Treat Prev Policy 9(1):15, 2014 24679108

Vaez-Azizi L, Netherland J, Hansen H: Social determinants of the opioid epidemic, in Opioid Addiction: An American Crisis. Edited by Compton M, Manseau M. Washington, DC, American Psychiatric Association Publishing, 2019

PART V
Conclusion

CHAPTER 28
CONCLUSION

Toward a Revised Vision of Black Mental Health

Billy E. Jones, M.D., M.S.
Ezra E.H. Griffith, M.D.
Altha J. Stewart, M.D.

READERS WILL JUDGE for themselves how to define the general tone of the discourse presented in this text, as they take note of what individual chapter authors have said. For example, in Chapter 14, Patricia Newton introduces us to the problem of adult attention-deficit/hyperactivity disorder (ADHD) among blacks and makes a plea for attending to the effects of the disorder on blacks. She notes how the disorder obviously exacerbates the mundane life of disadvantaged blacks. It is an invitation to doctors everywhere to recognize the existence of the entity within the black population. Yet it is different from the indictment of the racialized culture in the United States that Williams and McAdams-Mahmoud present in Chapter 24. They outline a plethora of scholarship that highlights the malignant effects of racism on the general medical and psychiatric health status of blacks in this country. These subtleties and differences among the authors make for interesting reading and highlight the complexity of the subject.

Yes, there is noticeable improvement in many areas since this subject was visited by Dr. Jeanne Spurlock in 1999. However, it is clear there remains much to be done. There is a continuing need to expand the presence and availability of affordable mental healthcare to black Americans and to make the provision of these services more user friendly. At the same time, there is an ongoing need for more and better consumer/patient education. As with patient care, there has been some progress made with training and research issues related to black Americans, with much still to be accomplished.

The illustrious chapter authors invited to participate in this text have provided distinctive scholarship, not only because of their expertise but also because of their abiding interest in the subject and commitment to the black healthcare constituency. We are grateful they joined this arduous effort and we thank them for their hard work.

Part I: Reflections

This first part of the text consists of five chapters. The first three reflections are written by the editors of this text and the fourth by a noted senior black female psychiatrist whose professional career has spanned more than six decades. Three of these authors were born and grew up in different parts of this country (the South, Midwest, and New England), and one was a product of the British West Indies. They were reared for the most part in middle-class families who placed a premium on obtaining a good education. Those growing up in the United States did so in different decades but experienced racism early and learned to expect it and cope with it in integrated situations. They discuss their interests and experiences in college that led to medical school and how they became interested in psychiatry. A theme here emphasizes the role that strong role models have played in the selection of psychiatry.

Each of the first four reflections shows a different pathway to individual career development. The pathways relate the intensity of primary interest to the centrality of their special areas of focus—namely, administration, public service, training, and organizational leadership. Of course, these are overlapping rather than separate or distinct categories, and, in fact, each of the careers shows participation in all four focus areas to a greater or lesser extent. The authors maintained involvement with academic institutions and steadily progressed up the academic ladder because of their contributions to psychiatry. The experiences and efforts related in these stories eventually led to the kind of success in their professional activities that may be characterized by visibility, recognition, reputation, and even a certain influence in their work sectors. Yet the stories also reveal an involvement with discrimination of different sorts. They highlight the ubiquitous nature of this struggle even for individuals blessed with distinctive educational advantages and working to conquer mundane life difficulties.

The last chapter of reflections, "Black Psychiatrists of 1969 Survey the Scene, Then and Now," reports interviews of several black psychiatrists who attended the

American Psychiatric Association (APA) meeting in 1969. Some of those interviewed were APA members who actively participated in the meetings with APA officers. Others were black APA attendees who cheered on the militants. Those interviewed comment on differences then and now, point out the changes, and recommend current needed actions.

The few common themes from this part of our book include the role of supportive parents and families in motivating and assisting the authors in striving toward reaching their potential. Although discrimination placed obstacles in their way, they persisted and ultimately succeeded in reaching their goals. Several authors stressed that public-sector positions were of greater interest to them, a preference that emanated from their desire to be of service and assistance to black people. A substantive worry of the informants is their conclusion that racism against black psychiatrists and black patients is still palpably present.

One significant recommendation in Chapter 5 bears repeating here. It is that a national entity in the form of a think tank/alliance/consortium/forum should be developed and funded by black psychiatrists and other professionals across multiple disciplines. This entity would have educational and research capabilities with implications for clinical practice. It would study the multiple dimensions of racism/white supremacy and the coping mechanisms required to manage racism/white supremacy in all areas of civil discourse. This recommendation centers on a dynamic, vital matter that requires continued attention and review. An assessment of progress regarding the implementation of this recommendation should be initiated within 5 years.

Part II: Patient Care

This part of the text comprises 12 chapters (6 through 17) relating to different aspects of patient care. These chapters illustrate the complexity of delivering mental healthcare to the black population.

System Concerns

The first subgroup of chapters (Chapters 6, 7, and 8) addresses some systems or delivery issues. Chapter 6 focuses on the public system of care, its payment mechanisms, and the impact of the "recovery" and "citizenship" movements; Chapter 7 examines the role of the criminal justice system in accounting for the predominant presence of blacks in prisons across the country and the role of psychiatric care in that system; and Chapter 8 concentrates on black international medical graduates and their contributions to the care of black patients. It also highlights the adaptation of these black psychiatrists to the task of caring for their patients in the unique American context so prominently defined by the structural features of poverty and racism.

Chapter 7, "African Americans and the Criminal Justice System," starts with the alarming notion that African Americans are overrepresented in the criminal justice system. Blacks are incarcerated at more than five times the rate of whites, and in some state prison systems the disparity is more than 10 to 1. The author then examines reasons, internal to the criminal justice system, for this drastic difference. Implicit bias, distorted perceptions of and responses to African Americans, and the role of racial bias in forensic mental health evaluation account for some of the causes. In the latter category he points out how intellectual disability and other cognitive deficits are often missed and, if seen, sometimes considered normal for blacks. The effects of childhood trauma are often not understood or not connected to later psychopathology in blacks. He also points out the overdetermined finding of antisocial personality disorder in blacks. He closes with the message that even with good, bias-free evaluations, there is a need to educate the final decision makers during the trial or hearing so as to include compassion and fairness in the outcome.

Chapter 8, "Black International Medical Graduates and the Care of Black Patients," raises issues that are not widely known, even in medical/psychiatric communities and groups. Black international medical graduates (IMGs) are rarely the topic of discussion among most psychiatrists, even black psychiatrists. While the need for support in finding and securing training programs is known, other facets—assistance with acculturation and help in understanding the realities of being black in this country and understanding and overcoming the inherent disadvantages linked to color, standing, and status they face—are hardly addressed. We hope that the author's discussion sparks some advocacy work to address some of these problems, to include linkages not only to underserved populations but to areas that clearly have physician/psychiatrist shortages.

Clinical Concerns

The second subgroup of chapters, Chapters 9 through 14, in Part II emphasizes the significance of social determinants of mental illness, intersectionality (as seen with black women and black LGBTQ patients), and the presence of multiple medical problems in black elderly patients. The psychiatrist/therapist must be aware of the accompanying illnesses or problems and ensure they get addressed. Another major theme is the need for additional knowledge when treating black patients.

Chapter 9, "Providing High-Quality Psychiatric Care for Black Children and Youth," argues that practitioners should have some understanding of black children and their families, and of their values and lifestyles, as well as the general health and behavioral health difficulties they face when seeking mental health treatment. This includes incorporating positive identity strategies when working with children and adolescents and using objective, validated tools to identify and address clinician and treatment bias related to blacks. The authors' insight and practical tips for handling the therapeutic encounter in a culturally competent manner will be helpful to all practitioners working with black children and families.

The authors point out that research findings indicate that black youth as young as 10–12 years of age are significantly more likely to receive harsher judgments, punishments, and disciplinary action, as well as to be perceived more negatively when compared to their white peers exhibiting similar behaviors. The authors recommend the use of evidence-based assessment tools that are useful in providing information about a child's or adolescent's functioning compared with normative data. They caution, however, that clinicians should be aware that the reliability and validity of these measures with black youth vary from poor to superior. Clinicians must know the psychometrics of the assessment tool used to diagnose black youth, if the assessment measures are to be used in a clinically and culturally appropriate way. In this work, clinicians should recognize their own biases, the cultural variation in symptomatology, and a black client's possible mistrust during the assessment process.

Chapter 10, "Black Women and Mental Health," reviews how the checkered past of the United States, with slavery, misogyny, racism, and poverty, has affected black women and their mental health. The authors also point out the impact of the social determinants of mental health—the societal, environmental, and economic conditions that impact mental health outcomes among black women. Yet black women have endured these negative forces and survived, striving in the face of tremendous odds to raise their children and support their families while holding out hope for the promise of a brighter future. Despite tremendous historical adversity and trauma, black women have collectively demonstrated powerful resilience and a capacity not only to endure but also to thrive. Regardless of a black woman's psychological and trauma burdens, clinicians can help mitigate risk factors and determinants of poor mental health by employing cultural humility as well as their understanding of the permutation of psychosocial challenges black women face, as a group and individually.

In Chapter 11, "Young Minority Fathers," the authors document the positive impact that men and fathers can have on the child; the family, including the mother of their child; and the community. As this research area has developed, attention has been paid to adolescent paternity. This attention is an outgrowth of the documented negative effects adolescent paternity has been shown to exert on the development of young men, their partners, and children.

There is evidence that teen fatherhood occurs more often among individuals in the inner city, where the population is mostly composed of ethnic minority young men. Estimates in these settings range from 15% to 20%, and there is some evidence that neighborhoods with greater environmental physical risk factors, such as those found in inner cities, are significantly more predictive of adolescent fatherhood. A group that is often neglected in discussions and considerations of adolescent paternity is young men involved with child welfare systems. When the risk factors associated with adolescent paternity and child welfare involvement are considered, there is significant overlap.

There are several risk factors that predispose young men to fathering a child. The most frequently studied risk factors include family demographic variables, delinquency, low educational attainment, substance use, and psychological factors. What remains elusive and may be an area ripe for intervention are longitudinal studies that are able to make causal inferences about these risks.

While national rates of adolescent paternity have consistently declined, there continue to be pockets of significant intransigence: minority individuals (especially black and Latino/Hispanic young men) and those involved in the child welfare and juvenile justice systems. Young minority men are a vulnerable group who experience disparate "system contact." These systems have limited information, interest, and services to support young minority fathers. Early paternity is a marker of risk for poor physical and mental health outcomes, as well as for substance use and delinquency. Fathering may include motivation to learn new skills in preparation for the role, and these skills can position their children for future success.

In Chapter 12, "Black Elders of the Twenty-First Century," the author provides a detailed picture of elders at the start of this century, paying specific attention to baby boomers. Her comparison of black and white elders is critical to understanding their unique needs. Born before the end of the segregation of the Jim Crow era, they lived to see a black man serve 8 years as U.S. president and the rise of a social justice movement that uses Twitter instead of mimeographed flyers and hand-painted placards to protest injustices, including those in the healthcare arena. Mental illness, substance abuse, and dementia are problems for this group, but they are also experiencing less retirement security and are often returning to rearing their grandchildren. The situation for rural black elderly is more severe than that for urban black elderly.

Black elders in general are more at risk for cognitive impairment from multiple causes, including multiple medical problems, the prescription of multiple medications, and psychosocial stressors involving finances and family concerns. Because of a long history of hypertension beginning in their 20s, the black elderly in their 60s and older are at increased risk to develop vascular dementia. As they age, they enter cohorts that are at increased risk to develop major neurocognitive disorder of the Alzheimer's type. Thus, black elders are at an increased risk to have more than one type of dementing illness as they age. Reliance on church and the role of a faith community are discussed; both church and faith community are a significant source of support for many in this cohort, providing not only spiritual counseling but financial and social support as well.

In Chapter 13, "Black Lesbian, Gay, Bisexual, Transgender, and Queer [LGBTQ] Identities and Mental Health," the authors point out that just as there is no monolithic black community, the black LGBTQ community is diverse. However, black LGBTQ persons share the lived experience of having multiple stigmatized racial, sexual, and gender identities. While there is some work assessing the mental health of black LGBTQ persons, more remains to be done. The literature is particularly sparse on transgender men, nonurban populations, bisexually identified men and women separate from gay men and lesbian women, and those younger than 18 years. While the impact of HIV on black men who have sex with men (MSM) cannot be overstated, studies also need to be done on the mental health issues in this community that do not focus on HIV. More research is necessary to determine risk factors for mental illness, resources for resilience, and effective interventions. That research should be done using an intersectional approach to appreciate the various roles of the multiple identities.

Clinicians need to be aware of some significant problems in addition to the health disparities among black LGBTQ patients to be able to address them, whether the problem be gender dysphoria in transgender persons, HIV in black MSM, or substance use in black sexual minority women. Mental healthcare providers should be aware of the discrimination black LGBTQ individuals may experience—racism in the majority LGBTQ community, and bias against sexual minorities in the black community—and the role these experiences may have on the lives of their patients.

Studies have shown that, contrary to what the minority stress model would have predicted, black LGBTQ persons have generally lower rates of mental illness relative to the white LGBTQ community. Various sources of resilience have been proposed, most often identifying the role of spirituality or religion and a connection with the black community (e.g., family, social network). Clinicians should be aware of what psychosocial supports exist for their patients and should work to strengthen them when present and help create them when absent. Black LGBTQ persons are also generally less likely to be open about the sexual minority status in many situations, including with providers. In most cases, their decision not to disclose does not appear to decrease their acceptance of this status but functions as a way to maintain connection with the black community. Clinicians should provide an open, safe, and nonjudgmental space where patients may feel comfortable sharing all aspects of their identity.

Chapter 14, "Adult Attention-Deficit/Hyperactivity Disorder in African American Populations," emphasizes that ADHD in adult African Americans is often unrecognized and underdiagnosed. The author points out that reports in the United States estimate a prevalence rate of about 4.4%. However, in African American populations, this rate falls to around 2.2%. Several factors contribute to this lack of recognition of the disorder in this population: presence of comorbid conditions such as alcohol and substance use disorders, mood disorders, anxiety disorders, trauma- and stressor-related disorders (including posttraumatic stress disorder and historical trauma); implicit bias among healthcare providers; cultural factors; and general disparities relative to the healthcare delivery system. Social stigma regarding mental health treatment among African Americans, coupled with fear and distrust of psychiatry, also contributes to the failure to seek treatment.

Clinicians should now be committed to improving the lives of African American patient populations through the recognition and treatment of a disorder that has far too long plagued the social fabric of this community. The public health implications are significant. In terms of costs and morbidity to the entire nation, ADHD in adults should not be disregarded or marginalized any longer.

Treatment Modalities and Black Patients

The last three chapters in this part of the text (Chapters 15, 16, and 17)—about psychotherapy, psychopharmacology, and the role the church can play in healthcare—address unique treatment issues of black patients. A major common theme is that black people will utilize certain therapeutic approaches, such as psychotherapy and medication, if they find the approaches relevant to their well-being, affordable, and delivered with cultural competency.

Chapter 15, "Psychotherapy With African Americans and People of African Descent," emphasizes that psychotherapy is an important intervention in mental health treatment for black people. Access to and utilization of psychotherapy are a function of how it is perceived as a credible curative intervention. The author points out that health disparities mirror the continued second-class citizenship of the black community and persistence of discrimination and racism. This is reinforced by the underrepresentation of blacks in psychotherapy research and clinical trials for empirically supported treatments. There is need for greater inclusion and sophistication in sampling and recognizing demographic and health variables (e.g., intergroup ethnic variation and socioeconomic status) in highly differentiated and stratified black populations within the African diaspora. Psychiatrists and psychologists should sustain and advance cultural competency in their professional training and for the broad mental health workforce. Social policy should allow affordable access to psychotherapy and mental health services. The perception of psychotherapy by black people remains tied to the legacy of health and mental health treatment as well as experiences of mental healthcare in the community. The author stresses that race matters in psychotherapy and emphasizes the significance of asking for a black therapist.

In Chapter 16, "Biological Therapies and Black Patients," the author reports that while black psychiatrists who are primarily researchers are only a minority among minorities, they have played a key role in reducing mental health misinformation for patients and served as their advocates in directing research to their needs. Moreover, they have clearly influenced policy. Their research findings are leading to better treatments and access to treatment. The numbers remain small, but we are now seeing emerging leadership in research funders. The awareness of the problem and the creativity of committed individuals suggest a bright future.

In Chapter 17, "The Black Church and Mental Health," the authors report that increasing mental healthcare among African Americans is a complex issue for which there is no single solution. The authors argue that the black church can play a central role in mental health service provision but point out the current literature is extremely limited. They highlight how two innovative mega-churches in Los Angeles are addressing the mental health needs of their congregations and surrounding communities. Additional work, especially that which utilizes participatory approaches, is needed to explore opportunities and limitations of church-based mental healthcare for African Americans.

Part III: Training of Black Mental Health Care Providers

Part III addresses training and workforce issues regarding blacks. Integrating black cultural differences into curriculum while understanding the various cultures in the groups being trained is a theme. Workforce issues include the fact that the general black population is younger, whereas the psychiatric provider group is aging—a trend that further creates a discordance in the respective understanding and skill in the use of today's technology, especially regarding the role of social networking sites. The use of feeder programs to attract black youth to medicine/psychiatry is also discussed.

Chapter 18, "Psychiatric Training and Black Mental Health," discusses the evolution of medical and psychiatric education in the context of treatment of underserved populations or what was once called "cross-cultural psychiatry." The authors review literature regarding rates of mental illness in blacks compared with other groups and reports regarding engagement by nonminority providers and black patients' trust in receiving care from these providers in treatment settings. Their review indicates that providers are more effective when all likely cultural stressors are considered and that the needed skills can be taught to improve this understanding by trainees and practicing psychiatrists alike.

The chapter includes an account of the history of psychiatric treatment of blacks in America and includes the inclusion in DSM-IV (American Psychiatric Association 1994) of "culture-bound syndromes." The authors acknowledge the challenges faced in training environments as trainees bring their own cultural histories and experiences that must be integrated into the didactic as well as the clinical teaching. Differences in patient care in a variety of treatment settings (e.g., inpatient, outpatient) and using different modalities (e.g., psychotherapy, psychopharmacology, family therapy) must be accommodated in the curriculum, and both trainees and faculty must be open to the challenges they will face in adapting their individual ideas, beliefs, and values when in a treatment setting with someone from another culture about whom they have limited knowledge.

Chapter 19, "A Seat at the Psychiatric Table," addresses the workforce development challenges facing psychiatry and the rest of medicine as we work to address health disparities, treatment access, and the provision of culturally appropriate services. The author uses his own story to encourage us to recognize ways in which we can support young blacks entering medicine. The importance of inclusive medical associations is highlighted as one of the value-added components in understanding the culture of medicine and creating the needed pipeline to ensure that those young blacks who wish to become physicians enter the profession and are supported through their training and early career period. Model pipeline programs, some sponsored by the APA, are described, as well as the role of organized medicine and medical/psychiatric societies in reducing health disparities and achieving health equity.

Chapter 20, "Addressing the Mental Health Needs of African American Youth in the New Millennium," begins with a review of the difficulties confronting black youth and young adults in the context of the sociocultural framework in which they live. The author provides a detailed picture of how mental healthcare and social justice intertwine. The importance of social media in their lives and its impact on their health and well-being, as well as its role in help-seeking behavior, is discussed. As noted earlier in this section, the general black population is younger, while the psychiatric provider group is aging, and there is a discordance in their respective understanding and skill in use of today's technology, especially regarding the role of social networking sites for their engagement with psychiatric treatment providers and services. Many readers will come away with an appreciation of the need for more understanding of these tools and applications and for more research in this area. Online discussions of everything from mental health concerns to social justice advocacy regarding microaggressions, police harassment and violence, and the media's stigmatizing perceptions of black youth can be harmful, especially for those with mental illness. Disclosure of personal information and the ability to remain isolated from family, friends, and face-to-face supports create challenges to treatment and recovery for young people. Providers must learn more about how the use of social networking sites encourages this and how the "digital lives" of black youth compare with their real ones, especially as these relate to intersectionality. The author concludes with recommendations for how practitioners can incorporate this understanding of youth's interactions online into their treatment to achieve improved outcomes.

In Chapter 21, "Training in the Effects of Implicit Racial Bias on Black Health," the authors define *implicit bias* and acknowledge that it affects health. They offer a detailed history of implicit racial bias in healthcare and medicine. Such bias has gained substantial attention and has become an ever-growing area of research. The Institute of Medicine report *Unequal Treatment* (Smedley et al. 2002) stated that minorities receive lower quality of care than whites, even when controlling for certain factors. The report also suggested that bias on the part of the healthcare provider may lead to disparate care among nonwhites and whites. The report sparked new dialogue regarding the role of the provider.

While implicit bias in healthcare is a relatively new concept, the presence of bias in Western medicine dates back centuries. As a result, a separate, substandard system of care was formed. In the post–Civil Rights era, while advances in medical care and technology have improved, health disparities for blacks persist and, in some cases, have worsened. The literature has shown that most physicians, with the exception of African American doctors, hold significant pro-white bias. Implicit bias has significant impact on patient health outcomes, treatment decisions, treatment adherence, and patient-provider interactions, which means provider implicit bias has the potential to negatively impact the health of blacks and perpetuate disparities. The authors describe the unique impact of implicit bias in specific populations, including health outcomes among black patients in children's behavioral health, adult and elderly behavioral health, correctional health, and HIV/AIDS care.

There is a growing literature on the impact of provider implicit bias on the health outcomes of black children (also discussed elsewhere in this book). The case is made for why we must engage trainees in implicit bias training as part of the medical school curriculum. The authors encourage trainees and providers to make individualized assessments of a person. Current providers should advocate for adequate physician-patient time to avoid the unconscious bias that is more likely to occur under time constraints. This is key in a time when insurance and clinical mandates limit contact between patients and providers. Time constraints coupled with implicit bias can lead to poor patient-physician communication, subsequent dissatisfaction with care, and lower likelihood of engagement.

Chapter 22, "Historically Black Colleges and Universities and African American Psychiatry," offers a detailed history of four historically black colleges and universities (HBCUs) and their important role in the training of many black doctors. The departments of psychiatry in these four institutions— Howard, Meharry, Drew, and Morehouse—have similar missions, programs, and challenges. The author gives the history of these departments and notes they have been responsible for many treatment innovations that have advanced the practice of psychiatry, especially with respect to blacks. He reports that several psychiatrists affiliated with them are legends in the field. The importance of these departments is not just historical; they have a continuing role in ensuring culturally appropriate access to care for many underserved populations and training for underrepresented minority groups. As more is learned about the important role of behavioral interventions in improving overall health and well-being, the role for HBCUs will continue to be important. Awareness of what practitioners of the future must know about providing services to black patients and families beyond the twenty-first century is an important part of their work going forward.

Part IV: Psychiatric Research and Blacks

The five chapters (23 through 27) of Part IV address scholarship related to blacks and behavioral health. They highlight thematic emphasis on the need for more inquiry into these topics, especially concerning racism, its mental health consequences for blacks and whites, and the emotional, economic, and social trauma it causes. They also raise questions about how to increase the number of black scholars interested in participating in this kind of work.

Chapter 23, "The Importance of 'Bent Nail' Research for African American Populations," proposes a different approach to research on African Americans. While recognizing the importance of pristine, formal academic research, the author advocates for "bent nail," or rudimentary, basic clinical research, as a solution to the paucity of knowledge about African American mental health. However, he stresses that there is also a need for large-scale public health research on African American matters to confirm and validate the "bent-nail" research. The author argues that it is not enough to find answers to public health problems of African Americans. Black scholars have an additional obligation to thrust their evidence-based strategies into the public eye to create the political will to enact the solutions into public policy. That is how the public health of African Americans will benefit. This approach to the national research program is intriguing, although there is still the nagging problem that many scholars find their choice of academic inquiry being determined by what money is available to them in the marketplace. In other words, the availability of funds often dictates the direction of a scholar's scientific interests.

Chapter 24, "Racism and Mental Health," provides an overview of empirical research that delineates the multiple mechanisms by which racism, by unfairly advantaging some groups and disadvantaging others, can adversely affect community and individual mental health. First, institutional racism can lead to societal policies that reduce access of the socially stigmatized to desirable opportunities and resources in society. Second, a large and growing body of evidence indicates that experiences of racial discrimination are an important type of stressful life experience that can adversely affect mental and physical health. Third, cultural racism can initiate and sustain negative racial stereotypes that can lessen support for egalitarian policies, trigger health-damaging psychological responses such as internalized racism and stereotype threat, and facilitate explicit and implicit biases that restrict access to desirable resources, including medical care.

One research priority for the authors is to understand better the mental health consequences of racial hostility that is embedded in the larger societal environment. Another is the importance of understanding the ways in which racism can affect the mental health of whites. The other side of this research agenda is the need to understand the resilience resources and protective factors that insulate the mental health of blacks and other minorities from at least some of the negative effects of racism. This chapter reinforces the scholarship available to undergird the principle that racism, given that it is alive and well in the United States, must be understood as a public health pollutant. Thus, it demands continuing scholarly examination.

In Chapter 25, "Toward a Liberation Psychiatry," the author proposes that the development of liberation psychiatry requires an exploration of "place," the locations in which people live, work, and love, and that the psychology of place becomes a fundamental, albeit often overlooked, part of human psychology. The author and her team have a dynamic model of the injuries of oppression, which occur across systems and at multiple levels of scale. Liberation psychiatry, by incorporating the psychology of place, will be well positioned to implement complex ecological interventions that are sensitive to time, place, and culture. Place psychology often helps to track and interpret an often overlooked narrative of forced displacements that have had devastating effects on inner-city communities. In the last half-century, medical geographers and anthropologists have pointed out some essential connections between place and health. Thus, we now recognize the health implications of links between individuals and their place of residence. Community structure and integration can help forge the strength of racially segregated communities. Deterioration of that structure and the uprooting of citizens from their geographic reference points can weaken connectedness and a sense of identity.

Liberation psychiatry presupposes that the world around us is influencing our mental health. This basic premise represents a unique basis of the author's political application of the scholarly work on health and place. She argues that the psychology of place can help us understand the ways in which the social, economic, and political processes actually become embodied in our hearts and minds. Mental health professionals can make an important contribution to people's awareness that mental well-being requires a world, with individuals and institutions within the community spaces working together to accent fairness and justice based on mutual respect.

Chapter 26, "The 'New' Epidemic: Trauma Among Urban Adolescents Living in Poverty," reports that 52% of poor black children, 50% of poor Hispanic children, and 36% of poor white children are being raised by single mothers. In this chapter, the authors remind us that living in poverty presents a multiplicity of challenges in communities plagued by social, economic, and environmental disadvantage. This is a concretization of the relationship between place and health as much as it is a powerful exemplar of a social determinant of health. The theorem unfolds with solid logic. Urban minority youth are placed at high risk for engagement in risky behaviors that have implications for their healthful adjustment along cognitive, social, emotional, and behavioral domains of functioning. Youths' prolonged exposure to stressful life conditions (e.g., violence, drugs, food insufficiency, housing insecurity) severely compromises the functioning and development of emergent brain and body systems that help regulate the body's response to stress. Trauma in this context is anything but new. What may be novel is the now explicit acknowledgment that there is scientific evidence demonstrating a link between adverse childhood experiences and long-term health consequences in adulthood.

This chapter endorses a specific locus of activity, schools, where trauma affects the lived experience of urban adolescents and where prolonged exposure to toxic stress affects their health and well-being. Although targeted interventions have demonstrated positive effects for alleviating students' symptoms of trauma, there are often challenges in implementing these types of programs in school settings. Urban public schools are woefully under-resourced and therefore lack the ability to meet the demand of providing high-quality behavioral health services to students, particularly those affected by trauma. In a climate of ever-shrinking educational funding, school districts are often forced to cut mental health services to students in desperate need of support. This translates into fewer mental health practitioners in schools, who struggle to manage large caseloads and long waitlists while students' behavioral health needs are neglected.

Fortunately, research has demonstrated that stable and responsive relationships with caring adults can protect youth from the damage done by toxic stress and promote resiliency. Adopting a trauma-informed approach and implementing evidence-based clinical interventions provide behavioral health support to students affected by trauma. Schools working in collaboration with university partners can provide critical resources to promote adolescents' academic, social-emotional, and behavioral development.

In Chapter 27, "Addiction, Drug Policy, and Black Clinical Innovations," the authors describe how the legal, moral, and biological distinctions between licit and illicit narcotics use have served as American sociopolitical technologies of racial segregation and racial violence for more than a century. They examine the past and future role of black psychiatrists in challenging and reframing the cultural logic embedded in clinical practice, research, and popular understanding of addiction. The chapter illustrates how cultures of poverty and of spiritual renewal, biological predisposition and heredity, intergenerational trauma, structural racism, and mass incarceration have been deployed to support policy initiatives and community resistance.

The authors use pointed language to emphasize how public officials and popular media have for decades magnified racial stereotypes of narcotic users. This has perpetuated misconceptions of those who abuse substances, which in turn has influenced public policy in problematic directions. These authors raise significant concerns about the political and biomedical bases of public policies in this arena. They advocate a shift in targeted directions from individuals to communities and institutions, reminding us of arguments previously made by Williams, Fullilove, and Ward and their colleagues in their respective chapters.

Concluding Thoughts

As we have reviewed the chapters produced in this new volume, one clear finding is that scholars are vibrantly preoccupied with the concerns of the black U.S. population. There is a palpable commitment to their mental healthcare, and that commitment is demonstrated on different levels. Healthcare professionals are thinking about the traditional use of time-honored interventions such as psychotherapy and psychopharmacology. Others want to make sure that we appreciate the unique concerns of black women, black elders, the LGBTQ community, children and adolescents, and those who make use of their connections to faith-based communities. The inescapable reminder here is that race matters and that discrimination has a powerful effect on the interventions used with these populations. Yet some of our authors have shown that ingenuity and scholarship can lead to unique developments in areas such as implicit racial bias and the care of substance users.

It is a striking observation that the editors of this text have led lives of leadership in public systems of care. In addition, the authors of Chapter 4 and Chapter 5, and several of the individuals interviewed in the latter chapter, have consistently been influential in the execution of public policy. The authors of Chapter 6 invited us into the real and present world of policy making, showing how the thoughtful application of public resources to the task of improving the mental health of blacks and other disadvantaged minorities in this country can make a difference.

We editors hope that through this text, we have made effective witness to the state of black mental health in this country.

References

American Psychiatric Association: Diagnostic and Statistical Manual of Mental Disorders, 4th Edition. Washington, DC, American Psychiatric Association, 1994

Smedley BD, Stith AY, Nelson AR (eds): Unequal Treatment: Confronting Racial and Ethnic Disparities in Health Care. Washington, DC, National Academies Press, 2002

INDEX

Page numbers printed in **boldface** *type refer to tables or figures.*